BONE

Volume 7: Bone Growth — B

BONE

Volume 7: Bone Growth — B

Brian K. Hall
Department of Biology
Dalhousie University
Halifax, Nova Scotia
Canada

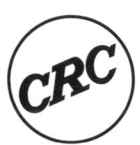

CRC Press
Boca Raton   Ann Arbor   London   Tokyo

Library of Congress Cataloging-in-Publication Data

(Revised for vol. 7)

   Vols. 3-   have imprint: Boca Raton : CRC Press.
   Includes bibliographical references and index.
   Contents: v. 1. The osteoblast and osteocyte --
[etc.] -- Fracture repair and regeneration --
v. 7. Bone growth - B.
   1. Bones. I. Hall, Brian Keith, 1941-   .
[DNLM: 1. Bone and Bones. WE 200 B7113]
QP88.2.B58   1990   599'.01852   89-20391
ISBN 0-936923-24-5 (v. 1)

Developed by Telford Press

© 1993 by CRC Press, Inc.

International Standard Book Number 0-8493-8827-9

Library of Congress Card Number 89-20391

Printed in the United States of America   1   2   3   4   5   6   7   8   9   0

Printed on acid-free paper

Preface

The impetus for initiating this series was to fill the need for an up-to-date, comprehensive, and authoritative treatment of all aspects of bone. Cartilage has been covered in the three-volume series, *Cartilage* (Hall, 1983), and in *Cartilage: Molecular Aspects* (Hall and Newman, 1991) published by CRC Press.

The volumes in this series are organized thematically, each volume integrating structure, function, biochemistry, metabolism, and the molecular and clinical aspects of a particular aspect of the biology of bone. The chapters are written by authors actively engaged in basic, applied, and/or clinical research upon bone, ensuring that each chapter is both authoritative and up-to-date.

Bone-forming cells were covered in *Volume 1: The Osteoblast and Osteocyte.* The second volume, *The Osteoclast,* dealt with bone-resorbing cells, both multicellular osteoclasts that resorb the mineral and organic phases of bone, and mononuclear cells that resorb only the latter. The third volume, *Bone Matrix and Bone Specific Products,* extended coverage from bone-forming and -resorbing cells to the synthesis of bone-specific products and their deposition into the extracellular matrix. Volume 4, *Bone Metabolism and Mineralization,* summarized the current status of knowledge on bone metabolism and mineralization of the bone matrix. Volume 5, *Fracture Repair and Regeneration,* treated the dual processes of repair of complete fractures of bones and the potential for regeneration of lost skeletal units, from regeneration of microfractures to the replacement of complete skeletal elements. Volume 6, *Bone Growth-A,* was the first of two volumes devoted to bone growth, concentrating on the growth of major regions of the skeleton. This volume, *Bone Growth-B,* concentrates on the relationship of bone growth to the mechanical properties of bone and relates the growth of bone to physiological and ecological aspects of the life cycle and to evolutionary change.

Both the first and the last chapters in this volume deal with the mechanical properties of bone, the first in the context of long bone growth at different sites and at different times during the life cycle and the effects of disuse on cortical bone growth, and the last (Chapter 10) in the context of the differing material properties of trabecular and cortical bone, their behavior in response to repetitive loading, and how fatigue and fracture relate to the mechanical properties of bone as a material. Together these chapters provide authoritative and thoroughly up-to-date analyses of the best current thinking on the mechanical properties and mechanical loading of bone.

The second chapter utilizes *in vitro* organ culture systems to analyze how mechanical factors influence bone formation, resorption, and growth. Although work in this area is half a century old, it is the pioneering work of the authors of this chapter that has provided the best available data on the actual mechanical forces applied, and to which bone cells respond, *in vitro.*

The theme of the importance of mechanical loading and biomechanical factors is continued in Chapter 3 in the context of the effects on bone growth of physical inactivity, paralysis, or weightlessness. Clinical studies on bedrest and paralytic diseases such as poliomyelitis are combined with analysis of the data from U.S.A. and U.S.S.R. space flights (Skylab, Cosmos) to highlight that bone loss from decreased loading is a local process that is not directly mediated by systemic hormones.

In Chapter 4 we move from mechanical influences on bone growth to an applied subject, the effect of miniaturization of body size on the skeleton. The adaptiveness of the skeleton is emphasized in this treatment; the skeleton can compensate for, or adapt to, body size decrease by reduction, hyperossification, increased variability, or the appearance of morphological novelties. That many dwarfed taxa display one or more of these features attests to the significant effect that decrease in body size can have on skeletal growth.

The theme of the adaptiveness of the skeleton is continued in Chapters 5 and 6 in the context of the effect of domestication of animals on bone growth (Chapter 5) and primate evolution (Chapter 6). Here the effects are primarily on scaling or allometric growth, discussed in the context of ontogenetic allometry, effects evident over the whole lifetime, and effects evident on the evolutionary time scale.

The evolutionary theme is further developed in Chapter 7, which deals with knowledge of bone growth that can be gleaned from the field of paleopathology of human skeletal material. Three conditions (infection, anemia, and congenital/metabolic diseases) are treated as case studies to illustrate the wealth of information that can be retrieved from such "dry-bone, biomedical research materials".

In Chapter 8 we move to an extensive treatment of the effects of drugs on bone growth, which analyzes and synthesizes a vast amount of information on the effects on bone growth of analgesic, anesthetic, anticonvulsant, anti-infective, chemotherapeutic, diuretic, and psychotropic drugs. Nowhere else is such information gathered and synthesized.

Chapter 9 completes a series of superb chapters produced for this series by the French workers in the Equipe de Recherche "Formations squelettiques" of the Université Paris 7. In this chapter they provide a masterly synthesis of the use of growth marks preserved in bone to age individual organisms, the discipline of skeletochronology. This chapter will be valuable to workers in many specialities who deal with the problem of having to age individuals or to measure the temporal aspects of processes recorded in bone. Zoologists, ichthyologists, paleopathologists, anthropologists, clinicians working with metabolic bone diseases, paleontologists; all will find much of practical utility in this chapter.

In summary, Volume 7, in combination with Volume 6, provides an authoritative overview of the most important factors affecting bone growth.

In its treatment of the mechanical and material properties of bone, the consequences for bone growth of variation in body size, domestication, and evolutionary changes, and its analysis of how paleopathology, skeletochronology, and pharmacology instruct us about bone growth and the temporal changes in bone over individual or species lifetimes, it represents the starting point for the next phase of research into bone growth.

Brian K. Hall

The Editor

Brian K. Hall, Ph.D., D.Sc., is Izaak Walton Killam Research Professor in the Department of Biology, Faculty of Science, Dalhousie University, Halifax, Nova Scotia, Canada. He also holds an appointment as Professor of Physiotherapy, Faculty of Health Professions, Dalhousie University.

Professor Hall received his B.Sc. (Hons.) degree in 1965, his Ph.D. in Zoology in 1969, and a D.Sc. in Biological Sciences in 1978 from the University of New England (UNE), Armidale, New South Wales, Australia. He was appointed a Teaching Fellow in the Department of Zoology, UNE in 1965, Assistant Professor in the Department of Biology, Dalhousie University in 1968, Associate Professor in 1972, Professor in 1975, and Killam Research Professor in 1990. He served as Chair of the Biology Department, Dalhousie University, from 1978 to 1985.

Professor Hall is a Fellow of the Royal Society of Canada and a member of the American Society of Zoologists, International Society for Differentiation, British Society for Development Biology, International Society for Developmental Biology, Society of Vertebrate Palaeontology, The Bone and Tooth Society, and the British Connective Tissue Society. He is an editor of *Anatomy and Embryology*, member of the editorial board of the *Journal of Craniofacial Genetics and Developmental Biology*, member of the international advisory board of the *Croatian Medical Journal*, past associate editor of the *Canadian Journal of Zoology*, and past member of the advisory editorial board of *Bone*.

Professor Hall has worked on the development and differentiation of cartilage and bone for 25 years. He has presented 64 invited lectures at international meetings and symposia and 102 guest lectures at universities and institutes. He is the author or co-author of 5 books, the most recent of which is *Evolutionary Developmental Biology* (1992), 127 papers in refereed scientific journals, and author of 35 chapters in edited works or conference proceedings. He edited a three-volume series on cartilage (1983) and was co-editor of *Cartilage: Molecular Aspects* published by CRC Press in 1991. The current focus of his research is on the development and evolution of neural crest-derived craniofacial cartilage and bone.

Contents

1

Mechanical Loading and Bone Growth *In Vivo*

ANDREW A. BIEWENER and JOHN E. A. BERTRAM
Department of Organismal Biology and Anatomy
Division of Biological Sciences
The University of Chicago
Chicago, Illinois

Introduction

The post-natal development and growth-modeling processes of bone represent extensions of tissue interactions and processes established early in skeletal differentiation and embryogenesis. As a bone increases in length and size during this period, its shape must be continually remodeled to maintain a form appropriate to its biomechanical function. Post-natal growth often involves more than an order of magnitude increase in size of individual bone elements. Hence, bone growth modeling involves the coordination of vigorous processes of both bone deposition and resorption initiated at differing times, rates, and sites within the bone. While most work has focused on hormonal and biochemical factors that influence skeletal growth, recent studies indicate that mechanical factors may also play an important role in the post-natal growth of bone. The perceived importance of mechanical function stems in part from studies showing that mature bone is capable of responding to alterations in its normal loading environment (see Volume 3, Chapter 2). Frequently referred to as "functional adaptation", the remodeling response of bone to changes in physical usage has also had a long history, initiated by Wolff's (1892) pioneering work hypothesizing that the maintenance and transformation of skeletal form is greatly influenced by the mechanical forces acting on a bone during its use. If mechanical function has a similar effect on the growing skeleton, bone growth modeling likely reflects the complex interplay of not only epigenetic, hormonal, and bio-chemical factors during ontogeny (Hall, 1982; Raisz and Bingham, 1972; Rodan and Rodan, 1983) but mechanical factors as well.

Our goal in this chapter is to evaluate the extent to which mechanical factors associated with physical activity have been shown to affect the postnatal growth of the skeleton, which in turn may provide some insight into the mechanism by which this interaction is mediated. Given that growth modeling processes of the skeleton involve both a rapid increase in bone mass and change in cortical geometry, it is often presumed that the sensitivity and reponse of the skeleton to changes in mechanical loading are greater during growth than at maturity (Carter, 1982; Fig. 1). On the other hand, it has also been argued that extreme loading associated with strenuous exercise may be detrimental to skeletal growth (Booth and Gould, 1975). Finally, given the overriding importance of genetic and epigenetic regulation of skeletal tissue differentiation early in development (Fell, 1956), a third possibility is that physical exercise exerts little influence on the growth of the skeleton, during which time the skeleton is constrained by developmental processes to follow a particular growth trajectory.

The view that the response of growing bone to changes in mechanical loading parallels that of mature bone, but at a heightened level (Fig. 1), is likely oversimplified and misleading. During growth, changes in bone mass and shape associated with changes in mechanical loading must be super-imposed on modeling processes underlying the normal growth of the bone. Consequently, overall changes in bone mass and shape during growth in relation to mechanical loading history must be distinctly different from those of mature bone. Whereas the mature skeleton may respond very little to differences in mechanical loading within its normal physiological range, by definition a growing bone is always in a state of net bone formation. Similarly, whereas disuse promotes net bone loss in the mature skeleton, disuse presumably retards, but does not prevent, net bone formation during growth. These responses are more realistically depicted in Fig. 2 (solid curve), in contrast to those shown in Fig. 1. The relevant question is whether changes in bone formation rate with changes in loading history (the slopes of these curves) are similar for growing and mature bone at specific regions of their loading history range. Given the basic difference in bone growth modeling

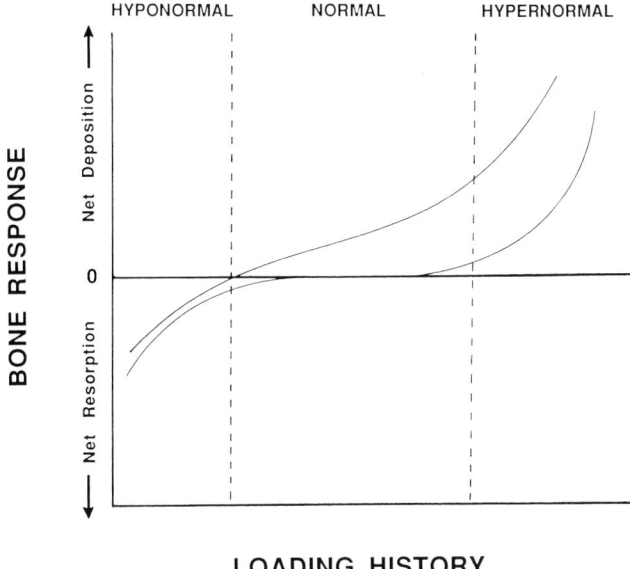

Fig. 1 A diagram showing a recently portrayed view of the differences between the response of mature vs. growing bone to changes in mechanical loading history (modified from Carter, 1982). The abscissa represents the loading history of the bone, characterized by the accumulation of loads experienced by the bone in terms of strain (or stress) magnitude, frequency, rate, and number of loading cycles. The curve for mature bone indicates that its response (shown on the ordinate) is minimal over most of the physiological range, being most pronounced at either extremes of disuse (bone loss) or intense physical activity (bone formation). Growing bone is generally viewed as exhibiting a similar, but heightened (steeper slope), response to changes in loading history, compared to mature bone.

to maintain active net bone formation (the level of which will generally decline as growth progresses) vs. the normally balanced state of bone turnover in mature bone, the remodeling processes by which these tissues respond to altered loading histories may be expected to differ as well.

A key difficulty of existing work that impedes attempts to distinguish the relationship between skeletal growth and physical activity is that different studies have examined the effects of exercise, or lack thereof, on bone growth at quite different stages of skeletal maturity and in different species. Few studies, in fact, have investigated the response of the skeleton to exercise early in post-natal growth. As skeletal growth varies considerably among species that differ in size and other life history traits, interpretations of skeletal modeling observed in relation to influences such as physical exercise are confounded by differences in the period of growth studied and rate of tissue maturation. Finally, it seems likely that skeletal elements comprising different portions of the skeleton, which are subjected to quite different

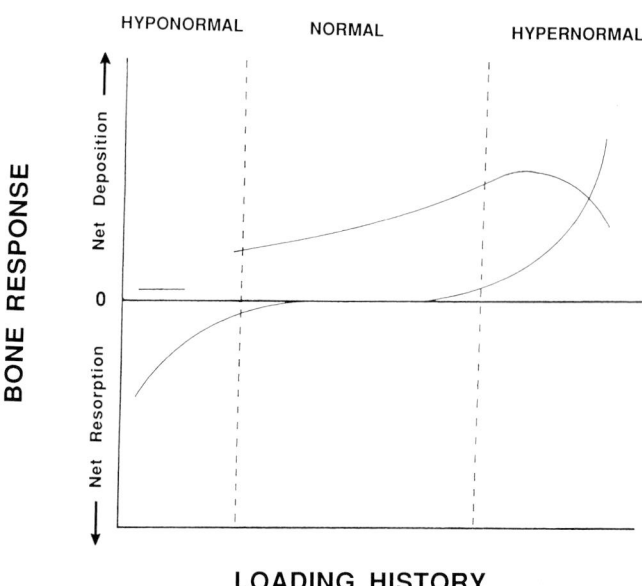

LOADING HISTORY

Fig. 2 A more realistic comparison of growing vs. mature bone in response to mechanical loading history. The curve for growing bone takes into account that changes in bone modeling associated with mechanical loading are superimposed on the normal growth trajectory of the bone to increase its size and mass. The vertical position of the curve for growing bone varies with age, shifting toward zero (i.e., bone turnover balance) as growth progresses to maturity. The response curve for growing bone within the normal physiological loading range may still have a steeper slope than that of mature bone (as depicted in Fig. 1) , reflecting a heightened responsiveness of growing bone to changes in loading history. Very high loading intensity (right of graph) may retard normal growth, whereas growth still continues even when functional loads are removed (left of graph). The gap in the growing bone curve from normal to hypo-normal loading indicates our present lack of understanding of the changes that occur in this range. The differing shapes of these curves suggests that modeling processes underlying adaptation to changes in mechanical loading may be different for growing vs. mature bone.

loading environments (e.g. dermal bone elements of the skull vs. long bones of the limbs; Hall and Herring, 1990), may themselves differ in their sensitivity and capacity to respond to extrinsic mechanical loading during growth.

Given these potentially confounding effects, we confine our discussion here to the post-natal growth of long bones in an attempt to clarify the role of physical exercise in relation to this particular aspect of skeletal growth. At present, the great majority of data (summarized in Tables 1 and 2) are based on measurements of skeletal mass and shape in comparatively few species, with little or no information on how physical activity actually affects tissue-modeling dynamics of growing long bones.

Overview of Growth Modeling in Long Bones

Much of our current understanding of bone growth modeling stems from comparative studies of post-natal growth of the mammalian skeleton (Enlow, 1962, 1964). Little systematic descriptive work has been carried out on the post-natal growth of non-mammalian bone. Because of its mineralized extracellular matrix, bone is an extremely rigid tissue with a high elastic modulus. As a result, bone modeling to alter bone shape and size must occur on preexisting surfaces of the bone. Growth proceeds therefore by a continual process of bone formation and resorption on periosteal, endosteal, and intracortical (osteonal) surfaces of the bone, the historical pattern of which can be observed by histological examination of the bone at different levels along its length (Enlow, 1964).

Overall increases in bone diameter are achieved by the simultaneous processes of periosteal deposition to expand the bone's external diameter and endosteal resorption to enlarge its medullary cavity. Increases in cortical thickness, therefore, are mediated by a greater rate of bone formation at the periosteal surface vs. bone resorption along the endosteal surface. This simple scheme of diameter increase, however, is only observed within the midshaft diaphysis of a growing long bone. At more proximal or distal locations, changes in bone shape associated with remodeling of the metaphysis, as well as the development and maintenance of a bone's longitudinal curvature, substantially alter this simple scheme of diameter increase (Fig. 6; see below). Changes in cross-sectional shape and curvature frequently alter this scheme at the midshaft as well.

Early in development when growth is most rapid, bone deposited at the periosteal surface is woven or fibrous in nature, being comprised of irregularly oriented collagen fibers that are imbedded in a less highly mineralized matrix than other forms of primary bone (Currey, 1984). As growth begins to slow, more organized bone tissue (increased alignment of collagen fibers) is layed down at the periosteal surface. The deposition of primary osteonal or lamellar bone characterizes most of the period of size increase during post-natal growth in endothermic species (Enlow, 1962, 1964). More slowly growing ectothermic species, in contrast, generally deposit poorly vascularized circumferential lamellar bone at the periosteal surface (Enlow and Brown, 1957; de Ricqles, 1979).

Generally, in species that grow rapidly (such as gallinaceous birds) primary osteonal bone constitutes the majority of newly deposited bone at the periosteal surface (Fig. 3). A high density of primary vascular canals provides increased surface area for lamellar infilling of the newly formed osteons, facilitating the overall rate of bone growth. Later in age, as growth continues to slow, or in less rapidly growing species (large mammals), newly formed periosteal bone is less vascularized and is deposited in a plexiform arrangement or as circumferential lamellae at the surface.

Table 1.
Bone Growth in Response to Increased Mechanical Loading

Species	Age (Weeks)	% Mature Body Mass	Exercise/Loading Regime	Strain History	Bone Response Structural (%)	Histological	Ref.
Mouse	2–7	25–75	Treadmill running [moderate] 1 h at 0.3 m/s, 5° incline		nc / L +19 / M		Kiiskinen (1977)
			Treadmill running (strenuous) 3 h at 0.3 m/s, 5° incline		– 4 / L nc / M		
	7–12	75–100	Treadmill running (moderate)		– 3 / L nc / M		
			Treadmill running (strenuous)		– 3 / L nc / M		
Rat	4–14	15–100	Treadmill running 3 h (2 km/d)		+ 4 / M nc / σ_f + 5 / Ca		Saville and Whyte (1969)
	4–10	15–75	Treadmill running (to fatigue)		+ 4 / L + 5 / D + 12 / M		Steinberg and Trueta (1981)
	1–12.5	5–100	Centrifugation at 1.1 g		+ 5 / L nc / BMC		Simon et al. (1985)
			Centrifugation at 1.5 g		nc / L – 8 / BMC		

Key
L: bone length
M: bone mass or weight
D: cortical diameter
A: cortical area
I: second moment of area
C: bone curvature
Ca: calcium content
BMC: bone mineral content
U_f: energy at failure
σ_f: failure stress
nc: no change

Animal			Loading regimen	Strain	Response	Notes	Reference
Chicken	3–8	12–50	Centrifugation at 2.0 g		-3 / L, nc / BMC		Matsuda *et al.* (1986)
			Treadmill running 40 min at 0.7–1.1 m/s (75% aerobic maximum)		-17 / D, -21 / A, -38 / I, nc / U_f		
	8–12	50–75			-11 / D, $+15$ / A, nc / I, -25 / U_f		
	2–4	8–14	Treadmill running 15 min at 60% maximum speed (0.9–1.7 m/s), loaded at 1.2× body mass	$+53\%$ peak ϵ, 1800 cycles per day	nc / L, $+12$ / A, $+29$ / I, nc / % ash		Biewener and Bertram (unpublished)
	4–8	14–50			nc / L, $+30$ / A, $+45$ / I, nc / % ash		
	8–12	50–75			nc / L, $+20$ / A, $+30$ / I		
Yucatan swine	26–52	?–?	Track running 1 h at 1.55 m/s		$+23$ / A, $+26$ / I	Increased endosteal deposition	Woo *et al.* (1981)
Pig	12–26		Radius overstrain via ulnar osteotomy	$+28\%$ peak ϵ	$+35$ / A	Periosteal deposition of woven bone	Goodship *et al.* (1979)

Table 2.
Bone Growth in Relation to Disuse or Paralysis

Species	Age/Duration (Weeks)	% Mature Body Mass	Disuse Method	Bone Response		Ref.
				Structural (%)	Histological	
Rat	4–64	15–100	Sciatic denervation and patellar tenotomy	nc / L −13 / M −13 / Curv	Change in normal cross-sectional shape	Lanyon (1980)
	4–10	15–75	Immobilization	−3 / L −5 / D −16 / M	Decreased vascularity (change in normal cross-sectional shape)	Steinberg and Trueta (1981)
	4–19	15–95	Brachial plexus denervation	−4 / L −12 / D −23 / M nc / % ash −3 / L nc / BMC		Armstrong (1946)
	3.5–7.5	15–66	Brachial plexus denervation	−2 / L −17 / D		Dysart et al. (1989)
	9–11.7	50–80	Spaceflight—19.5 d (Cosmos 782)		−40% periosteal bone formation rate; nc endosteal resorption	Morey and Baylink (1978)
	9–11.6	50–80	Spaceflight—18.5 d (Cosmos 936)	nc / L nc / ρ −33 / Torque$_{\text{failure}}$ −31 / U_f		Spengler et al. (1983)

Animal			Treatment	Result	Effect	Reference
Chicken	9–11.6	50–80	Spaceflight—18.5 d (Cosmos 936) Sciatic denervation	nc / L −18 / M −12 / A nc / I nc / % ash	−44% periosteal bone formation rate −27% periosteal bone formation rate	Turner *et al.* (1985)
	2–4	8–14	Sciatic denervation and patellar tenotomy	−2 / L −17 / M −5 / A nc / I nc / % ash −85 / C		Biewener and Bertram (unpublished)
	4–8	14–50		−2 / L −11 / M −12 / A −16 / I nc / % ash −135 / C		
	8–12	50–75				
Cat	?–+8	75–100	Lumbosacral paralysis	−18 / M nc / σ_f nc / E nc / ρ	More circular cross-sectional shape of femoral and tibial cortices	Gillespie (1954)
Dog (1–3 year)	?–+6 +6–+12 12–60	?–?	Immobilization	−16% / A −10% / A −38% / A	Increased trabecular and periosteal bone resorption; followed by decreased periosteal deposition	Uhthoff and Jaworski (1978)

Table 2 (continued).
Bone Growth in Relation to Disuse or Paralysis

Species	Age/Duration (Weeks)	% Mature Body Mass	Disuse Method	Bone Response		Ref.
				Structural (%)	Histological	
Rhesus monkey (4 year)	?– + 2	75–80	Immobilization		−16% osteonal bone formation rate nc frequency of active osteons −98% frequency of trabecular bone formation	Wronski and Morey (1983)

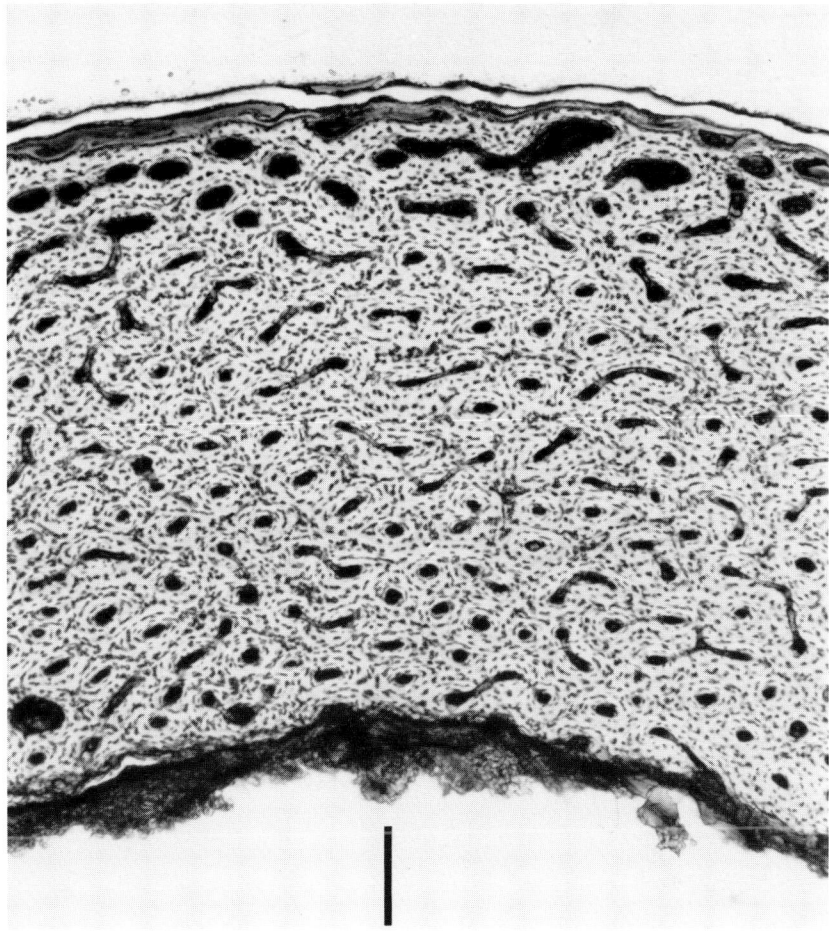

Fig. 3 Light micrograph (× 30) of an undecalcified section of a chick tibiotarsus at 8 weeks of age, showing primary osteonal bone deposition associated with periosteal expansion of the posterior midshaft cortex. Note the high density of primary vascular canals. As the osteons form near the periosteal surface (at top), the vascular canals are initially large and subsequently infilled to form mature primary osteons deeper within the expanding cortex. Endosteal surface is at bottom. Scale bar: 100 μm.

To maintain its characteristic shape and, hence, functional integrity during growth, the cortices of a long bone must be continually reshaped to accomodate increases in length (Fig. 4). Because the articular ends of long bones are enlarged relative to the diaphysis to reduce stress within the articular cartilage and underlying subchondral bone (by distributing joint reaction forces over a wider area of contact; Currey, 1984), as a long bone

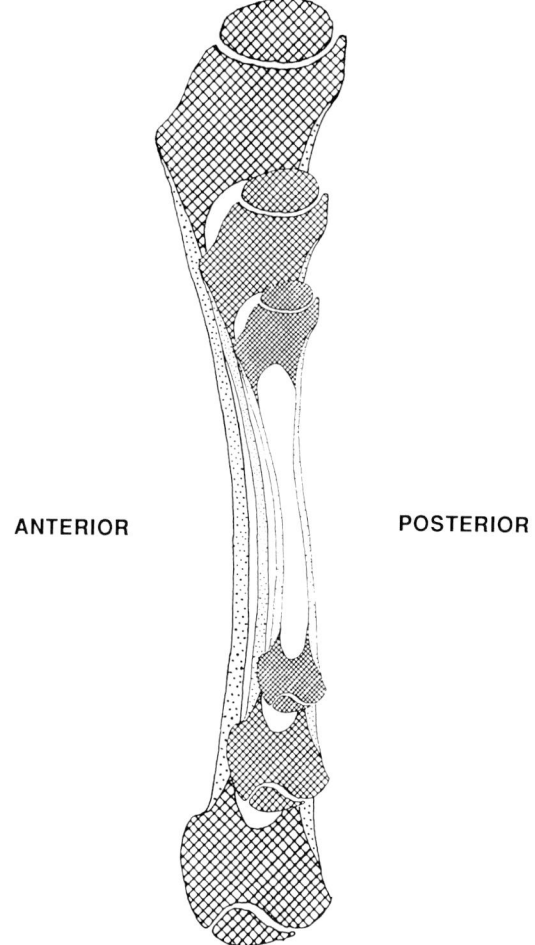

ANTERIOR   POSTERIOR

Fig. 4 Diagramatic representation of long bone growth (patterned after the canine tibia; anterior is left and posterior is right). A twofold increase in length requires substantial modification, replacement, and generation of bone volume due to the appositional nature of bone growth. These changes are particularly pronounced within the metaphysis. Cross-hatched areas indicate cancellous bone and stippled areas indicate compact, cortical bone. See text for details.

grows in length, the metaphysis must be reduced in size as the bone formed behind the advancing growth plate progressively shifts toward the diaphysis. This metaphyseal reduction or "waisting" (Enlow, 1962) of the bone's cortex typically involves resorption at the periosteal surface and endosteal deposition of new bone along surfaces of cancellous trabeculae formed behind the advancing growth plate. This process gradually fills in the spaces among

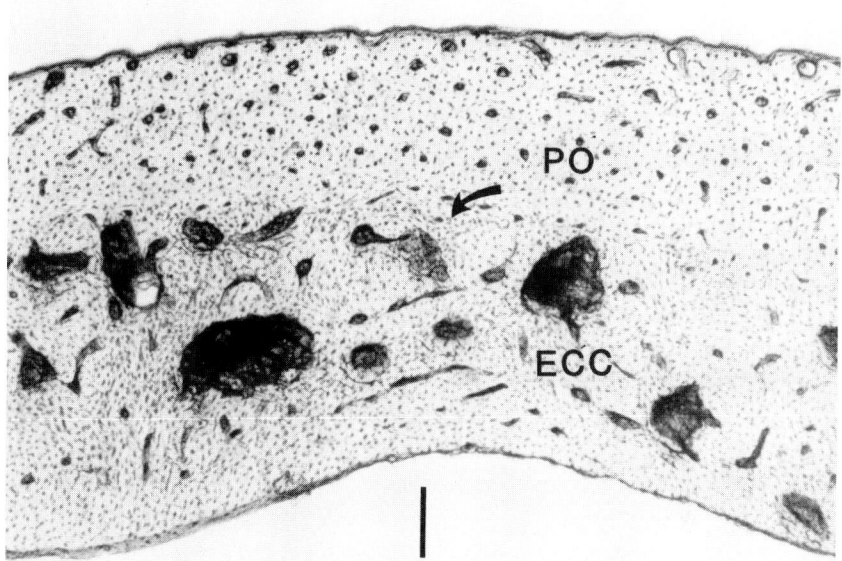

Fig. 5 Light micrograph of endosteally compacted cancellous (ECC) bone in the anterior midshaft cortex of the chick tibiotarsus at 12 weeks of age (× 30, undecalcified), formed during metaphyseal reduction. The endosteal compacted cancellous bone is located deep to primary osteonal (PO) bone formed at a later age. Periosteal surface is at top and endosteal surface is at bottom. Arrow shows reversal 'line' indicating transition from periosteal resorption of endosteally compacted cancellous bone, associated with metaphyseal reduction, to periosteal deposition of primary osteonal bone, associated with subsequent radial expansion of the bone's diaphysis.

the trabeculae to form a distinct histological zone, termed "endosteally compacted" (Enlow, 1962) or "coarsely compacted cancellous" (Currey, 1984) bone (Fig. 5). Endosteally compacted cancellous bone is often found in the diaphysis of older bones as they near the limit of their longitudinal growth. In some cases, narrowing of the medullary cavity associated with metaphyseal reduction or cortical drift (see below) occurs by additional lamellar deposition of bone on the inner surface of endosteally compacted cancellous bone. As the metaphysis grades into the diaphysis, the process of metaphyseal reduction eventually reverses at the level where cortical diameter is increasing via periosteal deposition. At this site a 'reversal line' frequently remains, reflecting the shift from periosteal resorption of previously formed endosteally compacted bone to lamellar or osteonal bone deposited on the external surface (Fig. 5).

In addition to modeling processes associated with length and diameter increases of the bone during growth, shifts in bone formation and resorption also occur to maintain the longitudinal curvature of a bone and change its cross-sectional shape. Most long bones change shape along their length. Such changes in cross-sectional shape, in fact, are most relevant to bone-remodeling responses to altered mechanical loading. Studies of bone loading *in vivo* during locomotion (Biewener *et al.*, 1983, 1986; Lanyon and Bourn, 1979; Lanyon and Baggott, 1976; Lanyon *et al.*, 1982; Rubin and Lanyon, 1982) show that, by promoting bending in a given plane, a bone's longitudinal curvature can greatly affect the distribution of strains (local tissue deformations produced by forces acting on the bone) developed in its cortex during physical activity. Although the functional significance of long bone curvature is not fully resolved, it has been argued to reduce the variability of functional strains engendered within the bone during activity (Bertram and Biewener, 1988) or to provide increased space for muscle attachment to the bone and packaging near its longitudinal axis (Lanyon, 1980). Available evidence indicates that the curvature of most long bones augments, rather than diminishes, externally applied bending moments and, thus, does not function to maintain a bone in overall axial compression (Biewener *et al.*, 1983; Biewener and Taylor, 1986; Lanyon and Baggott, 1976; Lanyon and Bourn, 1979; and see below).

Growth modeling associated with maintaining or altering the curvature of a long bone, or changing the cross-sectional shape of its cortex, involves "cortical drift" (Enlow, 1962; Frost, 1964). Cortical drift describes relative shifts in the position of compact bone in a transverse plane relative to the bone's longitudinal axis. Hence, a shift in the bone's diaphysis to produce a posteriorly convex curvature involves periosteal deposition and endosteal resorption on the posterior cortex vs. periosteal resorption and endosteal deposition on the anterior cortex (Figs. 6 and 7). As with metaphyseal reduction, cortical drift involves shifts in the relative position of bone tissue layed down at an earlier time. Not only does cortical drift underlie the capacity of long bones to straighten defects in alignment after fracture (Friberg, 1979a, b; Frost, 1964), it is fundamental to adaptive remodeling in response to changes in mechanical loading. As this capacity is more limited in the mature skeleton (Frost, 1964; Currey 1984), adaptive remodeling via cortical drift may be expected to be more prevalent in growing animals.

In contrast to the fairly uniform drift observed in the midshaft cortices of the chick tibiotarsus (Figs. 6 and 7), cortical drift can be asymmetric, involving radial expansion of the bone's shaft in only one direction. ^{45}Ca labeling of the tibia of growing dogs indicates that the posterolateral aspect undergoes remarkably little drift, either endosteally or periosteally (Figs. 8 and 9; Ponlot, 1960; Dhem and Vincent, 1965). Expansion of the shaft over a 4-week period involves drift (with periosteal deposition and endosteal resorption) primarily in the anteromedial direction. *In vivo* bone strain recordings from the tibiae of adult dogs (Rubin and Lanyon, 1982) indicate

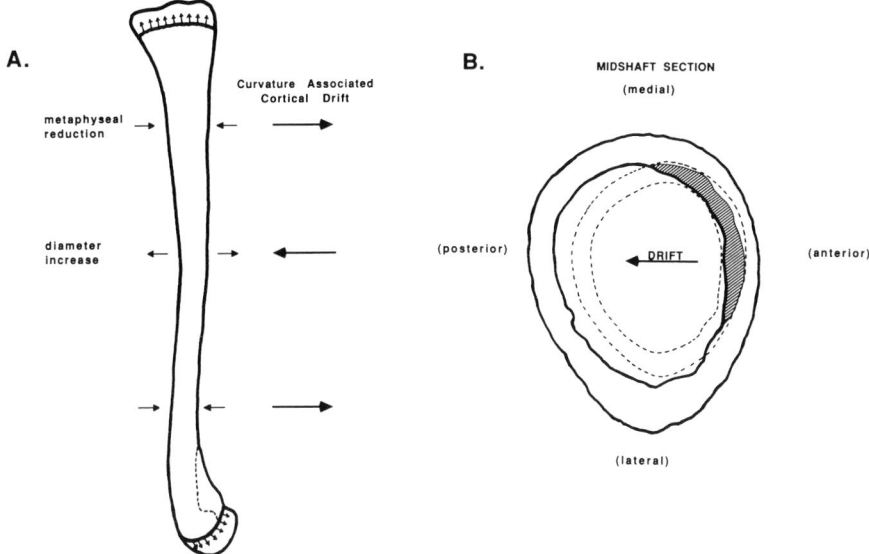

Fig. 6 (A) A diagramatic representation of cortical drift (large arrows) in the chick tibiotarsus associated with maintenance of the bone's longitudinal curvature. Smaller arrows show periosteal surface modeling changes associated with either metaphyseal reduction or diameter increase at the midshaft. The direction of longitudinal growth at the epiphyseal growth plates is also shown. Note that the direction of epiphyseal growth does not necessarily parallel the bone's shaft; this is particularly so at the distal growth plate. Patterns of drift must be interpreted in light of these processes of diameter change in the bone's shaft and the growth trajectories of the physes. (B) Drift occurs in the posterior direction at the midshaft level, corresponding to the shift in curvature of the bone from its proximal to distal level (proximal: anteriorly convex to distal: posteriorly convex). As a result of this posterior drift, endosteally compacted cancellous bone (hatched region) is retained in the anterior cortex (see Figs. 5 and 7A) and periosteal deposition of osteonal bone is disproportionately greater on the posterior vs. the anterior cortex of the bone. Dashed lines show shape of bone at 4 weeks of age compared to that at 8 weeks of age (solid lines).

that this growth modeling drift of the tibia does not represent a change in bone architecture to reduce bending-induced strain, as the principal plane of bending in this bone is anteroposterior during locomotion, with maximal tensile strain developed in the anterior (cranial) cortex and maximal compressive strain developed in the posterior (caudal) cortex. Under these loading conditions, the lateral and medial cortices presumably experience intermediate levels of axial strain and higher levels of shear strain. As with this bone and other bones studied (see below), therefore, the correlation between bone growth modeling and patterns of bone strain during activity remains obscure.

It is worth noting that the processes of bone modeling described above involve distinct "envelopes" of the bone. Frost (1969) distinguishes three surfaces or envelopes on which bone can be added or removed from cortical bone: (1) periosteal, (2) endosteal, and (3) intracortical (with a fourth involving trabecular bone). Long bone growth involves bone formation and removal within each of these envelopes. Generally, bone removal within the intracortical envelope involves osteoclastic tunneling of previously existing bone and subsequent lamellar infilling to form secondary osteons, or Haversian systems, which typically do not occur until relatively late in growth, or at maturity, and may not occur at all in many smaller, short-lived species (Enlow and Brown, 1958). The endosteal envelope is continuous with that of cancellous bone located in the metaphysis. Although bone modeling within these three envelopes is coordinated to achieve the overall shape and function of bone, factors and mechanisms that regulate bone turnover within each envelope may not be the same (Uhthoff, 1982).

Functionally Equivalent (Homotypic) Sites in Growing Bone

The importance of the particular pattern of mechanical loading in relation to the structural form of a bone during its growth is supported by data that show a uniform pattern of bone strain at functionally equivalent sites on the surface of a bone's shaft during exercise (Biewener et al., 1986). In this study, functionally equivalent, or "homotypic" sites on the chick tibiotarsus were defined with respect to a percentage of the bone's length and orientation about the perimeter of the cortex. A similar shift in muscular, tendinous, and ligamentous attachments to the bone occurs in relation to a fixed percentage of the bone's length as it grows (Dorfl, 1980; Grant et al., 1980), supporting this definition of functional equivalence at specified sites on a growing bone. Bone strains recorded at such sites during treadmill locomotion did not vary significantly in magnitude, sign (tension vs. compression), or orientation from 4 to 17 weeks of age, during which time the bone increased tenfold in mass and threefold in length. Functional strains, however, varied both in magnitude and sign among the differing bone sites within an individual, suggesting that the remodeling response of local bone cell populations to exercise-induced strain may be site specific, responding to the state of strain within local regions of the bone.

Though the maintenance of a uniform pattern of locomotor bone strain during much of the post-natal growth of this bone suggests that mechanical factors may play a role in regulating bone growth modeling, this need not be the case. Since normal functional strain patterns are experienced by a bone throughout the animal's lifetime and over a range of activity, the ontogeny of bone form may be largely constrained by selection for epigenetic processes (tissue interactions) that govern its development along a given growth trajectory. To distinguish between these two possibilities it is necessary to show that known changes in the loading history of a growing bone *produce* a change in bone mass *and shape* that structurally matches the new loading conditions. Clear evidence of such a response has been demonstrated in few cases.

Mechanically Induced Changes in Longitudinal Growth

The transformation of cartilage to bone and its subsequent remodeling to produce a bone's final form ultimately depends on the kinetics, distribution, and orientation of cartilage formation at the growth plate. Consequently, the effect of mechanical loading on the biology of the growth plate is fundamental to a broader understanding of how physical activity influences skeletal form. As cartilage grows by hyperplasia and interstitial hypertrophy, changes in bone length and width at the growth plate can result from changes in the division rate of proliferative cells (Kember, 1985), the number of proliferative cells (zone thickness; Kember, 1972, 1973), the rate or extent of cellular hypertrophy (Kember, 1985), the amount of matrix production, and the longevity of chondroprogenitor cell division (or their replenishment from perivascular undifferentiated cells). Although their relative importance differs, all of these mechanisms likely influence to some degree the rate and overall extent of longitudinal bone growth. As many of these processes are reviewed in detail elsewhere in this series (Volume 6, Chapter 8), we limit our discussion here to studies of how the longitudinal growth of long bones may be influenced by mechanical loading associated with physical activity.

For well over a century, interpretations of the effect of mechanical loading on the growth plate have been dominated by the Heuter-Volkmann Law of Epiphyseal Pressures, which states that a bone's growth rate is inversely related to the magnitude of static (compressive) force transmitted across the growth plate parallel to the axis of growth (Heuter, 1862; Volkmann, 1862). More recently, this relationship has led to the hypothesis that changes in tensile stress within the periosteum (produced by active growth of the proximal and distal growth plates of a bone) affect long bone growth, with decreased tension (associated with decreased compression across the growth plate) stimulating increased growth (Crilley, 1972; Harkness and Trotter, 1978). Studies of circumferential division of the periosteum producing overgrowth and compensatory growth of one growth plate following inhibition of the opposite growth plate (Dawson and Kember, 1974; Hall-Craggs, 1968) support this view.

Although extreme physical loading (increased compression) may indeed inhibit longitudinal bone growth, other studies indicate that the relationship between longitudinal growth and mechanical loading is more complex at moderate load levels in which the responsiveness of the growth plate likely depends not only on the nature (tension, compression, or shear) and magnitude of the load applied but the animal's age as well. Moreover, it is important to recognize that changes in bone length may be caused by

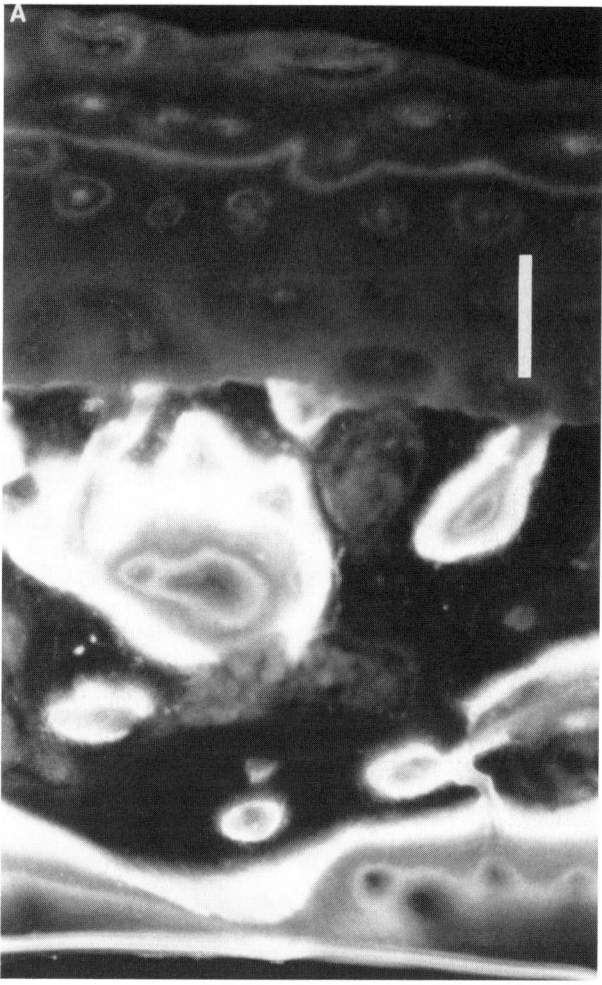

Fig. 7 Fluorescent micrographs of the (A) anterior and (B) posterior cortices of the chick tibiotarsus at 8 weeks of age ($\times$ 40, undecalcified 70-μm section). Periosteal surface is at top and endosteal surface is at bottom. Two fluorochrome labels are seen; the first label (calcein, bright in contrast) was administered at 5 weeks of age and the second (xylenol orange, less bright) at 7 weeks of age. The reversal from periosteal resorption and endosteal compaction associated with metaphyseal reduction to subsequent periosteal deposition associated with diameter increase of the diaphysis is clearly seen in the anterior cortex (A). The calcein label shows the process of endosteal compaction in the anterior cortex at 5 weeks of age, whereas in the posterior cortex (B) it is associated with the formation of primary osteons involved in rapid periosteal expansion. The second label (xylenol orange) shows a similar contrast of the patterns of bone deposition in the anterior vs. posterior cortex, associated with the posterior drift that occurs in the bone at this level. Note the much broader zones of labeled bone in the posterior cortex (B) compared to the anterior cortex (A), reflecting its much greater expansion via periosteal osteonal bone formation. Scale bars: 100 μm.

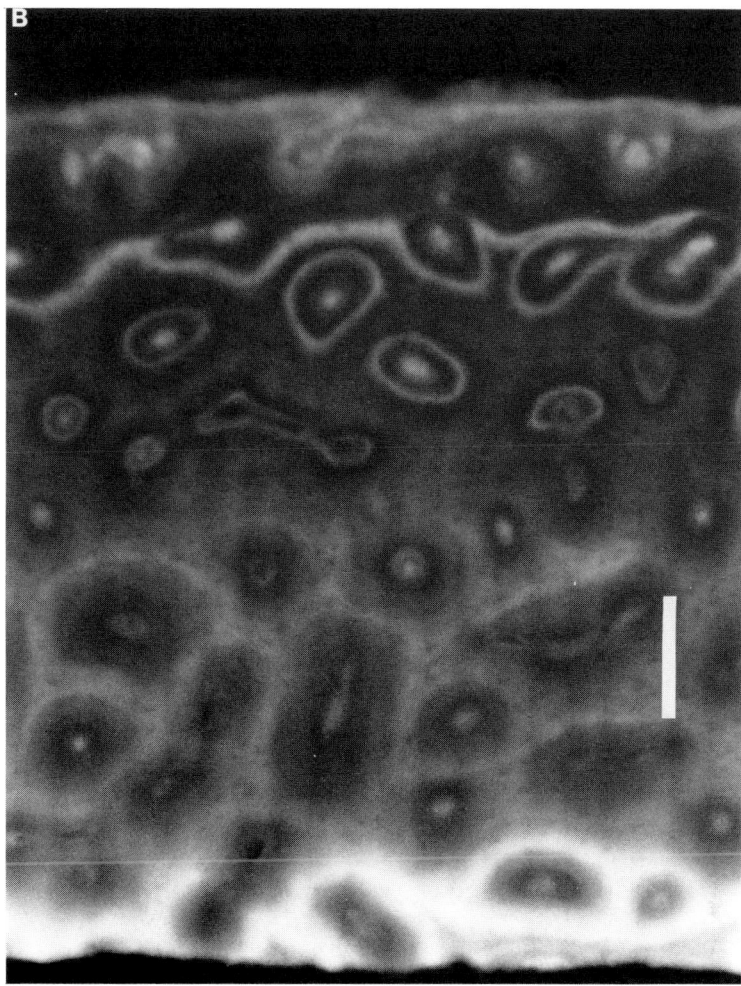

Fig. 7B

changes in either the rate or the duration of cartilage production at the physes. Early studies (reviewed by Murray, 1936) show a broad spectrum of both negative and positive growth responses to increased loading. The conflicting and highly variable results of these early studies is likely due, in part, to physiological and/or surgical trauma experienced by the bone under study.

In a more recent study, using mechanical spring distractors (producing static tension) to reduce exercise-related compression loads transmitted across the proximal epiphyseal plate of the rabbit tibia, Hert *et al.* (1969) found that a 25 to 50% decrease in force relative to that estimated during limb support at moderate exercise (no speed or force data were reported) resulted

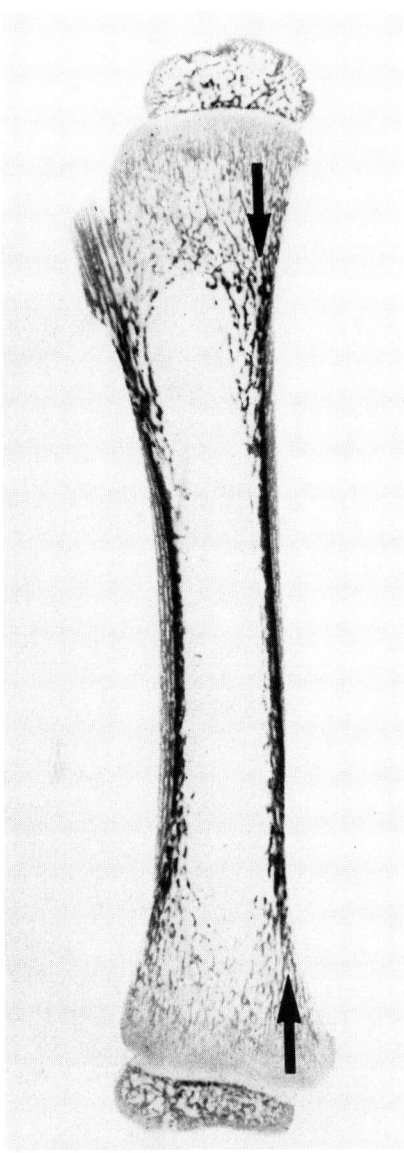

Fig. 8 Lateral autoradiograph of a 7-week-old canine tibia that had been labeled with ⁴⁵C 3 weeks prior to recovery of the bone. Deposition overlaps the labeled cortex exclusively on the anterior aspect (left). The posterior cortex (right) has undergone some intracortical remodeling but remains largely unchanged from the time that the label was administered. (Autoradiograph courtesy of Prof. A. Dhem.)

ANTERIOR

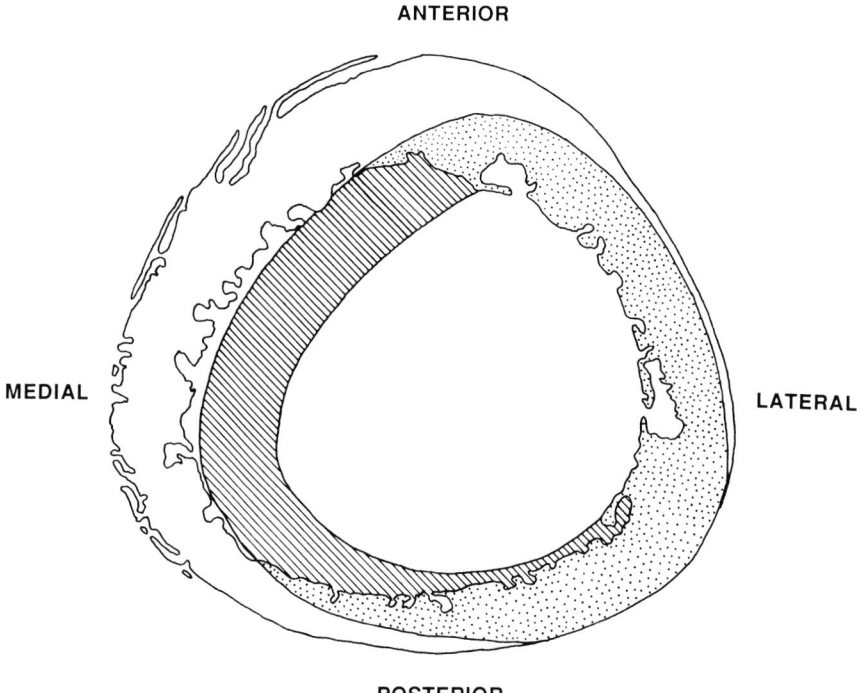

MEDIAL

LATERAL

POSTERIOR

Fig. 9 Line drawing from an autoradiograph of a midshaft transverse section of the canine tibia shown in Fig. 8, illustrating two growth stages at ages 4 and 7 weeks. Stippled area is original bone present at 4 weeks, which has undergone only intracortical Haversian remodeling. Hatched area is reconstruction of original cortex based on remaining label in the bone and its known dimensions at 4 weeks of age. Unmarked cortex is bone deposited between 4 and 7 weeks of age. (After Ponlot, 1960.)

in a substantial (13 to 27%) increase in longitudinal growth at the proximal plate. The distracted proximal plate also closed at a younger age than normal, however, resulting in no *final* difference between the experimental and control limb lengths in fully mature animals. This finding raises the intriguing possibility that changes in the rate of longitudinal growth by extrinsic factors may be compensated for by an opposing change in the duration of growth, reflecting a relatively fixed intrinsic potential of the epiphyseal plate for longitudinal growth. Although Hert *et al.*, interpreted the bone's length increase as resulting from a decrease in compressive load transmitted across the proximal epiphysis, their method of distraction does not distinguish between the alternative effects of decreased compression (during limb support) vs. net tension (at other times in the step cycle) produced by distraction of the plate. Using a similar approach to increase, rather than decrease, compressive loading of the epiphyseal plate, Strobino *et al.* (1952) found that increased compressive stress, estimated to be as high as 60 lb/in^2 (or 2.7 MPa) at the end of the experimental period, had no effect on the longitudinal growth of the proximal tibial plate of cattle following 4 months of growth (beginning at 6 to 8 weeks of age).

Consistent with the view that excessive compressive stress may exert an inhibitory effect on the growth plate, however, Kiiskinen (1977) found that intensive (5° incline at 0.3 m/s, 3 h/d) treadmill exercise in young mice (2 to 12 weeks of age) resulted in a 1 to 4% decrease in the longitudinal growth of the femur (Table 1). At moderate exercise (1 h/d), no consistent differences in bone length were observed between exercise and control animals.

On the other hand, Steinberg and Trueta (1981) reported a 4% increase in long bone growth in rats following 6 weeks of daily treadmill exercise to fatigue (no speed or duration was reported). Because the body mass of exercise animals was 26% greater than age-matched controls, however, it is unlikely that the observed increase in bone length would have been statistically significant had the data been normalized for the difference in body mass. A similar difficulty arises in interpreting the results of a study of young rats (5 weeks of age) that were swum for 1 h/d (Swissa-Sivan *et al.*, 1989), in which it seems unlikely that the reported 2-3% increase in humeral length following 20 weeks of exercise would have been found had the data been normalized for differences in size (experimental animals were 17% heavier than controls). When normalized for differences in body mass, no significant effect of intensive treadmill exercise (60% of maximum speed, or 1.54 m/s at 12 weeks of age, carrying a weight equal to 20% of body mass) on the longitudinal growth of the white leghorn chick tibiotarsus (2 to 12 weeks of age) is observed (Table 1; Biewener and Bertram, unpublished). Finally, in a study of 9 d-old rats subjected to 81 d of centrifugation, Simon *et al.* (1985) reported that increased gravitational loading produced a modest increase in long bone length. However, their data are difficult to interpret as the greatest increase (5%) occurred at only 1.1 *g* acceleration and was inconsistent among the different long bones examined and with respect to the magnitude of gravitational loading experienced (increments between 1.0 and 2.0 *g* acceleration were studied).

As with the conflicting and modest growth responses observed following exercise, studies of disuse or paralysis also demonstrate little definitive effect of the absence of physical loading on longitudinal bone growth. In a study of young growing rats (4 to 64 weeks of age), Lanyon (1980) found no difference in the length of the tibia following denervation and patellar tenotomy to remove functional load bearing (at 4 weeks of age) when compared to the contralateral control limb. Dysart *et al.* (1989) found only a slight, but significant, decrease (2%) in the length of the humerus of rats denervated from 4 to 7 weeks of age compared to contralateral controls. In a similar study of young growing chicks (2 to 12 weeks of age), Biewener and Bertram (unpublished) also found a slight (1 to 2%) but significant decrease in length of the chicken tibiotarsus following denervation and patellar tenotomy compared to the contralateral tibiotarsus. When normalized for differences in body mass and compared to a control sedentary population, however, tibiotarsal length was found to be 10 to 15% less in the denervated limb. Given that the length of the contralateral control bone of the denervated group was also shorter, the observed difference between control and denervated animals likely reflects differences in the nutritional status of the two groups (denervated animals grew less rapidly than control animals). The absence of significant changes in bone length following limb paralysis is consistent with earlier findings of bone growth in young adult cats and rats (Gillespie, 1954).

It seems likely that, in addition to decreased loading of the plate itself, decreased blood flow or muscle atrophy associated with limb denervation may also be contributing factors to differences in bone growth. Steinberg and Trueta (1981) found that within 1 week bone vascularity was substantially decreased following paralysis of the femur of growing rats, noting that this may have contributed to the observed decrease in bone formation.

Following hindlimb suspension of Wistar rats for 22 d (begun at ages 1, 2.5, and 6 months), Novikov and Ilyin (1981) found a 5% decrease in femur length in the 1-month old rats and a 4% decrease in the 2.5-month old rats. No significant difference was found in the 6-month old group. While these animals were matched for weight and age with controls at the beginning of the study, comparisons were not made with controls at later ages to evaluate the effect of the experimental procedure on the general growth of the animals. Following 7 d of spaceflight, Shaw *et al.* (1988) found no difference in the tibial length of 30-d-old rats, but did note a slight depression in longitudinal growth of the humerus compared to ground-based controls. Similarly, Spengler *et al.* (1983) found that 18.5 d exposure to microgravity had no significant effect on the longitudinal growth of the femur in 9-week-old rats (Table 2).

In summary, little experimental evidence exists to indicate that the longitudinal growth rates of long bones are substantially altered by extrinsic mechanical loading, provided that the magnitude and manner in which the loading is applied does not cause physical or physiological trauma. When measured in the same individual, slight length changes may occur following the total removal of load, but these are of only a few percent of the bone's length. It appears, therefore, that the interaction between physical activity and epiphyseal growth has far more bearing on the correction of angular deformities (Friberg, 1979a, b; Frost, 1964) than it does on determining the ultimate length achieved by the growing bone. This latter observation suggests that the growth plate may be more responsive to changes in loading orientation (causing increased shear strain within the plate) than simply to the magnitude of axial compressive load. Consequently, available data indicate that post-natal longitudinal growth of long bones is strongly controlled by intrinsic genetic and epigenetic factors that are largely independent of mechanical stimuli experienced over a wide range of normal physical exercise.

Cortical Bone Growth in Response to Increased Mechanical Loading

Although a substantial number of studies have examined the influence of physical exercise on cortical bone growth, the majority of these have either only qualitatively assessed the mechanical loading environment of the bone under study or have examined bone growth fairly late in post-natal growth. Few studies have actually attempted to quantify the strain-loading history of the bone under study. Underlying the changes in bone mass and form that occur during growth are the manner in which changes in bone length, diameter, and overall shape are achieved and ultimately, then, the tissue-modeling processes upon which these changes depend. In most cases, the skeleton's response to physical exercise has been assessed in terms of bone mass and diameter, with little data presented regarding changes in bone shape, cortical area, and histology.

Several experimental approaches have been used to vary the mechanical loading of growing bones within the normal physiological range, including treadmill or track exercise (with or without weights), swimming, and chronic acceleration via centrifugation. More invasive procedures to remove one supporting element, causing overload of the intact element (as in radial overload following ulnar osteotomy in quadrupedal animals, see below), are also effective but introduce the potential confounding effects of physiological and mechanical trauma. An important advantage of chronic running exercise is the natural manner in which loads are dynamically applied to the skeleton. Loading can be varied in terms of magnitude, frequency, and the number of loading cycles, which can be quantified in terms of *in vivo* recording of localized surface bone strains (Biewener *et al.*, 1986; Lanyon, 1976). The range and precision of control of bone loading patterns, however, is limited using this approach.

Because differences in the growth stage of the species studied and the bone envelope examined can have an important effect on the results obtained and their interpretation, we distinguish between studies of animals early (defined as when the growing animals are less than 50% of mature body mass) vs. late in post-natal growth. We also attempt to evaluate how differences in loading technique may affect interpretation of the data obtained. In general, only modest changes in bone mass, cortical area, and diameter have been reported in growing animals following running exercise, with conflicting results obtained in regard to whether exercise exerts a positive or negative influence on bone growth (data are summarized in Table 1). Studies showing an inhibitory effect on bone growth most often involve more strenuous exercise training.

Early Growth

In a study of 4-week-old rats (corresponding to 15% of mature body mass), Saville and Whyte (1969) found a small (4 to 5%) increase in bone mass following 10 weeks of exercise (no speed or duration was reported). This difference was established within 2 weeks of exercise training and did not change during the remainder of the study. When normalized for differences in body mass, however, the significance of the reported change in bone mass is questionable. In a study of 3-week-old white leghorn chicks (12% of mature body mass), Matsuda *et al.* (1986) reported an inhibitory skeletal response to 5 or 9 weeks of strenuous daily treadmill exercise (40 min at 75% of maximal aerobic capacity; 0.7 to 1.1 m/s). Midshaft periosteal diameters of the tarsometatarsus were reduced by 17% at 8 weeks and by 11% at 12 weeks in exercise vs. control chicks. Endosteal diameters were also reduced in the exercise animals, producing a cortical shaft that was narrower both in external and internal dimensions. Overall, cortical area was reduced by 21% in 8-week animals, but was *increased* by 15% in 12-week animals. Similarly, the second moment of area (a measure of a bone's cross-sectional shape associated with its ability to resist bending) was significantly lower (38%) in runners compared to controls at 8 weeks but was not significantly different at 12 weeks of age. These results suggest an initial negative response to exercise that is reversed at a later stage of growth.

In contrast to the inhibitory effects of strenuous exercise observed by Matsuda *et al.* (1986) early in growth, in a similar study of white leghorn chicks (2 to 12 weeks of age; 8 to 80% of mature body mass, Biewener and Bertram, unpublished) we found that strenuous daily treadmill exercise (1800 loading cycles at 15 min/d), corresponding to an average 53% increase in measured peak bone strain levels, resulted in a 30% increase in cortical area and a 45% increase in second moment of area of the tibiotarsus following 6 weeks of exercise compared to controls (at 8 weeks of age). These data were normalized for differences in body mass. Significant differences in cortical A and I were observed within 2 weeks of exercise (at 4 weeks of age). The differences between exercise and control animals at 12 weeks of age were slightly less than those at 8 weeks of age, but remained statistically significant and were consistent at proximal, midshaft, and distal levels of the bone (Table 1). The main difference between the study by Matsuda *et al.* (1986) and our own was the duration of exercise (40 vs. 15 min/d, respectively). Consequently, exercise duration may be an important factor determining whether a given mechanical stimulus exerts a negative or positive effect on a growing bone.

The transient nature of the skeleton's growth response to exercise in certain cases may be even more profound, with only minor differences remaining between exercise and control animals at skeletal maturity. For instance, Kiiskinen (1977) reported a 19% increase in the dry weight of long bones of juvenile mice within 2 weeks of moderate exercise (begun at 2 weeks of age when the animals were 25% mature body mass) compared to controls. This difference was maintained throughout the middle period of growth (8 weeks of age), but at 12 weeks of age (95% of mature body mass) no difference in the dry weight of exercised vs. control long bones remained. Kiiskinen (1977) attributed the initial gain in long bone weight to an increase in the maturation rate of the skeleton induced by the moderate exercise program. While this interpretation is plausible, characterization of the bone's "maturation rate" based solely on length increase is likely overly simplistic.

Studies of the effect of exercise on the skeleton of young children are understandably rare and the findings of such studies have been contradictory. Some studies suggest that exercise stimulates growth (Van Dusen, 1939; Ekblom, 1969); however, these results could not be verified statistically. Other studies indicate a restriction in growth as a result of exercise (Bugyi and Kansz, 1970; Kato and Ishiko, 1966). Bugyi and Kansz (1970) found that the growth plates of highly active competitive swimmers were at a more advanced stage of development than their less-active age-matched counterparts. An increase in growth plate maturation and early closure is one possible explanation for shorter (and consequently more robust) limbs in children that have been highly active from an early age (Parizkova, 1968).

Late Growth

Later in growth, a more consistent, positive skeletal response to mechanical loading has been documented; but again, this is based on only a few studies. In a study of 1-year-old miniature Yucatan swine run at 1.55 m/s (80% of maximal heart rate) for 6 km/d (1 h) over a period of 1 year, Woo et al. (1981) found a 23% increase in femoral cortical area and a 26% increase in second moment of area compared to sedentary controls. The mechanical properties and mineral composition of the femur did not differ, however, indicating that increased activity evoked mainly a structural response in these animals. The increase in cortical area and thickness of the femoral shaft was achieved mainly through a decrease in the area of the medullary cavity rather than an increase in periosteal diameter, suggesting (although not stated by the authors) that the increase was mediated via reduced endosteal resorption relative to that associated with normal diaphyseal diameter increase during growth.

In a study of young pigs, ranging from 3 to 6 months in age, Goodship *et al.* (1979) increased functional strain levels in the growing radius by surgical removal of a segment of the ulna proximal to its attachment to the radius. The magnitude of overstrain produced within the radius was 28% (peak compressive strain). Within 3 months following ulnar osteotomy, the radius increased in size to compensate for the lost support of the ulna. *In vivo* strain measurements made at the radial midshaft after the 3-month period closely matched those measured in animals during normal locomotion (prior to ulnar osteotomy). The increase (35%) in cortical area of the radius constituted 80% of the combined cortical area of the radius and ulna of the contralateral limb and was mediated via a rapid periosteal expansion of radially oriented laminae, comprised primarily of woven bone during the initial 3 weeks of the bone's response. Flourochrome labeling indicated that the response was initiated within 1 week of overstrain in the radius. Subsequent remodeling over the next 2 months consolidated the periosteal bone into a dense cortex with additional circumferential lamellar bone deposited thereafter at the periosteal surface. In a similar study of mature sheep, Lanyon *et al.* (1982) found that even a smaller strain overload (a 10 to 20% increase) promoted adaptive remodeling of the radius to reduce the elevated strains to normal presurgical levels. The comparatively small increase in strain above those normally experienced by the bone during walking could easily have been engendered by a slightly higher activity level, such as moderate trotting or running. Physical exercise at these levels, however, does not generally elicit a remodeling response in the mature skeleton. The distribution of strains recorded *in vivo* at different sites about the midshaft of long bones, moreover, remains fairly uniform over a wide range of speed during normal locomotion, despite changes in strain magnitude (Biewener *et al.*, 1983, 1988; Biewener and Taylor, 1986; Rubin and Lanyon, 1982). These studies suggest, therefore, that disruption of the normal *distribution* of functional strain, not simply a change in strain magnitude, is most critical for eliciting adaptive remodeling of the bone.

It is noteworthy that the means by which skeletal adaptation to increased load was achieved in the studies of Woo *et al.* (1981) and Goodship *et al.* (1979) involved distinctly different tissue responses and bone tissue envelopes in the pig. Whereas Goodship *et al.* (1979) observed a dramatic periosteal expansion of the radius to overload, Woo *et al.* (1981) interpreted the femur's response to exercise as being via increased endosteal bone formation (or, as we note above, a retardation of endosteal resorption associated with diameter increase of the growing bone). In both cases, the net effect was to increase bone mass and cortical area. The differing tissue responses observed could reflect, in part, differences in the experimental approach used to increase skeletal loading. Surgical removal of the ulnar diaphysis adjacent to the radial diaphysis (Goodship *et al.*, 1979) may have caused local inflammation, evoking a response in the radius at its periosteal, rather than its endosteal, surface. The differing nature of the skeletal tissue responses reported in these two studies requires further explanation and study.

In their study of 5-week-old rats swum daily over a 20-week period, Swissa-Sivan et al. (1989) found a significant increase in the diameter of the proximal and distal humeral metaphyses of exercised vs. age-matched controls. No difference in diaphyseal diameter was found. As noted above, however, the difference in size between exercised (17% larger) and control animals was not accounted for, rendering the significance of these data suspect.

Although studies of animals subjected to long-term centrifugation generally indicate a positive response to increased gravitational loading, this approach suffers several potential problems. First, it is difficult to verify, let alone quantify, whether activity levels associated with increased acceleration are normal and increase proportionately with increases in acceleration. Indeed, there is evidence of muscle atrophy following centrifugation, indicative of decreased muscle loading (Smith and Kelly, 1963; Amtmann and Oyama, 1973). Generally, this is associated with a depression of the animal's overall growth rate following long-term centrifugation. This, in turn, suggests a second potential difficulty, namely, that animals subjected to long-term centrifugation may experience some degree of physiological and/or psychological stress, introducing the possible side effect of corticosteroid release (Morey and Baylink, 1978; Wronski and Morey, 1983; Amtmann and Oyama, 1973). A third and rarely considered complication is the change in blood pressure, particularly in the extremities, induced by centrifugation, which can also influence bone formation (Kelly, 1971; Dankwardt-Lilliestrom et al., 1972).

Effect of Disuse on Cortical Bone Growth

Whereas conflicting interpretations and results have been reported for the effects of increased loading on skeletal growth, there is general agreement that the absence of functional loads, or physical disuse, promotes bone loss. Indeed, the loss of bone resulting from disuse is often cited as evidence in favor of the view that the skeleton adaptively remodels in response to changes in its mechanical environment (Donaldson et al., 1970; Uhthoff and Jaworski, 1978). Although the loss of bone resulting from disuse is fairly well established for mature animals, comparatively few studies have examined its effect on the growing skeleton, particularly at an early age. The manner in which the absence of functional load bearing affects tissue-modeling processes associated with normal bone growth is, in general, therefore, not well known.

Although current studies indicate a similar net response (in terms of bone mass or bone area) of growing vs. mature bone to increased mechanical loading, the mechanism by which a growing bone adjusts its mass and shape may be quite different from a mature bone, involving different bone envelopes. It seems likely, therefore, that the removal of functional load bearing may also evoke a differing response in growing vs. mature bone. Available data indicate that this is the case.

The mature skeleton normally exists in a balanced state of bone turnover, with most of its surfaces quiescent. Loss of functional load bearing results in osteopenia (generalized bone loss) that progresses in a two-phase manner (Jaworski and Uhthoff, 1986; Uhthoff and Jaworski, 1978; Uhthoff et al., 1985). Initially, bone resorption increases and bone formation remains unchanged, or decreases only slightly (osteoclast proliferation has been documented within as short a time as 30 h following the onset of disuse, Weinreb et al., 1989). In older dogs (7 to 8 years of age), resorption is localized mainly in the trabecular envelope, but also occurs within the endosteal and intracortical envelopes Jaworski and Uhthoff, 1986). Subsequently, resorption rates return to near normal levels, during which time bone deposition rates fall, maintaining a state of progressive bone loss (for up to 60 weeks). This shift occurs after approximately 6 weeks of immobilization in the dog, but varies depending on the particular bone involved.

In young adult dogs, immobilization also exhibits a similar biphasic pattern of bone loss, affecting the trabecular and periosteal envelopes (Table 2, Jaworski and Uhthoff, 1986; Uhthoff and Jaworski, 1978). This is in contrast to older dogs, in which resorption occurs predominantly at the endosteal, rather than the periosteal, surface. A limitation of these studies in regard to the effect of disuse on bone growth, however, is that both sets of animals were skeletally mature during the period of study.

In much younger, actively growing animals, the diameters of the medullary cavity and outer cortex both decrease following paralysis or immobilization, resulting in a bone that is narrower and has thinner cortices compared to the bone of the normally functioning limb (Armstrong, 1946; Gillespie, 1954; Lanyon, 1980; Turner et al., 1985), as well as a diminution of characteristic features of its shape (Dysart et al., 1989). The removal of load, however, never reverses the growth process (i.e., the bone continues to increase in size, but at a slower rate; Fig. 2), nor does it substantially affect the mineralization and mechanical properties of newly formed bone (Armstrong, 1946; Gillespie, 1954). Relative to normal growth modeling, these morphological differences indicate a decrease in both the rates of periosteal deposition (Turner et al., 1985) and endosteal resorption within the diaphysis of growing bones.

The differing responses of mature vs. growing bone suggest that the sensitivity of bone remodeling to the complete removal of load depends both on the maturation level of the bone and its anatomic location. In general, functional loading appears to be required for the normal development of the subperiosteal external dimensions of long bones during growth. It remains unclear, however, whether functional loading during growth is a fundamental determinant of a bone's external morphology or whether it acts more to enable the acquisition of an intrinsically determined shape — in much the same way as calcium-regulating hormones are known to act.

This latter issue is of interest in relation to why and how most long bones develop their longitudinal curvature (Bertram and Biewener, 1988). In his study of paralysis in growing rats, Lanyon (1980) found that the longitudinal curvature of the rat tibia failed to develop following sciatic denervation at 4 weeks of age. Similarly, following denervation at 2 weeks of age (Biewener and Bertram, unpublished), the chicken tibiotarsus also fails to develop its characteristic curvature. These results are in contrast to those of Howell (1917), who found that longitudinal bone curvatures from the paralyzed limb of one young dog were equivalent to those of the functional limb, although other features of disuse during growth were evident (decreased bone mass and diameter at maturity).

In addition to the loss of characteristic features of overall bone shape, disuse or paralysis generally retards bone growth, leading to modest decreases (-5 to -15%) in bone mass, diameter, and cortical area compared to age-matched controls in young growing animals (Table 2). Consistent with the response to increased exercise, however, no significant effect on bone mineralization levels and mechanical properties is observed; indicating that the inhibition of bone growth occurs largely at a structural, rather than at a tissue, level. Interestingly, one of the more striking changes following limb paralysis is the increased variability in cortical bone geometry and thickness compared to normal control bones (Biewener and Bertram, unpublished; Steinberg and Trueta, 1981).

Considerable interest in the effects of physical disuse or microgravity on the growing skeleton has been stimulated by manned spaceflight. Most of these studies however have been limited to rodent species fairly late in their growth. In 12-week-old rats subjected to 18.5 d of spaceflight (Jee et al., 1983), osteoblast numbers were moderately reduced near the growth plate and their ultrastructure showed diminished bone forming activity. Osteoclast numbers were unaffected, however, suggesting no change in bone resorption. In addition, space-flown rats accumulated substantial marrow fat. Ground-based controls subjected to similar flight conditions, however, showed many of the same, but less extensive, skeletal changes as the space-flown animals, indicating that factors other than microgravity, such as systemic corticosteroid excess (Morey and Baylink, 1978), were involved. This view is supported by the observation of adrenal hypertrophy (Portugalov et al., 1976) and substantial bone resorption in non-weight-bearing bones of the skeleton, in regions free of muscle attachment (e.g., the mandibular ramus), of rats subjected to spaceflight (Simmons *et al.*, 1983). Bone loss, depressed longitudinal growth, and marrow fat increase are all consequences of exogenous administration of corticoids (Hulth and Olerud, 1963; Kawai *et al.*, 1985; Martin *et al.*, 1990; Storey, 1963). A similar increase in marrow fat content has also been noted in rats subjected to simulated weightlessness (Wronski and Morey, 1982).

Decreased periosteal bone formation (up to -44%) appears to be a major component of the modeling response underlying the retardation of bone growth following spaceflight and paralysis (Turner *et al.*, 1985). This decline may be associated with a decrease in primary bone vascularity (Steinberg and Trueta, 1981). Young adult rats (12 weeks of age) subjected to 18.5 d of spaceflight show a similar 33 to 40% decline in periosteal bone formation in the femur and humerus compared to ground controls (Wronski and Morey, 1983a). No effect on periosteal bone formation was observed within the rib, nor were changes in endosteal bone remodeling noted for any of these bone elements. In juvenile rhesus monkeys (about 4 years of age) subjected to 2 weeks of immobilization, these same workers (Wronski and Morey, 1983b) noted nearly a complete arrest of new bone-forming sites in trabecular bone, but only a slight decrease in cortical bone. Late in growth, therefore, decreased trabecular and periosteal bone formation appear to contribute to slowed bone growth. Data are unavailable to evaluate whether a similar change occurs in much younger animals following disuse. Finally, no evidence of increased endosteal resorption to slow bone mass increase was found in 9-week-old rats following 19.5 d of spaceflight (Morey and Baylink, 1978). In addition to these structural and modeling changes in bone growth following spaceflight, changes in bone mineral composition also occur (Patterson-Buckendahl *et al.*, 1987; Simmons *et al.*, 1986), indicating depressed or delayed mineralization of newly formed matrix following exposure to microgravity. This is in contrast to the general absence of such changes following disuse or paralysis.

Conclusions

In general, modest changes in bone mass and shape are observed following changes in bone loading *in vivo*. Evidence is generally lacking that significant changes in bone tissue composition occur in response to changes in mechanical loading, at least in terms of whether the reported changes are of functional significance. For the most part structural changes in bone are achieved at the extremes of a bone's loading history range, with decreased bone growth following periods of disuse or paralysis and increased bone formation generally following strenuous exercise. The response of growing bone to strenuous exercise remains unresolved, however, as some studies show an inhibition of bone growth at intense levels of exercise. The "intensity" of exercise in most cases, however, is only known in qualitative terms (which are usually inconsistent among studies). Over much of its normal physiological range, bone growth modeling appears to be primarily regulated by genetic, epigenetic, and other extrinsic factors, such as hormones and diet. Changes in longitudinal growth appear the least sensitive to changes in physical activity, again suggesting a central, intrinsically determined growth potential of the bone.

These interpretations, however, are based on a surprisingly limited set of experimental data. In nearly all cases, no quantitative evaluation of mechanical loading has been carried out for the bone(s) under study. Further, only a few studies have examined changes in the dynamics of bone modeling that underlie changes in bone geometry and mass associated with changes in mechanical loading, focusing instead on rather crude measures of the skeleton's response such as bone mass, diameter, and length. More comprehensive studies that integrate ultrastructural, microscopic, and mechanically relevant structural responses to experimentally quantified changes in loading history and compare these responses in different species are clearly needed. Finally, knowledge of an animal's stage of growth or level of maturity is important for a more complete understanding of the response of growing bone to mechanical loading *in vivo* as well as for properly evaluating the functional adaptation of growing bone to mechanical stimuli.

References

Alberts, J. R., Serova, L. V., Keefe, J. R., and Apansenko, Z. (1985). Early postnatal development of rats gestated during flight of Cosmos 1514. *Physiology,* **28**: S81–S82.

Amtmann, E. and Oyama, J. (1976). Effect of chronic centrifugation on the structural development of the musculoskeletal system of the rat. *Anat. Embryol.,* **149**: 47–70.

Armstrong, W. D. (1946). Bone growth in paralyzed limbs. *Proc. Soc. Exp. Biol. Med.,* **61**: 358–362.

Bertram, J. E. A. and Biewener, A. A. (1988). Bone curvature: sacrificing strength for load predictability? *J. Theor. Biol.,* **131**: 75–92.

Biewener, A. A., Thomason, J. J., and Lanyon, L. E. (1983). Mechanics of locomotion and jumping in the forelimb of the horse (*Equus*): *in vivo* stress developed in the radius and metacarpus. *J. Zool.,* **201**: 67–82.

Biewener, A. A., Swartz, S. M., and Bertram, J. E. A. (1986). Bone modeling during growth: dynamic strain equilibrium in the chick tibiotarsus. *Calc. Tiss. Int.,* **39**: 390–395.

Biewener, A. A. and Taylor, C. R. (1986). Bone strain: a determinant of gait and speed? *J. Exp. Biol.,* **123**: 383–400.

Booth, F. W. and Gould, E. W. (1975). Effects of training and disuse on connective tissue. *Exer. Sports Sci. Rev.,* **3**: 83–112.

Bugyi, B. and Kansz, I. (1970). Radiographic determination of the skeletal age of the young swimmers. *J. Sports Med.*, **10**: 269–270.

Cann, C. E. and Adachi, R. R. (1983). Bone resorption and mineral excretion in rats during spaceflight. *Am. J. Physiol.*, **244**: R327–R331.

Carter, D. R. (1982). The relationship between *in vivo* bone stresses and cortical bone remodeling. *Crit. Rev. Bioeng.*, **8**: 1–28.

Carter, D. R., Orr, T. E., Fyhrie, D. P., and Schurman, D. J. (1987). Influences of mechanical stress on prenatal and postnatal skeletal development. *Clin. Orthopaed.*, **219**: 237.

Crilley, R. G. (1972). Longitudinal overgrowth of chicken radius. *J. Anat.*, **112**: 11–18.

Currey, J. D. (1968). The adaptation of bones to stress. *J. Theor. Biol.*, **20**: 91–106.

Currey, J. D. (1984). In: *The Mechanical Adaptations of Bones*, Princeton University Press, Princeton, NJ.

Dankwardt-Lilliestrom, G., Gresten, S., Johansson, H., and Olerud, S. (1972). Periosteal bone formation on medullary evacuation. *Upsala J. Med. Sci.*, **77**: 1071–1084.

Dawson, A. and Kember, N. F. (1974). Compensatory growth in the rat tibia. *Cell Tissue Kinet.*, **7**: 285–291.

de Ricqles, A. (1979). Quelques remarques sur l'histoire evolutive des tissus squelettiques chez les vertebres et plus particulierement chez les tetrapodes. *Ann. Biol.*, **18**: 1–35.

Dhem, A. and Vincent, A. (1965). Analyse microradiographique du squelette. *Extrait Recipe*, **24**: 515–536.

Donaldson, C. L., Hulley, S. B., Vogel, J. M., Hattner, R. S., Bayers, J. H., and McMillan, D. E. (1970). Effect of prolonged bedrest on bone mineral. *Metabolism*, **19**: 1071–1084.

Dorfl, J. (1980). Migration of tendious insertions. I. Cause and mechanism. *J. Anat.*, **131**: 179–195.

Dysart, P. S., Harkness, E. M., and Herbison, G. P. (1989). Growth of the humerus after denervation. An experimental study in the rat. *J. Anat.*, **167**: 147–159.

Ekblom, B. (1969). Effect of physical training in adolescent boys. *J. Appl. Physiol.*, **27**: 350–355.

Enlow, D. H. (1962). A study of the post-natal growth and remodeling of bone. *Am. J. Anat.*, **110**: 79–101.

Enlow, D. H. (1964). In: *Principles of Bone Remodelling*. Charles C Thomas, Springfield, IL.

Enlow, D. H. and Brown, S. O. (1957). A comparative histological study of fossil and recent bone tissues. II. *Tex. J. Sci.*, **9**: 186–214.

Enlow, D. H. and Brown, S. O. (1958). A comparative histological study of fossil and recent bone tissues. III. *Tex. J. Sci.*, **10**: 187–230.

Eurell, J. A. and Kazarian, L. E. (1983). Quantitative histochemistry of rat lumbar vertebrae following spaceflight. *Am. J. Physiol.*, **244**: R315–R318.

Fell, H. B. (1956). Skeletal develpment in tissue culture. In: *The Biochemistry and Physiology of Bone*, Bourne, G. H., Ed., Academic Press, New York, 401–441.

Fielder, P. J., Morey, E. R., and Roberts, W. E. (1986). Osteoblast histogenesis in periodontal ligament and tibial metaphysis during simulated weightlessness. *Aviat. Space Environ. Med.*, **57**: 1125–1130.

Friberg, K. S. I. (1979a). Remodelling after distal forearm fractures in children. I. The effect of residual angulation on the spatial orientation of the epiphyseal plates. *Acta Orthop. Scand.*, **50**: 537–546.

Friberg, K. S. I. (1979b). Remodelling after distal forearm fractures in children. II. The final orientation of the distal and proximal epiphyseal plates of the radius. *Acta Orthop. Scand.*, **50**: 731–739.

Frost, H. M. (1964). In: *The Laws of Bone Structure*. Charles C Thomas, Springfield, IL.

Frost, H. M. (1969). Tetracycline-based histological analysis of bone remodeling. *Calc. Tissue Res.*, **3**: 211–237.

Frost, H. M. (1973). In: *Bone Modeling and Skeletal Modeling Errors*, Charles C Thomas, Springfield, IL.

Gillespie, J. A. (1954). The nature of bone changes associated with nerve injuries and disuse. *J. Bone Jt. Surg.*, **36B**: 464–473.

Goodship, A. E., Lanyon, L. E., and MacFie, H. (1979). Functional adaptation of bone to increased stress. *J. Bone. Jt. Surg.*, **61A:** 539–546.

Grant, P. G., Bushang, P. H., Drolet, D. W., and Pickerell, C. (1980). Invariance of the relative positions of structures attached to long bones during growth: cross-sectional and longitudinal studies. *Acta Anat.*, **107**: 26–34.

Hall, B. K. (1982). The role of tissue interactions in the growth of bone. In: *Factors and Mechanisms Influencing Bone Growth.* Dixon, A. D. and Sarnat, B. Eds., Alan R. Liss, New York, 205–215.

Hall, B. K. and Herring, S. W. (1990). Paralysis and growth of the musculoskeletal system in the embryonic chick. *J. Morphol.*, **206**: 45–56.

Hall-Craggs, E. C. B. (1968). The effect of experimental epiphysiodesis on growth in length of the rabbit's tibia. *J. Bone Jt. Surg.*, **50B**: 392–400.

Harkness, E. M. and Trotter, W. D. (1978). Growth of transplants of rat humerus following circumferential division of the periosteum. *J. Anat.*, **126**: 275–289.

Hert, J. (1969). Acceleration of the growth after decrease of load on epiphyseal plates by means of spring distractors. *Folia Morphol.*, **17**: 194–203.

Heuter, C. (1862). Anatomische Studien an den Extremitatengelenken Neugeborener und Erwachsener. *Virchows Arch. Pathol. Anat. Physiol.*, **25**: 572–599.

Howell, J. A. (1917). An experimental study of the effect of stress and strain on bone development. *Anat. Rec.*, **13**: 233–252.

Hulth, A., and Olerud, S. (1963). The effect of cortisone on growing bone in the rat. *Br. J. Exp. Pathol.*, **44:** 491–496.

Jaworski, Z. F. G. and Uhthoff, H. K. (1986). Disuse osteoporosis: current status and problems. In: *Current Concepts of Bone Fragility,* Uhthoff, H. K. and Stahl, E. Eds., Springer-Verlag, New York, 181–194.

Jee, W. S., Wronski, T. J., Morey, E. R., and Kimmel, D. B. (1983). Effects of spaceflight on trabecular bone in rats. *Am. J. Physiol.*, **244**: R310–R314.

Kato, S. and Ishiko, T. (1966). Obstructed growth of children's bones due to excessive labor in remote corners. Proc. Int. Congress of Sports Sciences, Japanese Union of Sports Sciences, Kato, K. Ed., Tokyo, 476.

Kawai, K., Tamaki, A., and Hirohata, K. (1985). Steroid-induced accumulation of lipid in the osteocytes of the rabbit femoral head. *J. Bone Jt. Surg.*, **67A**: 755–763.

Kelly, P. J. (1971). The effects of thyroid and parathyroid deficiency on bone remodelling distal to a venous tourniquet. *J. Anat.*, **110**: 349–361.

Kember, N. F. (1972). Comparative patterns of cell division in epiphyseal cartilages in the rat. *J. Anat.*, **111**: 137–144.

Kember, N. F. (1973). Patterns of cell division in the growth plates of the rat pelvis. *J. Anat.*, **116**: 445–451.

Kember, N. F. (1985). Comparative patterns of cell division in epithyseal cartilages in the rabbit. *J. Anat.*, **142**: 185–190.

Kiiskinen, A. (1977). Physical training and connective tissues in young mice — physical properties of Achilles tendons and long bones. *Growth.*, **41**: 123–137.

Lanyon, L. E. (1976). The measurement of bone strain *in vivo*. *Acta Orthop. Belg.*, **42 (suppl. 1)**: 98–108.

Lanyon, L. E. (1980). The influence of function on the development of bone curvature. An experimental study of the rat tibia. *J. Zool. London*, **192**: 457–466.

Lanyon, L. E., Goodship, A. E., Pie, C. J., and MacFie, J. F. (1982). Mechanically adaptive bone remodelling. *J. Biomech.*, **15**: 142–154.

Lanyon, L. E. and Baggott, D. G. (1976). Mechanical function as an influence on the structure and form of bone. *J. Bone Jt. Surg.*, **58B**: 436–443.

Lanyon, L. E. and Bourn, S. (1979). The influence of mechanical function on the development and remodeling of the tibia. *J. Bone Jt. Surg.*, **61A**:: 263–273.

Malina, R. M. (1969). Exercise as an influence upon growth. Review and critique of current concepts. *Clin. Pediatrics.*, **8**: 16–26.

Martin, R. B., Chow, D. B., and Lucas, P. A. (1990). Bone marrow fat content in relation to bone remodeling and serum chemistry in intact and ovariectomized dogs. *Calc. Tissue Int.*, **46**: 189–194.

Matsuda, J. J., Zernicke, R. F., Vailas, A. C., Pedrini, V. A., Pedrini-Mille, A., and Maynard, J. A. (1986). Structural and mechanical adaptation of immature bone to strenuous exercise. *J. Appl. Physiol.*, **60**: 2028–2034.

Morey, E. R. and Baylink, D. J. (1978). Inhibition of bone formation during space flight. *Science.*, **201**: 1138–1141.

Morey-Holton, E. R. and Arnaud, S. B. (1985). Spaceflight and calcium levels. *Physiology*, **28**: S9–S10.

Murray, P. D. F. (1936). In: *Bones: a Study of the Development and Structure of the Vertebrate Skeleton*, Cambridge University Press, Cambridge.

Novikov, V. E. and Ilyin, E. A. (1981). Age-related reactions of rat bones to their unloading. *Aviat. Space Environ. Med.*, **9**: 551–553.

Parizkova, J. (1968). Longitudinal study of the development of body composition and body build in boys of various physical activity. *Hum. Biol.*, **40**: 212–225.

Patterson-Buckendahl, P., Arnaud, S. B., Mechanic, G. L., Martin, R. B., Gindeland, R. E., and Cann, C. E. (1987). Fragility and composition of growing rat bone after one week in spaceflight. *Am. J. Physiol.*, **252**: R240–R246.

Ponlot, R. (1960). In: *Le Radiocalcium dans l'Etude des Os*, Editions Arscia S.A., Brussels.

Portugalov, V. V., Savina, E. A., Kaplansky, A. S., Yakovleva, V.I., Plakhuta-Plakhutina, G. I., Pankova, A. S., Katunyan, P. I., Shubich, M. G., and Buvailo, S. A. (1976). Effect of space flight factors on the mammal: experimental-morphological study. *Aviat. Space Environ. Med.*, **47**: 813–816.

Raisz, L. G. and Bingham, P. J. (1972). Effect of hormones on bone development. *Annu. Rev. Pharmacol.*, **12**: 337–352.

Rodan, G. A. and Rodan, S. B. (1983). Expression of the osteoblastic phenotypes. In: *Bone and Mineral Research, Annual 2*, Peck, W. A., Ed., Elsevier, Boston, 224–285.

Rubin, C. T. and Lanyon, L. E. (1982). Limb mechanics as a function of speed and gait: a study of functional strains in the radius and tibia of horse and dog. *J. Exp. Biol.*, **101**: 187–211.

Russell, J. E. and Simmons, D. J. (1985). Bone maturation in rats flown on the Spacelab-3 mission. *Physiology*, **28**: S235–S236.

Saville, P. D. and Whyte, M. P. (1969). Muscle and bone hypertrophy: positive effect of running exercise in the rat. *Clin. Orthop. Rel. Res.*, **65**: 81–88.

Shaw, S. R., Vailas, A. C., Grindeland, R. E., and Zernicke, R. F. (1988). Effects of a 1-wk spaceflight on morphological and mechanical properties of growing bone. *Am. J. Physiol.*, **254**: R78–R83.

Simmons, D. J., Russell, J. E., and Grynpas, M. D. (1986). Bone maturation and quality of bone material in rats flown on the space shuttle 'Spacelab-3 mission'. *Bone Miner.*, **1**: 485–493.

Simmons, D. J., Russell, J. E., Winter, F., Tran Van, P., Vignery, A., Baron, R., Rosenberg, G. D., and Walker, W. V. (1983). Effect of spaceflight on the non-weight-bearing bones of rat skeleton. *Am. J. Physiol.*, **244**: R319–R326.

Simon, M. R., Holmes, K. R., and Olsen, A. M. (1985). Bone mineral content of limb bones of male weanling rats subjected to 30 and 60 days of simulated increases in body weight. *Acta Anat.*, **121**: 7–11.

Smith, A. H. and Kelly, C. F. (1963). Influence of chronic acceleration upon growth and body composition. *Ann. N.Y. Acad. Sci.*, **110**: 410–424.

Spengler, D. M., Morey, E. R., Carter, D. R., Turner, R. T., and Baylink, D. J. (1983). Effects of spaceflight on structural and material strength of growing bone. *Proc. Soc. Exp. Biol. Med.*, **174**: 224–228.

Steinberg, M. E. and Trueta, J. (1981). Effects of activity on bone growth and development in the rat. *Clin. Orthop. Rel. Res.*, **156**: 52–60.

Storey, E. (1963). The influence of adrenal cortical hormones on bone formation and resorption. *Clin. Orthop.*, **30**: 197–216.

Strobino, L. J., French, G. O., and Colonna, P. C. (1952). The effect of increasing tensions on the growth of epiphyseal bone. *Surg. Gynecol. Obstet.*, **95**: 694–700.

Sweeney, J. R., Gruber, H. E., Kirchen, M. E., and Marshall, G. J. (1985). Effects of non-weight bearing on callus formation. *Physiology*, **28**: S63–S65.

Swissa-Sivan, A., Simkin, A., Leichter, I., Nyska, A., Nyska, M., Statter, M., Bivas, A., Menczel, J., and Samueloff, S. (1989). Effect of swimming on bone growth and development in young rats. *Bone Miner.*, **7**: 91–105.

Turner, R. T., Wakely, G. K., and Szukalski, B. W. (1985). Effects of gravitational and muscular loading on bone formation in growing rats. *Physiology*, **28**: S67–S68.

Turner, R. T., Bell, N. H., Duvall, P., Bobyn, J. D., Spector, M., Morey-Holton E., and Baylink, D. J. (1985). Spaceflight results in formation of defective bone. *Proc. Soc. Exp. Biol. Med.*, **180**: 544–549.

Uhthoff, H. K. (1982). The influence of mechanical factors in the activity of the three bone envelopes. *Acta Orthop. Belg.*, **48**: 563–575.

Uhthoff, H. K. and Jaworski, Z. F. G. (1978). Bone loss in response to long term immobilisation. *J. Bone Jt. Surg.*, **60B**: 420–429.

Uhthoff, H. K., Sekaly, G., and Jaworski, Z. F. G. (1985). Effect of long-term nontraumatic immobilization on metaphyseal spongiosa in young adult and old Beagle dogs. *Clin. Orthop. Rel. Res.*, **192**: 278–283.

Van Dusen, C. R. (1939). An anthropometric study of the upper extremities of children. *Hum. Biol.*, **11**: 277–284.

Volkman, R. (1862). Chirurgische Erfahrungen über Knochenverbiegungen und Knochenwachsthum. *Virchows Arch. Pathol. Anat. Physiol.*, **24**: 512–540.

Weinreb, M., Rodan, G. A., and Thompson, D. D. (1989). Osteopenia in the immobilized rat hind limb is associated with increased bone resorption and decreased bone formation. *Bone.*, **10**: 187–194.

Wolff, J. (1892). In: *The Law of Bone Remodelling (Das Gesetz der Transformation der Knochen)* (Translated by P. Maquet and R. Furlong, 1986), Springer-Verlag, Berlin.

Woo, S. L.-Y., Kuei, S. C., Amiel, D., Gomez, M. A., Hayes, W. C., White, F. C., and Akeson, W. H. (1981). The effect of prolonged physical training on the properties of long bone. A study of Wolff's law. *J. Bone. Jt. Surg.*, **63A**: 780–787.

Wronski, T. J. and Morey, E. R. (1982). Skeletal abnormalities in rats induced by simulated weightlessness. *Metab. Bone Dis. Rel. Res.*, **4**: 69–75.

Wronski, T. J. and Morey, E. R. (1983a). Effect of spaceflight on periosteal bone formation in rats. *Am. J. Physiol.*, **244**: R305–R309.

Wronski, T. J. and Morey, E. R. (1983b). Inhibition of cortical and trabecular bone formation in the long bones of immobilized monkeys. *Clin. Orthop. Rel. Res.*, **181**:269–276.

2

Influence of Mechanical Factors on Bone Formation, Resorption and Growth *In Vitro*

E. H. BURGER and J. P. VELDHUIJZEN
Department of Oral Cell Biology
Academic Center of Dentistry
Amsterdam, The Netherlands

Introduction

In humans and other vertebrates, bones act predominantly as structural organs, as the primary function of the skeleton is to provide mechanical strength. Bone tissue also serves as a calcium reservoir, but the amounts of mineral needed for this function are only a fraction of those needed for structural integrity. A wealth of studies in humans as well as animals has shown that reduction of mechanical loading of bone organs is followed by loss of bone mass, while additional mechanical loading leads to increased bone mass (Smith *et al.*, 1976; Uhthoff *et al.*, 1985; Li *et al.*, 1990; Goodship *et al.*, 1979; Lanyon *et al.*, 1982; Rubin and Lanyon, 1985; Jee *et al.*, 1990; Meade, 1989 for comprehensive reviews). However, the cellular response of bone tissue to changes in mechanical function is still poorly understood. More specifically, very little is known about the dose-response relationship between mechanical stimulation in terms of loading frequency, height and rate, and bone tissue metabolism. The increasing appreciation of mechanical stress as a factor determining skeletal quality has led to many studies of exercise as a means of preventing or even alleviating involutional bone loss in humans (Aloia *et al.*, 1978; Krolner *et al.*, 1983; Dalsky *et al.*, 1988; Smith *et al.*, 1989). *In vivo* studies on the relation between amount of mechanical loading and skeletal quality are however complicated by the complexity of the musculoskeletal apparatus. In addition, reactions at the cellular level remain largely unknown.

To study the processes whereby skeletal tissue reacts to mechanical stress, experimental systems are needed that allow direct measurement of cell proliferation, differentiation, and matrix metabolism under controlled loading conditions. Over the last 20 years several methods have been developed to apply some form of mechanical stress to cells, blocks of tissue or whole bone organs, kept in tissue culture. Starting from the simple technique of Glücksmann, (1939, 1941) increasingly sophisticated methods were developed, with the aim of applying in a reproducible fashion a mechanical stimulus of certain height, rate, and duration. Usually, however, the actual distribution of stress and strain over cell layer or tissue block during the *in vitro* experiment remained speculative. As a result, the feasibility of comparing the *in vitro* results with *in vivo* data is limited. The evidence emerging from *in vitro* studies indicates that osteoblasts, osteocytes, and chondrocytes respond to stress by a variety of actions. Osteoclast activity is also affected, as is the development of osteoclastic cells in bone marrow cultures. In addition, compilation of the results from different studies suggests that the relationship between stress and matrix metabolism is biphasic. Continuous stress of high magnitude may evoke a catabolic response while intermittent stress of moderate magnitude causes an anabolic response. Absence of mechanical stress, as in the usual tissue culture conditions, favors bone resorption.

Results from Organ Culture Studies

Bone tissue consists of cells embedded in a three-dimensional network of matrix macromolecules; see Volumes 1 and 3. As the extracellular matrix is the tissue component which carries mechanical load, its presence is an important argument for using tissue blocks or small bone organs rather than isolated cells for studies of mechanical effects. In addition, normal structural relations between different cells and cell types are maintained in organ cultures allowing for cellular interaction during the experiment. However, the presence of many cell types also precludes detailed analysis of the reactions of a specific cell type, unless a parameter is studied which may unequivocally be ascribed to a specific cell type.

Models Using Direct Force

The first observations of stress effects in bone organ cultures were made by Glücksmann (1939, 1941). He cultured several chick embryo bone rudiments together in such a position that because of their growth in length during culture they started to exert pressure on each other. Increased tension in the perosteum, caused by bending of the rudiment, seemed to enhance bone formation locally, while tension reduction on the concave side of the rudiment inhibited ossification. These observations indicated that skeletal cells are sensitive to mechanical stress and respond to altered stress by production of an altered intercellular matrix.

Bassett and co-workers (1961, 1962) subsequently studied the effects of compressive vs. tensile forces, at high and low concentration of oxygen, on the differentiation of the fibroblastic outgrowth of bone chips taken from near-term chick embryos. They showed that the differentiation of this fibroblastic outgrowth into cartilage, bone, or fibrous tissue was dependent on the locally prevailing amount of pressure or tension around the cell. Compaction of the tissue promoted the formation of cartilage or bone, depending on the oxygen concentration, while stretching of the cells promoted formation of a tendon-like tissue.

Although elegant in their simplicity, the studies of Glücksmann and Bassett did not allow any quantitation of magnitude and duration of the forces evoked *in vitro*. The importance of their observation is that they showed that bone cell differentiation does react to mechanical stress and that the type and, probably, magnitude of stress determine the type of tissue which develops.

Several other authors have applied direct force of known magnitude to skeletal organ cultures or blocks of tissue *in vitro*. Rodan *et al.* (1975) reported reduced glucose consumption and stimulated DNA synthesis in chick embryo tibiae submitted to 4 d constant pressure of physiological magnitude (80 g/cm^2). This effect could not be ascribed to a change in the rate of extracellular fluid equilibration which showed a half time of 2 min for both the pressed and the nonpressed bones. Thus the mechanical pressure itself was considered the cause of the cellular effects. In a study using isolated neonatal rat condyles clasped between two movable nylon strips, Copray *et al.* (1984a, b, 1985) found that a constant force of 3 g reduced, but intermittent (0.7 Hz) compressive force of 0.5 to 1.0 g stimulated, matrix synthesis. In addition, constant force reduced but intermittent force increased alkaline phosphatase activity in the calcifying hypertrophic cartilage zone (Copray *et al.*, 1985). Recently, a method was described for subjecting mature cancellous bone biopsies to mechanical load-bearing in short-term (24 h) tissue culture (El Haj *et al.*, 1990). Cell viability was maintained by simultaneous perfusion of the trabecular bone tissue block with medium. Intermittent loading at a frequency of 1 Hz for a single period of 15 min, by a load which produced a bulk strain across the core of 5000 microstrain,* induced a rise in glycolysis and RNA synthesis in osteocytes and endosteal lining cells.

In all three approaches, the applied force was calculated (Rodan *et al.*, 1975; Copray *et al.*, 1984a) or actually measured (El Haj *et al.*, 1990) to mimic maximal physiological magnitude. Thus, maximal physiological stress affected cellular energy metabolism as well as matrix synthesis. Interestingly, constant pressure reduced (Rodan *et al.*, 1975) while intermittent pressure stimulated (El Haj *et al.*, 1990) glucose consumption, in line with the opposite effects of constant vs. intermittent pressure reported by Copray (1984a, b, 1985) on matrix metabolism.

Collagen synthesis in fibrous joints subjected to tensile mechanical stress has been studied in explants of coronal sutures from newborn rabbits (Meikle *et al.*, 1979) and mature mice (Yen *et al.*, 1984). The latter group also developed a method to study collagen synthesis in stressed periodontal ligament during short-term organ culture of a piece of mouse mandible with three molar teeth (Yen and Melcher, 1978). In both systems direct tensile stress was applied by stainless steel open coil springs, inserted in the bony calvarial tissue on either side of the suture or, in the case of the mandible, around the molar teeth, thereby drawing them together. Forces of 30 to 50 *g* stimulated general protein as well as collagen synthesis in short-term (6 to 24 h) *in vitro* experiments. However, using a combined *in vivo-in vitro* system whereby stress was started *in vivo* and continued during short-term organ culture, it was found that collagen synthesis was specifically enhanced after 3 or more days application of stress (Yen *et al.*, 1984). In addition, type III collagen production was enhanced relative to type I (Meikle *et al.*, 1982). These studies indicate that in fibrous joints, as in bone and cartilage tissue, matrix synthesis is responsive to mechanical stress, not only in terms of quantity produced, but also in its macromolecular composition.

Models Using Hydrostatic Pressure

A major problem with all methods of applying direct force *in vitro* to tissue and organ cultures is the technical difficulty encountered when manipulating the small blocks of tissue. To resolve this problem Bourret and Rodan (1976) developed a relatively simple method to expose isolated cells and blocks of tissue to continuous pressure by compressing the gas phase of the culture system. This resulted in application of hydrostatic pressure to the cells.

*Mechanical strain is a measure of deformation as a result of stress. In one dimension, strain is defined as the change in length divided by the original length. Microstrain is a unit for small strains; 1 microstrain (μE) equals a deformation of 0.0001%.

The technique was further developed by Veldhuijzen *et al.* (1979, 1987) and Van Kampen *et al.* (1985), who used intermittent (0.3 Hz) hydrostatic compression of physiological magnitude (9.6 to 13 kPa) to study responses in embryonic chick epiphyseal explants and high-density chondrocyte cultures. Short-term (15 min to 24 h) intermittent hydrostatic compression increased cyclic AMP (cAMP) levels (Veldhuijzen *et al.*, 1979) and stimulated proteoglycan synthesis (Veldhuijzen *et al.*, 1987; Van Kampen *et al.*, 1985). The technique was further adapted by Klein-Nulend *et al.* (1986) to study effects on mineral metabolism in long-term (up to 5d) organ cultures of embryonic mouse bone. Intermittent (0.3 Hz) hydrostatic compression of 13 kPa, applied throughout the culture period, stimulated calcification of long bone rudiments as well as calvarial explants, and increased alkaline phosphatase activity (Klein Nulend *et al.*, 1986, 1987a). In addition, osteoclastic resorption of mineralized matrix was reduced (Klein Nulend *et al.*, 1990). Continuous 13-kPa hydrostatic pressure also stimulated calcification, but at a lower rate (Klein Nulend *et al.*, 1986). No effects were observed on the growth in length of the long bone rudiments. Intermittent compression increased the degree of sulfation of cartilage matrix proteoglycans and had opposite effects on sulfate metabolism in calcifying and noncalcifying cartilage while promoting mineralization (Klein-Nulend *et al.*, 1987b; Bagi and Burger, 1989).

The nature of the stimulus responsible for these effects was discussed by Wong and Carter (1990). They showed by computer simulation experiments using finite element analysis that in calcifying rudiments externally applied hydrostatic pressure produced significant shear stress at calcified/noncalcified tissue borders because of material mismatch along the interface. Pure hydrostatic pressure was created in the cartilaginous epiphyses. They concluded that the local shear stress in the ossifying bone center, as a result of hydrostatic compression, stimulated further osteogenesis, in line with earlier theoretical studies by Carter and collegues (Carter, 1987; Carter *et al.*, 1987; Carter and Wong, 1988). Experimental support for this explanation was obtained (Burger *et al.*, 1992b), using very early embryonic bones in which osteogenesis had not yet started. The osteogenesis-promoting effect of hydrostatic compression did not appear in homogeneous cartilage rudiments, but only after a hypertrophic center had appeared which allowed creation of shear stress.

Continuous hydrostatic compression of much higher magnitude, 100 to 200 kPa, designed to mimic orthodontic treatment, was used by Imamura *et al.* (1990) to study effects on mineral resorption and osteoclast formation in, respectively, embryonic mouse calvaria and mouse bone marrow cultures. Six days culture under 100-kPa continuous pressure increased mineral mobilization in the second part of the culture period. In addition, the formation of osteoclastic cells in the bone marrow cultures was increased. These effects were ascribed to enhanced prostaglandin E_2 (PGE_2) production. Interestingly, 13-kPa intermittent compression *inhibited* osteoclastic cell formation in similar bone marrow cultures (Klein-Nulend *et al.*, 1990). In addition, intermittent low (13-kPa) compression inhibited mineral resorption in calvaria (Klein-Nulend *et al.*, 1987b) by a mechanism which was antagonized rather than mediated by prostaglandin production (Burger *et al.*, 1991). Thus 100-kPa continuous pressure and 13-kPa intermittent pressure caused completely opposite effects, via different mediators. Application of 100-kPa (1000 millibar pressure above ambient) needed adequate reduction of O_2 and CO_2 concentration in the gas phase to maintain correct pO_2, pCO_2 and pH levels during compression (Ozawa *et al.*, 1990). When applying 13 kPa *intermittently*, correction was impossible; slight (13%) increases of pO_2, pCO_2 and consequently pH must have occurred during peak pressure. *Continuous* application of 13% increased pO_2 and pCO_2, without mechanical compression, however, had no effect on mineralization (Klein-Nulend *et al.*, 1986). A slight increase in pCO_2 and, consequently, a decrease in pH would have stimulated rather than inhibited mineral resorption (Arnett and Dempster, 1986). Thus it seems likely that in both systems, continuous high as well as intermittent low pressure, the tissue reactions indeed stemmed from mechanical stimuli.

Table 1 summarizes the studies using direct or hydrostatic compression of ossifying rudiments or bone biopsies. Although widely different organs, species, and ages were used, it is remarkable that intermittent compression of roughly physiological magnitude produced effects on extracellular matrix production and/or cell metabolism which may be considered anabolic. Continuous compression on the other hand, of high or physiological magnitude, usually had catabolic effects. Thus it seems that, in bone and ossifying cartilage cells, different regimes of mechanical perturbation (continuous vs. intermittent) evoke different responses. It is of interest that different responses of bone to intermittent and continuous mechanical stress *in vivo* have also been reported (Meade *et al.*, 1984; Lanyon and Rubin, 1984).

Studies Using Isolated Cells

For quantitative studies of cellular responses to mechanical force, the use of a homogeneous population of cells is a great advantage. For this reason many authors have used isolated cells from periosteum or growth plate cartilage, cultured as monolayers or as multilayered sheets. Because of the large variety of cell types as well as methods of applying mechanical force, we will first briefly discuss cell sources. Subsequently the methods of stress application and their results will be reviewed.

Table 1.

Mechanical Studies on Bone Organ Cultures

Authors	Material	Mechanical Stimulus	Cellular Response
Rodan *et al.* (1975)	Chick embryo tibia	80 g/cm,² continuous	DNA synthesis ↑ Glucose consumption ↓
Copray *et al.* (1984a, b, 1985)	Neonatal rat condylar cartilage	0.5–1 g, 0.7 Hz	Matrix synthesis ↑ Al.P. activity ↑
Copray *et al.* (1984a, b, 1985)	Neonatal rat condylar cartilage	3 g, continuous	Matrix synthesis ↓ Al.P. ctivity ↓
El Haj *et al.* (1990)	Mature dog cancellous bone biopsy	5000 µE, 1 Hz	RNA synthesis ↑ Glycolysis ↑
Veldhuijzen *et al.* (1979)	Chick embryo epiphysal explants	9.6 kPa hydrostatic, 0.3 Hz	cAMP ↑
van Kampen *et al.* (1985)	Chick embryo chondrocyte cultures	13 kPa hydrostatic, 0.3 Hz	Proteoglycan synthesis ↑
Veldhuijzen *et al.* (1987)	Chick embryo chondrocyte cultures	13 kPa hydrostatic, 0.3 Hz	Matrix volume ↑
Klein-Nulend *et al.* (1986, 1987a, 1990)	Embryonic mouse metatarsal bones	13 kPa hydrostatic, 0.3 Hz	Matrix calcification ↑ Matrix sulfation ↑ Mineral resorption ↓
Klein-Nulend *et al.* (1987b)	Embryonic mouse calvaria	13 kPa hydrostatic, 0.3 Hz	Matrix calcification ↑ Al.P. activity ↑ Mineral resorption ↓
Imamura *et al.* (1991)	Embryonic mouse calvaria	100 kPa hydrostatic, continuous	Mineral resorption ↑ PGE₂ production ↑

Al.P.: alkaline phosphatase; hydrostat.: hydrostatic pressure; ↑ : increase; ↓ : decrease.

Osteoblasts

A large body of information on the cellular responses to mechanical stress has been derived from primary cultures of osteoblasts, isolated from rat, mouse, or chicken calvaria. In most cases primary cell cultures were used, but sometimes cells were used after one or more passages (Yeh and Rodan, 1984; Hasegawa *et al.*, 1985; Buckley *et al.*, 1988; Reich *et al.*, 1990). Osteoblasts were usually isolated by sequential enzymatic digestion from embryonic or neonatal calvaria after removal of the periosteum. Only Reich *et al.* (1990) cultured chips of calvaria without the periosteum and used the cellular outgrowth as source of osteoblasts. In most studies the osteoblast-like character of the cells was demonstrated by their PTH responsiveness and expression of alkaline phosphatase activity. A few studies have used osteoblast-like cell lines. Among these are MC 3T3-E1 cells (Ozawa *et al.*, 1990; Imamura *et al.*, 1990; Burger *et al.*, 1992a) and UMR-106 cells (Sandy *et al.*, 1989).

Stress was always applied to monolayers which had not yet or had barely reached confluency. Thus, in contrast to the organ cultures discussed earlier, the matrix component was virtually absent in these studies.

Chondrocytes

Since epiphyseal cartilage is an essential cellular component of growing long bones, isolated chondrocytes have been used to study their response to mechanical stress. These cells were invariably derived from the growth plate of embryonic chick long bones.

Usually monolayers of primary cultures were used. Only De Witt *et al.* (1984), Van Kampen *et al.* (1985), and Veldhuijzen *et al.* (1987) used high-density (multilayered) cultures. In such cultures the cells rapidly produced a cartilaginous matrix, containing both proteoglycans and collagen.

Application of Stress by Deformation of the Culture Support

In vivo, mechanical loading of a skeletal element results in strain: a small deformation of the tissue under stress. Several authors have proposed that changes in bone structure, resulting from altered stress, are brought about by a feedback system in which changes in peak mechanical strain drive bone cells to change bone structure (Frost, 1988, 1990a, 1990b; Currey, 1984; Hart and Davey, 1989). Frost's "mechanostat" theory postulates a feedback control system where bone structure is maintained such that ordinary mechanical strains do not surpass a certain limit, called the minimum effective strain (or MES), which Frost speculates to be 1500 to 2500 μE. Only strains larger than the MES will cause a change in bone structure. As this change is brought about by cellular activity, it follows that strains above the MES should change bone cell metabolism.

In principle, *in vitro* methods which apply mechanical stress via deformation of the cell culture support allow measurement of the peak strain applied to the cells. As a result, comparison of strain effects observed *in vitro* with data obtained *in vivo* should be possible. However, in most studies strains were used which are many times higher than the physiological maximum of about 3000 μE which has been deducted from *in vivo* studies (Currey, 1984; Lanyon, 1984; Rubin, 1984; Bouvier, 1985). In addition, the devices often produced large variations of strain over the cell sheet, thereby precluding a careful dose-response study. Only the approach developed by

Murray and Rushton (1990) is an important exception, as it allowed more evenly distributed strains of both physiological and pathological range.

Among the first groups who reported effects of strain applied to a layer of isolated cells were Harell *et al.* (1977). Monolayers of osteoblasts were exposed to mechanical stress by deforming the bottom of a plastic petri dish. The device consisted of two pieces of acrylic connected with an orthodontic expansion screw, glued externally to the bottom of a petri dish by means of fast-curing epoxy glue. By turning the orthodontic screw (activation) the two pieces of acrylic are pulled apart, resulting in geometric deformation of the bottom. This creates tensile forces in the bottom which are not evenly distributed and which were calculated to reach a peak strain of 10,000 μE (Somjen *et al.*, 1980; Binderman *et al.*, 1984), although no data were presented on the strain rate. Cells were exposed for up to 60 min to continuous mechanical stress. The authors reported a rapid (five times) increase in PGE_2 synthesis reaching a maximum after 20 min. cAMP production also increased, reaching a maximum after 15 min. An increase in cellular calcium uptake was also reported (Harell *et al.*, 1977). In all experiments, ^{3}H-thymidine incorporation into DNA was increased when measured 24 h after exposing the osteoblasts to mechanical stretching. In line with the increased DNA synthesis, Somjen *et al.* (1982) reported that within a few hours the activity of the enzyme ornithine decarboxylase (ODC) was increased by stretching. Addition of indomethacin (5 μg/ml), which blocks the *de novo* synthesis of prostaglandins, abolished both the increased cAMP and DNA synthesis, suggesting that the reported increases were prostaglandin mediated (Harell *et al.*, 1977; Somjen *et al.*, 1980; Binderman *et al.*, 1984). More recently Binderman *et al.* (1988) suggested that, using the same experimental setup, mechanical forces exert their effect on bone cells via a chain of events involving the activation of phospholipase A_2, release of arachidonic acid, increase in PGE_2 synthesis, and augmentation of cAMP production. Interestingly, chondrocytes isolated from fetal rat condyles also showed an increased cAMP production and ^{3}H-thymidine incorporation into DNA, but the latter effect was not mediated by PGE_2 (Binderman *et al.*, 1984; Shimshoni *et al.*, 1984).

Based on the same principle of deforming the plastic culture support, Murray and Rushton (1990) developed a method using polycarbonate tissue culture slides. In contrast to the round plastic petri dish bottom, stretching of the slides produced a more even distribution of strain over the cell layer. Strains up to 28,000 μE, which is roughly the strain at which cortical bone fractures (Cowin, 1989), were repeatedly applied to neonatal mouse osteoblasts; the strain rate was 10,000 μE/s and stretching lasted for 1.5 to 5 h. A biphasic relationship was observed between strain magnitude and PGE_2 release. A peak response in which the PGE_2 release was about doubled was observed at 7000 μE. Subsequently, the response diminished, reaching control values at 14,000 μE, but went up again to two times control values at 28,000 μE and higher. Twelve hours after exposure to mechanical stress the PGE$_2$ production had returned to control values. No morphological changes were reported, nor did the cells show alignment to the strain direction. At lower strain (3000 μE) which is in the upper physiological range (Frost 1988), no effects on PGE$_2$ production were observed. In addition, varying the cycle time from 20 to 600 s did not modulate the response. This is in accordance with some *in vivo* experiments which indicate that bone remodeling is dependent on strain magnitude, rather than on strain frequency (Rubin and Lanyon, 1984).

Apart from these methods using a rigid cell culture support, specific culture plates with an elastic growth surface have been developed (Hasegawa *et al.*, 1985; Buckley *et al.*, 1988) and are now commercially available. Stress is applied by deforming the elastic bottom of the dish in two ways. Hasegawa *et al.* (1985) and Sandy *et al.* (1989a, b) used a curved, solid template, which was pushed against the petri dish bottom, thereby increasing the bottom surface by 4 to 5%, depending on the template used. This will give in one axis a strain of 20,000 to 25,000 μE, assuming that stretching is equivalent at each point of the surface. Buckley *et al.* (1988) deformed the elastic petri dish bottom by introducing a vacuum (5 in. of mercury) under the plates, which resulted in an elongation of the dish bottom radius from 24% at the edges to 0% in the center. Maximal strains were therefore 240,000 μE at the edges, declining to zero in the center.

Hasegawa *et al.* (1985) exposed monolayers of rat osteoblasts to 2 h continuous or intermittent (cycle time 10 min) uniform stretching of 20,000 μE. Under both experimental conditions the number of ^{3}H-thymidine-labeled cells increased. Twelve hours of intermittent or continuous stretching stimulated noncollagenous protein synthesis but not collagen. Using a similar stretching technique Sandy *et al.*, (1989a) exposed isolated mouse osteoblasts to intermittent (0.2 Hz) and continuous strains of 20,000 μE. They used a mouse calvarium assay to study the release of resorption-stimulating factors by osteoblasts submitted to stretching. Two hours intermittent, but not continuous, stretching increased the production of a low molecular weight factor, which stimulated bone resorption. The nature of the bone resorptive activity in the conditioned medium (CM) remained unclear. Although cAMP levels were increased in intermittently stretched cultures, the authors presented evidence (Sandy *et al.*, 1989b) that stretch-induced elevation of inositol phosphate production by osteoblasts might also account for the bone-resorbing activity in the medium.

Buckley *et al.* (1988, 1990) cultured chick osteoblasts and UMR-106 cells on a deformable petri dish bottom in such a manner that strains up to 240,000 μE were produced at the periphery of the dish. Intermittent (0.05 Hz) stretching, applied continuously, increased cell numbers after 2 d.

³H-thymidine incorporation was also increased. Microscopic inspection of the cultures showed that as early as 24 h after initiation of cyclic deformation the osteoblasts had aligned perpendicularly to the direction of the strain in the periphery of the bottom of the petri dish. Interestingly, Murray and Rushton (1990) using much lower strains of up to 20,000 μE found no changes in the orientation of the cells.

Yeh and Rodan (1984) exposed cells to tensile forces by culturing them on collagen ribbons which were mechanically stretched (eight times in a 2-h experimental period) to strains of 50,000 to 100,000 μE. This led to a 3.5-fold increase in PGE_2 synthesis. Using a mixture of epiphyseal and articular chondrocytes isolated from fetal chick femora and tibiae, DeWitt *et al.* (1984) produced multilayered sheets of chondrocytes surrounded by a considerable amount of extracellular matrix after 14 d of culture. These tissue-like sheets were removed intact from culture flasks, clamped between the two end plates of a stretching machine, and exposed for 24 h to intermittent (0.2 Hz) stretching, reaching 55,000 μE. After 24 h of treatment, ³H-thymidine incorporation was increased 2.4-fold and cAMP values 2.2-fold. The synthesis of important matrix components such as glycosaminoglycans (incorporation of $^{35}SO_4$ and ^{14}C-glucosamine) was increased after 4 and 24 h of stimulation. Total protein synthesis (³H-glycine incorporation) did not change. cAMP analogues could also induce increased matrix synthesis and thus mimicked the effect of mechanical stimulation.

Application of Stress by Hydrostatic Compression

Hydrostatic compression obtained by compressing the gas phase of the culture system, as discussed in the section on organ cultures, has also been applied to isolated bone and cartilage cells. Unfortunately, it is very difficult to relate results of these types of experiments, in which the force is expressed in kiloPascals and strains are not measured, to the stretching experiments. As in the stretching experiments, however, the response of skeletal tissue cells to a change in the mechanical environment is described, which may shed light on the mechanism of response of the cells.

Rodan *et al.* (1975) and Bourret and Rodan (1976) were the first to demonstrate that isolated embryonic chicken chondrocytes kept in Krebs-Ringer glucose solution responded to continuous hydrostatic compression of 6 kPa for 15 min. Chondrocyte response varied according to the area of origin in the epiphysis. In cells isolated from the proliferative zone of 16-d chick embryo tibiae epiphyses, continuous hydrostatic compression decreased cAMP but increased cGMP levels, whereas in cells from the hypertrophic zone no changes were found in cAMP and a decrease was found in the cGMP levels. The response in the proliferative cells could also be evoked by addition of the calcium ionophore A23187. The effects of the ionophore and pressure were not additive, suggesting a common mechanism. The different response of proliferative and hypertrophic cells was probably related to their different developmental stages, as membrane preparations of both cell types produced different cAMP responses to a calcium challenge (Bourret and Rodan, 1976).

Veldhuijzen *et al.* (1979) developed an experimental setup to expose isolated fetal chick tibia epiphyseal chondrocytes of the proliferative zone to intermittent (0.3 Hz) hydrostatic compression of up to 13 kPa. They demonstrated that intermittent compression increased the cAMP content both in whole epiphyses and in the isolated chondrocytes. The change in cAMP levels was followed by a reduction of cell proliferation. These authors were the first to demonstrate a dose-response relationship between magnitude of the mechanical stimulus and cellular response. The dose-response pattern indicated an all-or-none response with a threshold at 8 kPa, a pressure roughly equivalent to the *in vivo* weight-bearing pressure exerted on the newly hatched chick tibia.

Using high-density cultures instead of cell monolayers, Van Kampen *et al.* (1985) confirmed the results of Veldhuijzen *et al.* (1979) concerning the inhibition of cell proliferation by intermittent, 13-kPa hydrostatic compression. They also found that the synthesis of proteoglycans was increased by this regime. Gu-HCl extraction showed that, after exposure to intermittent compression for 24 h, proteoglycans had an improved aggregating capacity with hyaluronic acid and were more difficult to extract from the matrix, indicating a higher resilience of the matrix. The increased synthetic activity in chondrocytes was corroborated in histological studies (Veldhuijzen *et al.*, 1987). Opposite effects of intermittent hydrostatic compression on cell proliferation (inhibition) and matrix synthesis (stimulation) were also reported by Burger *et al.* (1991b) using monolayers of osteoblastic cell lines (MC3T3-E1 and Ros 17/2.8). After 3 or 4 d of exposure to pressure (13 kPa at 0.3 Hz) both cell cultures showed a decreased ^{3}H-thymidine uptake and a lower DNA content. In addition after 5 or 10 d culture under pressure amino acid uptake was increased, as was alkaline phosphatase activity.

A technique to apply much higher (200 kPa) pressure to cell cultures was developed by Ozawa *et al.* (1990). To avoid changes in the partial pressure of O_2 and CO_2 and, as a consequence, the pH of the medium, they used a $N_2:O_2:CO_2$ mixture adapted to the high pressure (91.3, 7.0, and 1.7%, respectively). Monolayer cultures of the osteoblastic cell line MC3T3-E1 showed a dramatic inhibition of alkaline phosphatase activity after exposure to 100 kPa continuous hydrostatic pressure, an effect which was reversible after removal of the pressure. Continuous pressure also suppressed collagen synthesis and calcification of the matrix. No effect was found on DNA synthesis or DNA content of the cells. After 2, 6, and 48 h of exposure to compression, *de novo* synthesis of PGE_2 was significantly increased. It seems plausible from their data that the increased PGE_2 synthesis caused the reduction in alkaline phosphatase activity. Thus, it seems that the expression of the osteoblastic phenotype was inhibited as a result of high PGE_2 synthesis under pressure.

Fluid Flow (Shear Stress)

One way by which mechanical loading of tissue may trigger cellular responses is by inducing flow of extracellular fluid (Seliger, 1969). To test this hypothesis, Reich *et al.* (1990) examined the reactions of osteoblasts to fluid flow *in vitro*. Osteoblasts isolated from rat calvaria were cultured on a glass coverslip in a polycarbonate chamber, designed to allow perfusion of medium. Cells were exposed to shear rates of 10 to 3500 s^{-1} (generating shear stresses of 0.1 to 35 $dyne/cm^2$). Increasing shear rates resulted in increased intracellular cAMP levels. To distinguish between effects of streaming potentials and mechanical perturbation of the cells as a result of fluid flow, they used fluids with various viscosity. For a given shear rate (as a result of fluid flow) streaming potentials are independent of viscosity, while the resulting shear stress is directly proportional to viscosity. Increasing the viscosity of the fluid medium (but not its ionic strength) further increased the cAMP response to a given shear rate, indicating that shear stress rather than streaming potentials mediates load-induced responses of bone cells.

Table 2 summarizes the studies on isolated bone and cartilage cells. Mechanical perturbation of cells *in vitro* by a variety of techniques stimulated cAMP production as well as PGE_2. In addition, cell proliferation was enhanced in several studies, all using strains of 10,000 μE and higher. On the other hand, hydrostatic pressure of physiological magnitude inhibited cell proliferation. Of the two dose-response studies, one observed a threshold value of 8 kPa hydrostatic pressure, which was near the physiological pressure. The other described a peak response at 7000 μE and another increase at 28,000 μE. A high pressure of 200 kPa inhibited collagen synthesis and matrix calcification, while near-physiologic low pressure stimulated matrix synthesis and alkaline phosphatase activity.

Conclusions

In vitro studies using cell and organ cultures have convincingly shown that skeletal cells do respond to mechanical stress by a number of reactions. However, because of the variation in stress-inducing devices, parameters studied, and magnitude and duration of the mechanical perturbation, generalized conclusions are limited.

Table 2.
Mechanical Studies on Bone Cell Cultures

Authors	Material	Mechanical Stimulus	Cellular Response
Harell et al. (1977) Somjen et al. (1980, 1982) Binderman et al. (1984)	Rat osteoblasts	Petri dish bottom expansion, 10,000 μE, continuous	PGE$_2$ production ↑ cAMP production ↑ DNA synthesis ↑
Shimsoni et al. (1984)	Rat condylar chondrocytes	Petri dish bottom expansion, 10,000 μE, continuous	cAMP production ↑ DNA synthesis ↑
Murray and Rushton (1990)	Mouse osteoblasts	Slide expansion, 3,000–28,000 μE, 0.05–0.002 Hz	PGE$_2$ production ↑ Biphasic dose-response pattern, peak at 7.000 μE
Hasegawa et al. (1985)	Rat osteoblast	Stretching of flexible support, 20,000 μE, 0.002 Hz	Cell proliferation ↑
Sandy et al. (1989a, b)	Mouse osteoblasts	Stretching of flexible support, 20,000 μE, 0.1 Hz	cAMP production ↑ Release of resorption- stimulating factors
Buckley et al. (1988)	Chicken osteoblasts	Stretching of flexible support, up to 240,000μE, 0.05Hz	Cell proliferation ↑ Cell alignment to minimize strain
Yeh and Rodan (1984)	Rat osteoblasts	Stretching of collagenous support, 50,000–100,000 μE, 0.001 Hz	PGE$_2$ production ↑
de Witt et al. (1984)	Chicken chondrocytes	Stretching of cultured cell sheet, up to 55,000 μE, 0.2 Hz	cAMP production ↑ Cell proliferation ↑ Proteoglycan synthesis ↑
Rodan et al. (1975)	Chicken chondrocytes, (proliferative zone)	6 kPa hydrostatic, continuous	cAMP level ↓ cGMP level ↑
Bourret and Rodan (1976)	Chicken chondrocytes, (hypertrophic zone)	6 kPa hydrostatic, continuous	cGMP level ↓
Veldhuijzen et al. (1979)	Chicken chondrocytes	2–10 kPa hydrostatic, 0.3 Hz	cAMP level ↑ Cell proliferation ↓ (threshold at 8 kPa)
Van Kampen et al. (1985)	Chicken chondrocytes	13 kPa hydrostatic, 0.3 Hz	Proteoglycan synthesis ↑
Burger et al. (1992a)	MC3T3E1 osteoblastic cells	13 kPa hydrostatic, 0.3 Hz	Cell proliferation ↓ Al.P. activity ↑ Protein synthesis ↑
Ozawa et al. (1990)	MC3T3E1 osteoblastic cells	200 kPa hydrostatic, continuous	PGE$_2$ production ↑ Al.P. activity ↑ Collagen synthesis ↓ Matrix calcification ↓
Reich et al. (1990)	Rat osteoblasts	Fluid shear stress 0.1– 3.5 dyne/cm^2	cAMP ↑

Al.P.: alkaline phosphatase; ↑: increase; ↓: decrease.

Nevertheless, comparison of the data leads to some interesting conclusions. Osteoblastic cells seem to respond differently to high and low stress compared with (control) culture in the absence of stress. At high stress, the cells respond with increased PGE_2 synthesis followed by increased cell proliferation. This occurs under continuous as well as cyclic (0.2 to 0.001 Hz) stimulation. In addition, release of resorption-stimulating factors is increased while alkaline phosphatase activity, collagen synthesis, and matrix calcification are reduced. Together these phenomena lead to a reduction of the amount of calcified extracellular matrix. At *low* cyclic stress of roughly physiological magnitude, however, cell proliferation is inhibited while alkaline phosphatase activity and protein synthesis are increased. In organ cultures matrix mineralization is stimulated while resorption is reduced. These activities lead to an *increase* in the amount of calcified matrix.

The question arises whether the biphasic relationship between stress magnitude and cellular response *in vitro* is related to phenomena which occur *in vivo*. Recently a theoretical model for mechanical adaptation of adult bone has been developed by Turner (1991), based on Frost's mechanostat postulate (Frost, 1988, 1990a,b) and simple feedback theory. The model assumes threshold levels of mechanical stress, above or below which bone adaptation is turned on. For young adult bone, a "physiological window" between 50 and 2500 μE is assumed in which no adaptation occurs. Only when mechanical usage causes strain levels that fall outside this physiological window will the bone be in a state of disuse or overuse, leading to an adaptive response. It is obvious that, for the *in vitro* cell and organ culture systems discussed above, such a model does not apply. First, the cultured cells are usually derived from rapidly growing embryonic or neonatal animals which are still actively modeling their skeleton. In addition, during the tissue culture experiment the cells are not in a steady state in terms of cell number and matrix volume. Therefore, a model which explains maintenance of a steady-state situation does not fit.

Rather, the *in vitro* results suggest the following: skeletal cells possess mechanoreceptors which inform them about their mechanical environment. Under control *in vitro* conditions, that is, in the virtual absence of mechanical stress, the cells behave in a manner which is reminiscent of early stages of tissue repair, that is, rapid cellular replication and little matrix production. Under these conditions, cyclic mechanical perturbation of low magnitude stimulates the cells to increase matrix synthesis at the expense of cell proliferation. The increased amount of matrix reduces the magnitude of strain resulting from the applied stress, thereby establishing a feedback loop, as has been postulated *in vivo* (Currey, 1984; Frost, 1988; Turner, 1991). Very high mechanical perturbation however leads to responses which reduce the amount of extracellular matrix. This catabolic type of response may be the *in vitro* equivalent of the effect of orthodontic tooth movement, where bone is resorbed in places of (very) high mechanical pressure (Imamura *et al.*, 1990). Alternatively, the inhibition of matrix synthesis by very high mechanical stress may have to do with another phenomenon. We speculate that the response may be related to the three-dimensional orientation of bony trabeculae in well-adapted bone tissue. Formation of bony trabeculae with a specific orientation means synthesis of bone matrix in one direction and not in another. Let us imagine a little trabecula being secreted and laid down fortuitously in any direction within the bone tissue. If it lies in the direction of one of the pressure or tension lines, it will be in a position of comparative strain equilibrium which means minimal mechanical disturbance of the cells. However, if it is inclined obliquely to the pressure or tension lines, it would be subjected to very high shearing stresses (D'Arcy Thompson, 1971). If such very high stresses inhibited bone matrix formation rather than stimulating it, we have a mechanism which might explain the well-known phenomenon of trabecular orientation along compression and tension lines. In this respect, the observation of Buckley *et al.* (1988), that osteoblasts under very high mechanical tension orient their shape to minimize the applied strain, is also important. However, the present studies are far from conclusive. There is clearly a need for extensive dose-response studies in which the magnitude, frequency, and rate of the applied stress are varied. These studies must be done using several devices and several different cell and tissue types. Together they may provide insight into the process of mechanical adaptation at the bone cellular level.

References

Aloia, J. F., Cohen, S. H., Ostuni, J. A., Cane, R., and Ellis, K. (1978). Prevention of involutional bone loss by exercise. *Ann. Intern. Med.*, **89**: 356–358.

Arnett, T. R. and Dempster, D. W. (1986). Effect of pH on bone resorption by rat osteoclasts *in vitro. Endocrinology*, **119**: 119–124.

Bagi, C. and Burger, E. H. (1989). Mechanical stimulation by intermittent compression stimulates sulfate incorporation and matrix mineralization in fetal mouse long-bone rudiments under serum-free conditions. *Calcif. Tissue Int.*, **45**: 342–347.

Bassett, C. A. L. and Hermann, L. (1961). Influence of oxygen concentration and mechanical factors on differentiation of connective tissue *in vitro. Nature*, **193**: 460–461.

Bassett, C. A. L. and Becker, R. O. (1962). Generation of electric potentials by bone in response to mechanical stress. *Science*, **137**: 1063–64.

Binderman, I., Shimshoni Z., and Somjen D. (1984). Biochemical pathways involved in the translation of physical stimulus into biological message. *Calcif. Tissue Int.*, **36** (suppl): 82–85.

Binderman, I., Zor, U., Kaye, A. M., Shimshoni, Z., Harell, A., and Somjen, D. (1988). The transduction of mechanical force into biochemical events in bone cells may involve activation of phospholipase A2. *Calcif. Tissue Int.*, **42**: 261–266.

Bourret L. A. and Rodan G. A. (1976). The role of calcium in the inhibition of cAMP accumulation in epiphyseal cartilage cells exposed to physiological pressure. *J. Cell Physiol.*, **88**: 358–361.

Bouvier, M. (1985). Application of *in vivo* bone strain measurement techniques to problems of skeletal adaptations. *Year. Phys. Anthropol.*, 237–248.

Buckley, M. J., Banes, A. J., Levin, L. G., Sumpio, B. E., Jordan, R., Gilbert, J., Link, G. W., and Tran, Son Tay. (1988). Osteoblasts increase their rate of division and align in response to cyclic, mechanical tension. *Bone Miner.*, **4**: 225–236.

Buckley, M. J., Banes, A. J., and Jordan, R. D. J. (1990). The effect of mechanical strain on osteoblasts *in vitro*. *Oral Maxillofac. Surg.*, **48**: 276–281.

Burger, E. H., Klein-Nulend, J., and Veldhuijzen, J. P. (1991). Modulation of osteogenesis in fetal bone rudiments by mechanical stress *in vitro*. *J. Biomech.*, **24** (suppl.): 101–109.

Burger, E. H., Gregoire M., Hagen J. W., and Veldhuijzen, J. P. (1992a). Osteogenic effects of mild mechanical stress on bone cell- and organ cultures. In: *The Biochemical Mechanisms of Tooth Movement and Craniofacial Adaptation.* Davidovitch, Z., Ed., Ohio State University College of Dentistry, Columbus, OH, 187–193.

Burger, E. H., Klein-Nulend, J., and Veldhuijzen, J. P. (1992b). Mechanical stress and osteogenesis *in vitro*. *J. Bone Min. Res.*, in press.

Carter, D. R. (1987). Mechanical loading history and skeletal biology. *J. Biomech.*, **20**: 1095–1109.

Carter, D. R., Orr, T. E., Fyhrie, D. P., and Schurman, D. J. (1987). Influences of mechanical stress on prenatal and postnatal skeletal development. *Clin. Orthop.*, **219**: 237–250.

Carter, D. R. and Wong M. (1988). Mechanical stresses and endochondral ossification in the chondroepiphysis. *J. Orthop. Res.*, **6**: 148–154.

Copray, J. C. V. M., Jansen, H. W. B., and Duterloo, H. S. (1984a). An *in vitro* system for studying the effect of variable compressive forces on mandibular condylar cartilage of the rat. *Arch. Oral Biol.*, **30**: 299–304.

Copray, J. C. V. M., Jansen, H. W. B., and Duterloo, H. S. (1984b). Effects of compressive forces on proliferation and matrix synthesis in mandibular condylar cartilage of the rat *in vitro*. *Arch. Oral Biol.*, **30**: 305–311.

Copray, J. C. V. M., Jansen, H. W. B., and Duterloo, H. S. (1985). Effect of compressive forces on phosphatase activity in mandibular condylar cartilage of the rat *in vitro*. *J. Anat.*, **140**: 479–489.

Cowin, S. C. (1989). The mechanical properties of cortical bone tissue. In: *Bone Mechanics.* Cowin, S. C., Ed., CRC Press, Boca Raton, 253–277.

Currey, J. D. (1984). *The Mechanical Adaptations of Bones.* Princeton University Press, Princeton, NJ.

Dalsky, G. P., Stocke, K. S., Ehsani, A. A., Slatopolsky, E., Lee, W. C., and Birge, S. J. (1988). Weight-bearing exercise training and lumber bone mineral content in postmenopausal women. *Ann. Intern. Med.*, **108**: 824–828.

D'Arcy Thompson, W. (1971). *On Growth and Form.* Cambridge University Press, Cambridge, England.

DeWitt, M. T., Handley, C. J., Oakes, B. W., and Lowther, D. A. (1984). *In vitro* response of chondrocytes to mechanical loading. The effect of short term mechanical tension. *Connect. Tissue Res.*, **12**: 97–109.

El Haj, A. J., Minter, S. L., Rawlinson, S. C., Suswillo, R., and Lanyon, L. E. (1990). Cellular responses to mechanical loading *in vitro*. *J. Bone Miner. Res.*, **5**: 923–932.

Frost H. M. (1988). Vital biomechanics: proposed general concepts for skeletal adaptations to mechanical usage. *Calcif. Tissue Int.*, **42**: 145–156.

Frost, H. M. (1990a). Skeletal structural adaptations to mechanical usage (SATMU). I. Redefining Wolff's Law: the bone modeling problem. *Anat. Rec.*, **226**: 403–413.

Frost, H. M. (1990b). Skeletal structural adaptations to mechanical usage (SATMU). II. Redefining Wolff's Law: the remodeling problem. *Anat. Rec.*, **226**: 414–422.

Goodship, A. E., Lanyon, L. E., and MacFie, H. (1979). Functional adaptation of bone to increased stress. *J. Bone Jt. Surg.*, **61**A: 539–546.

Glücksmann, A. (1939). Studies on bone mechanics *in vitro*. II. The role of tension and pressure in chondrogenesis. *Anat. Rec.*, **73**: 39–56.

Glücksmann, A. (1941). The role of mechanical stresses in bone formation *in vitro*. *J. Anat.*, **76**: 231–239.

Harell, A., Dekel, S., and Binderman, I. (1977). Biochemical effect of mechanical stress on cultured bone cells. *Calcif. Tissue Res.*, **22** (suppl.): 202–209.

Hart, R. T. and Davy, D. T. (1989). Theories of bone modeling and remodeling. In: *Bone Mechanics*, Cowin, S. C., Ed., CRC Press, Boca Raton, FL, 253–277.

Hasegawa, S., Sato, S., Saito, S., Suzuki, Y., and Brunette, D. M. (1985). Mechanical stretching increases the number of cultured bone cells synthesizing DNA and alters their pattern of protein synthesis. *Calcif. Tissue Int.*, **37**: 431–436.

Imamura, K., Ozawa, H., Hiraide, T., Takahashi, N., Shibasaki, Y., Fukuhara, T., and Suda, T. (1990). Continuously applied compressive pressure induces bone resorption by a mechanism involving prostaglandin E_2 synthesis. *J. Cell Physiol.*, **144**: 222–228.

Jee, W. S. S. and Li, X. J. (1990). Adaptation of cancellous bone to overloading in the adult rat: a single photon absorptiometry and histomorphometry study. *Anat. Rec.*, **227**: 418–426.

Klein-Nulend, J., Veldhuijzen, J. P., and Burger, E. H. (1986). Increased calcification of growth plate cartilage as a result of compressive force *in vitro*. *Arthritis Rheum.*, **29**: 1002–1009.

Klein-Nulend, J., Veldhuijzen, J. P., De Jong, M., and Burger, E. H. (1987b). Increased bone formation and decreased bone resorption in fetal mouse calvaria as a result of intermittent compressive force *in vitro*. *Bone Miner.*, **2**: 441–448.

Klein-Nulend, J., Veldhuijzen, J. P., Van de Stadt, R. J., Van Kampen, G. P. J., Kuijer, R., and Burger, E. H. (1987a). Influence of intermittent compressive force on proteoglycan content of calcifying growth plate cartilage *in vitro*. *J. Biol. Chem.*, **262**: 15490–15495.

Klein-Nulend, J., Veldhuijzen, J. P., Van Strien, M. E., De Jong, M., and Burger, E. H. (1990). Inhibition of osteoclastic bone resorption by mechanical stimulation *in vitro*. *Arthritis Rheum.*, **33**: 66–72.

Krolner, B., Toft, B., Nielsen, S. P., and Tondevold, E. (1983). Physical exercise as prophylaxis against involutional vertebral bone loss: a controlled trial. *Clin. Sci.* **64**: 541–546.

Lanyon, L. E., Goodship, A. E., Pye, C. J., and MacFie, J. H. (1982). Mechanically adaptive bone remodeling. *J. Biomech.*, **15**: 141–154.

Lanyon, L. E. (1984). Functional strain as a determinant for bone remodeling. *Calcif. Tissue Int.*, **36** (suppl): 56–61.

Lanyon, L. E. and Rubin, C. T. (1984). Static versus dynamic loads as an influence on bone remodeling. *J. Biomech.*, **17**: 897–905.

Li, X. J., Jee, W. S. S., Chow, S. Y., and Woddbury, D. M. (1990). Adaptation of cancellous bone to aging and immobilization in the rat: a single photon absorptiometry and histomorphometry study. *Anat. Rec.*, **227**: 12–24.

Meade, J. B., Cowin, S. E., Klawitter, J. J., van Buskirk, W. C., and Skinner, H. B. (1984). Bone remodeling due to continuously applied loads. *Calcif. Tissue Int.*, **36** (suppl): 25–30.

Meade, J. B. (1989). The adaptation of bone to mechanical stress: experimentation and current concepts. In: *Bone Mechanics*. Cowin, S. C., Ed., CRC Press, Boca Raton, FL.

Meikle, M. C., Reynolds, J. J., Sellers, A., and Dingle, J. T. (1979). Rabbit cranial sutures *in vitro*: a new experiment model for studying the response of fibrous joints to mechanical stress. *Calcif. Tissue Int.*, **28**: 137–144.

Meikle, M. C., Heath, J. K., Hembry, R. M., and Reynolds, J. J. (1982). Rabbit cranial suture fibroblasts under tension express a different collagen phenotype. *Arch. Oral Biol.*, **27**: 609–613.

Murray, D. W. and Rushton, N. (1990). The effect of strain on bone cell prostaglandin E_2 release: a new experimental method. *Calcif. Tissue Int.*, **47**: 35–39.

Ozawa, H., Imamura, K., Abe, E., Takahashi, N., Hiraide, T., Shibasaki, Y., Fukuhara, Y., and Suda, T. (1990). Effect of continuous applied compressive pressure on mouse osteoblasts-like cells (MC3T3-E1) *in vitro*. *J. Cell Physiol.*, **142**: 177–185.

Reich, K. M., Gay, C. V., and Francos, J. A. (1990). Fluid shear stress as a mediator of osteoblast cyclic adenosine monophosphate production. *J. Cell. Physiol.*, **143**: 100–104.

Rodan, G. A., Bourret, L. A., Harvey, A., and Mensi, T. (1975). 3′,5′ Cyclic AMP and 3′,5′ cyclic GMP: mediators of the mechanical effects on bone remodeling. *Science*, **189**: 467–469

Rubin, C. T. and Lanyon, L. E. (1984). Regulation of bone formation by applied dynamic loads. *J. Bone Jt. Surg.*, **66A**: 397–402.

Rubin, C. T. (1984). Skeletal strain and the funtional significance of bone architecture. *Calcif. Tissue Int.*, **36** (suppl.): 11–18.

Rubin, C. T. and Lanyon, L. E. (1985). Regulation of bone mass by mechanical strain magnitude. *Calcif. Tissue Int.*, **37**: 411–417.

Sandy, J. R., Meghji, S., Scutt, A. M., Harvey, W., Harris, M., and Meikle, M. C. (1989a). Murine osteoblasts release bone-resorbing factors of high and low molecular weights: stimulation by mechanical deformation. *Bone Miner.*, **5**: 155–168.

Sandy, J. R., Meghji, S., Farndale, R. W., and Meikle, M. C. (1989b). Dual evaluation of cyclic AMP and inositol phosphates in response to mechanical deformation of murine osteoblasts. *Biochim. Biophys. Acta*, **110**: 265–269.

Seliger, W. G. (1969). Tissue fluid movement in compact bone. *Anat. Rec.*, **166**: 247–256.

Shimshoni, Z., Binderman, I., Fine, N., and Somjen, D. (1984). Mechanical and hormonal stimulation of cell cultures derived from young rat mandible condyle. *Arch. Oral Biol.*, **29**: 827–831.

Smith, D. M., Khairi, M. R. A., Norton, J., and Johnson, C. C., Jr. (1976). Age and activity effects on rate of bone mineral loss. *J. Clin. Invest.*, **58**: 716–721.

Smith, E. L., Gilligan, C., McAdam, M., Ensign, C. P., and Smith, P. E. (1989). Deterring bone loss by exercise intervention in premenopausal and postmenopausal women. *Calcif. Tissue Int.*, **44**: 312–321.

Somjen, D., Binderman, I., Berger E., and Harell, A. (1980). Bone remodeling induced by physical stress is prostaglandin E_2 mediated. *Biochim. Biophys. Acta* **627**: 91–100.

Somjen, D., Yariv, M., Kaye A. M., Korenstein R., Fischler, H., and Binderman I. (1982). Ornithine decarboxylase activity in cultured bone cells is activated by bone-seeking hormones and physical stimulation. *Adv. Polyamine Res.*, **4**: 713–718.

Turner, C. H. (1991). Homeostatic control of bone structure: an application of feedback theory. *Bone*, **12**: 203–217.

Uhthoff, H. K., Sekaly, G., and Jaworski, Z. F. G. (1985). Effects of long term nontraumatic immobilization on metaphyseal spongiosa in young adult and old beagle dogs. *Clin. Orthop. Relat. Res.*, **192**: 278–286.

Van Kampen, G. P. J., Veldhuijzen, J. P., Kuijer R., van de Stadt, R. J., and Schipper, C. A. (1985). Cartilage response to mechanical force in high density chondrocyte cultures. *Arthritis Rheum.*, **28**: 419–424.

Veldhuijzen, J. P., Bourret, L. A., and Rodan, G. A. (1979). *In vitro* studies of the effect of intermittent compressive forces on cartilage cell proliferation. *J. Cell Physiol.*, **98**: 299–307.

Veldhuijzen, J. P., Huisman, A. H., Vermeiden, J. P. W., and Prahl-Andersen, B. (1987). The growth of cartilage cells *in vitro* and the effect of intermittent compressive force. *Connect. Tissue Res.*, **16**: 187–196.

Wong, M. and Carter, D. R. (1990). Theoretical stress analysis of organ culture osteogenesis. *Bone*, **11**: 127–131.

Yeh, C. and Rodan, G. A. (1984). Tensile forces enhance PGE synthesis in osteoblasts grown on collagen ribbon. *Calcif. Tissue Int.*, **36** (suppl.): 67–71.

Yen, E. H. K., Duncan, G. W., and Suga, D. M. (1984). Biological response to orthodontic and orthopedic forces *in vitro*. In: *Malocclusion and the Periodontium*. McNamara, J. A., Jr. and Ribbens, K. A., Eds., Monograph 15 in Craniofacial Growth Series, University of Michigan, Ann Arbor, 149–164.

Yen, E. H. K. and Melcher, A. (1978). A continuous-flow culture system for organ culture of large explants of adult tissue: effect of oxygen tension on mouse molar periodontium. *In vitro*, **14**: 811–818.

3

Effects of Physical Inactivity, Paralysis, and Weightlessness on Bone Growth

G. DONALD WHEDON
Shriners Hospitals for Crippled Children
International Shrine Headquarters
Tampa, Florida

AND

ROBERT P. HEANEY
John A. Creighton University Professor
Creighton University
Omaha, Nebraska

Introduction

The question of what happens to bone under varying loads was answered in a general way by Wolff a century ago in an expression that has come to be known as Wolff's law: "Every change in the function of a bone is followed by certain definite changes in internal architecture and external conformation . . . " (Wolff, 1892). While Wolff was interested more in form than in mass, *per se*, we believe that mass is included, at least implicitly, in his "law". In any event, changes in mass that follow altered bony loading have a practical significance that pervades many areas of physiology and medicine—including treatment of, and convalescence from, trauma and serious illness involving bed rest in otherwise fit individuals; management of paralytic and chronic debilitating diseases; recommendations for maintaining physical ability during normal aging; and maintenance of function of multiple systems in long-flying astronauts. Much has been observed about the kind and degree of changes in bone associated with long disuse, somewhat less about the effects of increased exercise. Much remains to be learned about the mechanisms of both changes, particularly about the potentially serious consequences of disuse and how to prevent or reverse them. A limited review of these considerations appeared in 1984 (Whedon). At a more general level, Currey (1984) and Smith and Gilligan (1989) have extensively reviewed the basic features of the bony response to altered loading.

Mechanical Control of Bone Mass

Bone form and mass have strong genetic determinants which express themselves most prominently during development. Additionally, bone possesses an endocrine/homeostatic function, serving as a reservoir and sink for both calcium and phosphorus. In this regard, calcium deficiency, even in fully mature adults, will reduce bone mass. These considerations aside, however, bone is predominantly a structural organ, and its mass and form are determined to a substantial extent by mechanical stresses sustained in use. All mechanical forces applied to a bone, whether acting as a lever arm or resisting gravity, result in minute structural deformations known technically as "strain". Strain is defined as a reversible fractional change in a dimension, and for stiff materials, such as bone, it is expressed in units that are millionths of the initial dimension (i.e., microstrain).

Bones, both in different regions of a single skeleton, and even across different species, exhibit a remarkably constant pattern of strain under loading. Peak loads typically result in 2500 to 3500 microstrain and routine loading typically produces 1000 to 1500 microstrain (Rubin and Lanyon, 1982). Yield strength—the point at which a physiologically applied load produces an irreversible deformation—is typically at values in the range of 7000 microstrain or above. Thus, even at peak stresses, bone has a built-in mechanical reserve of about 2 to 3×. Because the loads sustained by various

BONE MASS FEEDBACK LOOP

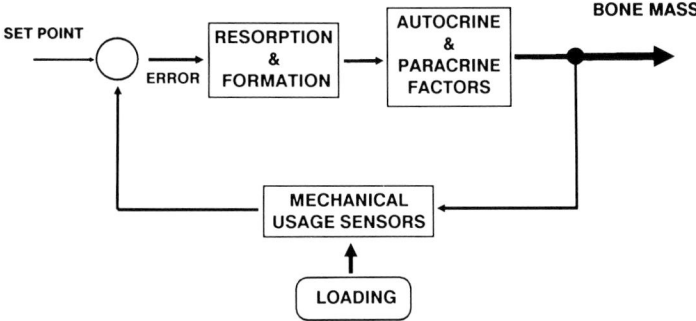

Fig. 1 Suggested feedback loop controlling bone mass. The quantity optimized is strain produced under routine use of the skeletal member. Strain values different from the set-point value result in an error signal that alters remodeling balance. Bones with greater values for mass density are stiffer, and thus bend or deform less (i.e., undergo less strain) when loaded. Rubin and Lanyon's data (see text) suggest that the cross-species set point is in the range of 1000 microstrain. (Copyright Robert P. Heaney, M.D., 1990; used with permission.)

bones differ over several orders of magnitude, this constancy of strain means that mass density of each bone is matched to the loads to which it is typically exposed.

This remarkable adjustment of bone mass is achieved through a classical feedback loop such as described by Turner (1991) or by Beaupré and associates (1990) and represented in Fig. 1. In this model the level of strain under loading is somehow monitored and then compared against a reference level (the "set point"). Any difference between the stimulus and the reference level generates an error signal which controls the local balance between the resorptive and formative phases of bone remodeling. (Probably, also, these error signals are important in localizing bone remodeling by altering the activation threshold at specific surface sites where remodeling will occur.) The resulting change in bone mass makes the bone more or less stiff, i.e., the bone bends more or less under the same loads. The cells monitoring strain detect this change in deformation and adjust their output accordingly. Thus the loop is closed.

Although much remains to be learned about the details of how the model operates, the best candidate for the monitoring system, and possibly for the location of the set-point apparatus itself, is the osteocyte. The processes of this cell ramify through the volume of bone surrounding it, and at the same time each osteocyte maintains cell-to-cell linkage with lining cells at anatomical bone surfaces. Thus the osteocyte is in an ideal position both to detect strain occurring in the course of musculoskeletal activity and to relay signals to the remodeling apparatus in the vascular spaces of bone.

Strain, as it occurs, forces fluid through the microscopic pores of bone—certainly through the canaliculi surrounding osteocyte processes, and possibly through even smaller channels in the calcified matrix between the osteocyte processes. The dissolved electrolytes in bony fluids are charge carriers, and as the fluid moves electrical phenomena called "streaming potentials" result. These in turn have been shown to alter the charge on the large proteoglycan molecules that are embedded in the cell membranes of the osteocyte processes and attached to the osteocyte cytoarchitecture (Skerry *et al.*, 1988). The charged polysaccharide component of the proteoglycans projects into the extracellular space. The streaming potentials alter the charge densities on these molecules; an increase causes them to repel one another and they thereby tug on the cytoarchitecture of the cell. Exactly what happens next in the interior is uncertain, but several biochemical changes have been identified which suggest that the cells both detect and respond to the streaming potentials in the fluid that bathes them. This sequence provides a very satisfying, if still incomplete, bridge between the world of biomechanics and the world of cell biology. Lanyon and colleagues have contributed much to the building of this bridge (Pead *et al.*, 1988a, 1988b; Skerry *et al.*, 1988, 1989).

One of the most satisfying aspects of the foregoing scheme arises from another set of observations by Rubin and Lanyon (1984, 1985). Using an isolated turkey ulna preparation, they showed that bone mass could be preserved by comparatively few loading cycles (in some experiments as few as a total of only four cycles), and in any case involving no more than 1 to 2 min of loading each day. What mechanism might explain an enduring response to such brief stimulation? It turns out that the polysaccharide portions of the proteoglycans act as electrical capacitors, and leak their charge away very gradually. Thus a brief burst of physical activity produces a persisting alteration on the surfaces of the very cells that are probably most involved in mediating the response to mechanical loading. Incidentally, this same experiment illustrated the operation of the feedback loop which adjusts bone mass to produce a constant level of strain under load. Variable loads were applied externally; strain levels below 1000 microstrain were found to result in bone loss from this isolated ulna preparation. Above 1000, there was a linear increase in bone mass, proportionate to strain, despite the complete isolation of this preparation from ordinary muscular pulls and environmental forces throughout the rest of the day.

O'Connor and Lanyon (1982) have also shown that the rate of strain is more important than its magnitude. Thus impact loading—resulting in rapid deformation—is more osteogenic than the same force applied slowly. This is consistent with the early impressions that, for the same expenditure of energy, swimming has less effect on skeletal mass than jogging.

The foregoing feedback system is quite site specific, not pan-skeletal. Thus, heavily loaded bones increase their mass density without any appreciable effect on other skeletal regions—at least so long as calcium intake is sufficient to permit the mass increase. (When it is not, less-used bones or regions will be decreased in density to provide the calcium needed to strengthen the bone subject to increased load.) Thus, the density of the radius is increased in the dominant arm of tennis players (Montoye *et al.*, 1980; Huddleston *et al.*, 1980) and the leg bones in weight lifters (Nilsson, 1971). Conversely, bed rest and space flight (see below) result in specific decreases in density of the bones resisting gravity in walking—as measured in the os calcis (Vogel and Whittle, 1976; Donaldson *et al.*, 1970).

Decreased Loading

Bedrest/Immobilization Studies

Because of the great number and complexity of factors potentially involved in the reaction of the skeleton in patients confined to bed with various diseases or disorders, it is important to analyze those observations which attempted to eliminate or minimize such complicating influences by studying the effects of physical inactivity in normal, healthy human beings. The first such study was in 1929 by Cuthbertson, who placed a group of medical students in bed, with activity restricted by splints and sandbags, for 10 to 14 d while on constant dietary intakes; this brief immobilization resulted in an increase in urinary calcium and nitrogen. Keys in 1944 performed a similar study, but the changes noted were of limited value because activity in bed was unrestricted and dietary intake was reduced during the bed-rest phase.

A more detailed study was carried out in 1944 through 1947 by Deitrick and associates (1948), who maintained constant dietary intakes in four subjects before, during, and following 6 to 7 weeks in plaster casts from waist to toes. Both urinary and fecal calcium were increased, the urinary calcium being doubled by the 4th to 5th week to a mean level of 312 mg/d, by which time calcium balance became significantly negative (mean balance: -0.182 g/d; mean change from control: -0.308 g/d) and continued so (Fig. 2). Serum calcium rose by 0.8 to 2.1 mg %. Urinary nitrogen and phosphorus were also considerably increased, nitrogen particularly during the first 3 weeks. This change was reflective particularly of loss of muscle mass. During the 4-week ambulatory recovery phase, urinary calcium subsided gradually to levels below those of the ambulatory pre-bed rest control phase.

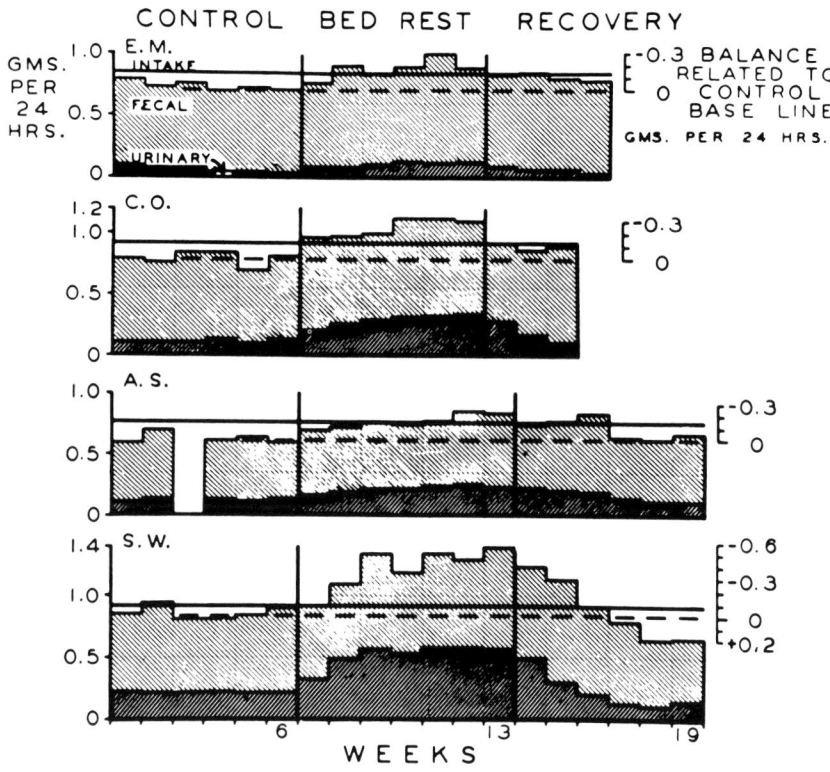

Fig. 2 Effect of immobilization on the calcium metabolism of four normal male subjects. In each subject the daily calcium intake was kept constant throughout all periods of the experiment. For each subject the control baseline (interrupted horizontal line) is an average of the total outputs of the last four control weeks. In this graph the intake and output are plotted upward from the zero baseline. (Reproduced by permission of *Medical Clinics of North America*, **35(2)**, 545, March 1951.)

In addition to the elevated urinary calcium during bed rest, several factors were noted which would favor precipitation of calcium phosphate in the urinary tract: excessive excretion of phosphate, slight alkaline shift of pH, and a failure of urinary citric acid to rise compensatorily with calcium as would be expected in ambulatory individuals. The high incidence of urinary tract calculi in immobilizing conditions is well known and is given as 5 to 15% (Flocks, 1945).

Subsequent bed-rest studies of normal subjects have confirmed these substantial metabolic derangements. Birkhead *et al.* (1963) observed sustained increases in urinary calcium over several weeks in bed. The longest bed rest (not immobilized) observations to date, 7 months by Donaldson and associates (1970), showed negative calcium balance of 200 mg/day throughout bed rest; the elevated (doubled) urinary calcium levels declined partially during the 3rd and 4th months of bed rest but did not fall to normal until many days after the bed-rest phase was over.

These same bed-rest studies showed extensive bone loss from the os calcis, where 25 to 40% of the bone originally present was lost over periods of 6 to 7 months (Hulley et al., 1971; Vogel and Anderson, 1972). Extrapolation of bone loss curves to the origin suggests that bone loss begins when the immobilization begins, or shortly thereafter. Fortunately, the lost bone was essentially completely restored within a few months of starting ambulation. How much bone needs to be lost, or for how long, before some of the loss becomes irreversible, is unknown. Presumably in the bed-rest studies trabecular structure remained intact, despite the substantial loss of trabecular mass. If whole trabecular elements had been resorbed, it is doubtful that full bony integrity could have been restored on reambulation.

Calcium Metabolism and Bone Loss in Paralytic Diseases

In extension of the Deitrick studies of immobilized bed rest, Whedon and Shorr (1957a) performed metabolic balance studies of 11 patients with paralytic acute anterior poliomyelitis, which in 4 patients were begun within the 1st week of illness. The pattern of severe calcium loss was very similar to that in the immobilization of normal individuals but the degree was greater, the mean maximal urinary calcium excretion being 67% higher than in the immobilized normal subjects. Hypercalcemia (>11.5 mg%) occurred repeatedly in the two of the four patients studied during the acute phase who had the greatest measured calcium loss. In these extensively paralyzed patients, the magnitude and particularly the duration of calcium loss were in proportion both to the degree of muscle paralysis and to the degree and duration of immobilization by the disease.

Accompanying such substantial calcium losses, X-ray detectable bone rarefaction developed. The initial evidences were in localized areas in the ends of the long bones of the lower extremities as early as 2 months after onset and associated with a measured loss of calcium (by balance study) equal to 2.0% of total body calcium. The sharp band of rarefaction in the submetaphyseal area of the distal tibiae of three patients indicated extremely rapid bone loss in a location where bone turnover is normally particularly active. As mineral losses continued, rarefaction became apparent in the pelvis and, in one instance, in the humerus of an extremely paralyzed upper extremity. No evidence of bone loss in the spine appeared although total body calcium losses ranged as high as 9.4%. That early stages of loss were present in this region is suggested by observation of other patients with poliomyelitic paralysis in whom bone loss from the spine was detected after approximately 1 year.

As would be expected, there were prodigious losses of nitrogen associated with the progressive decreases in muscle mass over the first 2 months after onset of paralysis; these nitrogen losses were accompanied by high creatinuria and a gradual decline in urinary creatinine. As a major component of both muscle and bone, phosphorus was also excreted in large amounts; a disproportionately highly negative phosphorus balance (relative to calcium and nitrogen) during the 2nd week suggested the possibility that it reflected destruction of sizeable amounts of nervous tissue.

Bloomfield *et al.* (1990) and Kiratli and associates (1989) have measured bone mass in various skeletal regions in patients with a variety of paralytic syndromes, from polio to spinal cord injury. In summary, they found striking reduction in bone mass in various regions of the femur and tibia in patients with lower extremity paralysis, with values in the proximal tibia and lower femur less than 40% of age-matched normals. Upper femoral sites were also reduced, though less severely. Interestingly, spinal cord injury patients showed no loss of vertebral bone density, presumably because the stimulus of wheelchair sitting was sufficient to maintain spinal bone mass. (Certainly, in many of the cases, paraspinal muscles were involved in the paralytic situation, so muscle pulls on the vertebrae would certainly have been reduced.)

Early Space Flight Observations

The first attempt at controlled metabolic observations in space flight was performed in conjunction with the 14-d Earth-orbital U.S. Gemini-VII flight in 1965. That relatively short study (Lutwak *et al.*, 1969) revealed quite modest losses of calcium and phosphorus and varying changes in the metabolism of other elements. During the Apollo series of flights to the Moon, urine and stool specimens were collected, but dietary intake was not controlled, and the flights were too short (up to 11 d) to detect significant calcium metabolic changes.

In early Soviet reports of metabolic observations, elevated urinary calcium levels were observed in periodic measurements on two cosmonauts during an 18-d flight on a Soyuz spacecraft (Biryukov and Krasnykh, 1970). Since then the Soviets have given little research attention to changes in mineral metabolism, except for pre- and postflight measurements of bone mineral density. After space flights of from 75 to 184 d, losses in density from the os calcis ranged from 0.9 to 19.8%, in rough correlation to the duration of the flight; the mean was 1.35% per month (Stubakov *et al.*, 1984). Recently CT scan measurements have been made of the spinal vertebrae of cosmonauts before and after flights of 187 and 211 d; losses in density from the bodies of the vertebrae were variable and small, whereas, curiously, significant changes were noted in the posterior elements of the vertebrae (Oganov *et al.*, 1989).

Skylab Studies of Calcium Metabolism

The first opportunity to study comprehensively the possible effects of weightlessness on calcium metabolism came in the U.S. Skylab program in 1973 and 1974. The series of three manned flights in Skylab were successively for 28, 59, and 84 d. The mineral and nitrogen metabolic balance studies (Whedon *et al.*, 1974, 1979) required the three astronauts on each flight to comply with nearly constant dietary intake, continuous 24-h urine collections, and total fecal collections for 21 to 31 d before each flight, throughout each flight, and for 17 to 18 d postflight for a total of 909 man-days of metabolic study. Only by these exacting methods can one observe a week-to-week pattern of change in calcium or nitrogen excretion and balance, and obtain a near accurate determination of the quantitative degree of change in the whole body content of the element being measured.

In flight, calcium excretion in the urine increased quite consistently in a pattern of gradual rise over the first 2 to 4 weeks to a plateau level varying from 60% to more than 100% greater than the control level. Fig. 3, displaying the data for the 84-d flight, shows the pattern and to some extent the individual variation. In addition, it indicates the persistence of a high level of calcium excretion over the nearly 3 months of weightlessness. Fecal calcium excretion showed an unusual but fairly consistent pattern of a decrease during the first few weeks in flight, followed by a gradual rise to levels greater than in the preflight control phase. This pattern probably indicated changes initially in colonic motility, with a later decrease in intestinal calcium absorption and possibly also an increase in endogenous fecal calcium. Calcium balance shifted from positive during preflight to negative inflight, with much interindividual variation.

Urinary hydroxyproline increased in flight with considerable interindividual differences; the mean increase for the nine crewmen was 30%. There was also a significant increase in total and nonglycosylated hydroxylysine. The increase in plasma calcium in flight averaged 0.6 mg/dl and was consistent from subject to subject. Plasma phosphorus was increased on average by 0.4 mg/dl. Phosphorus balance data showed a distinct increase in urinary phosphorus during flight, a small increase in fecal phosphorus, and negative balance in all crewmen.

Bone mineral content measurements by photon absorptiometry were made before and immediately after flight under the direction of Vogel (Vogel and Whittle, 1976). Significant losses were limited to the os calcis and occurred in the science pilot of SL-3 and science pilot and pilot of SL-4 (-7.4, -4.5, and -7.9% losses, respectively). These three astronauts had the greatest increases in urinary calcium and greatest negative shifts in calcium balance.

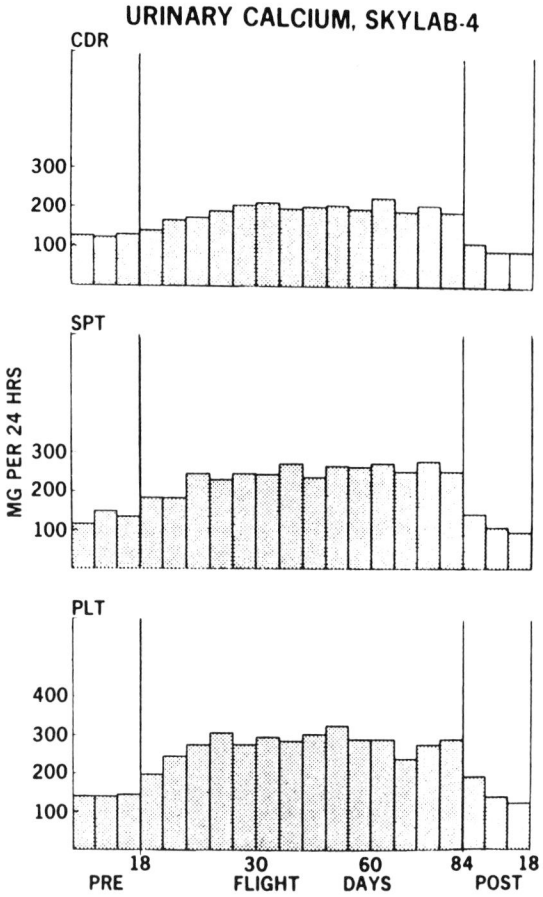

Fig. 3 Effects of space Skylab flight on urinary calcium excretion in the astronauts on the 84-day flight (SL-4). (Whedon *et al.*, 1979.)

Studies on Cosmos Flights

In the series of flights of the Cosmos program, which the Soviets began in 1966, various animals have been sent into space. As reported in 1976 by Yagodovsky *et al.* (1976), when the Wistar rats aboard the 22-d Cosmos-605 returned to Earth, their femora, tibiae, and humeri revealed decreased metaphyseal trabecular bone mass.

The invitation of the Soviets to put a number of U.S. animal experiments aboard some of their Cosmos biosatellite flights led to interesting results with respect to effects on bone. Cosmos-782 in November 1975 and Cosmos-936 in August 1977, both orbiting for about 19 d, carried two studies of 50-d-old, growing rats. In histological observations of bone, including tetracycline labeling, Morey and Baylink (1978) noted, immediately after flight, almost complete cessation of bone formation on the periosteal surfaces of the tibiae. Flight rats allowed to readapt to Earth gravity for 25 d resumed bone formation at a rate similar to that of control animals. In the second of these two Cosmos flights, a group of flight rats was subjected to artificial gravity by centrifugation at 1 g; in this group, decrease in bone formation was not quite as great as in the weightless group without centrifugation, recovery of bone mass after flight was more rapid, and decrease in femur-breaking strength was prevented.

In subsequent Cosmos studies, Wronski and Morey (1983) and Jee et al.(1983) saw cessation of bone formation in the humerus as well as in the tibia. There was less bone mass relative to 1-g controls, with the differences being more pronounced in trabecular bone than in cortical, and less vertebral crush strength and tibial trabecular bone mass as well; the latter did not return to normal in 29 d after the flight. Simmons et al. (1980) found changes in the mandible which indicated a defect in maturation in bone formation, and Roberts et al. (1981) similarly noted a defect in conversion of progenitor cells to preosteoblasts.

Countermeasures

The initial effort to find and test a means to suppress or prevent the losses of mineral resulting during the inactivity or immobilization associated with incapacitating disease was by Whedon et al. (1949) using a slowly oscillating bed. In an extension of the Deitrick immobilization study (1948), using three of the same four normal subjects similarly body casted, losses of calcium, phosphorus, and nitrogen during bed rest were halved. The partial weight bearing of the slowly rocking motion of the bed probably was the principal factor in producing this result.

The same Cornell investigators subsequently studied use of the oscillating bed in patients with paralytic poliomyelitis (Whedon and Shorr, 1957b). They found no protection from the major losses of mineral and nitrogen related to paralysis; this result suggested the importance of muscle pull on periosteum for assistance in maintaining the normal integrity of bone mass.

NASA over several years has been supporting efforts to develop ways which would protect astronauts' skeletons in future, long-duration space flights. Bed-rest metabolic studies of normal male subjects have been the practical Earth model for observing the effects of possible means of countering the mineral losses of weightlessness (Hulley et al., 1971; Hantman et al., 1973; Lockwood et al., 1975; Schneider, 1981; Schneider and McDonald, 1984). Initially a series of physical measures was tested on the young men in bed, none with significant effect. These included exercise with a pulley apparatus for 80 min daily, static and intermittent compression around the shoulders to the feet at a force of 80% of body weight 4 h/d, lower body negative pressure both statically and intermittently for 4 h/d, and impact loading at the heels for 6 to 8 h/d. In an effort to determine how much loading was required to maintain bone mass, Schneider found that 3 h of quiet standing plus 20 min of bicycle ergometry exercise were not sufficient to protect against bone loss. It took 4 h/d of walking to prevent loss of mineral if the remaining 20 h were spent in bed (Schneider, V.S., unpublished observations).

Exercise countermeasures including bicycle ergometry were implemented on all three Skylab flights, and, on Skylab-4, a simulated treadmill was used for 10 min daily (Thornton and Rummel, 1977). While lower extremity muscular deconditioning was less severe on Skylab-4, bone loss, as reflected in urinary calcium and in os calcis densitometry, was not clearly different from earlier flight experience or from bed rest. If some osseous benefit might have occurred, the conditions were not suitable for its experimental demonstration. Further, the negative experience with exercise countermeasures for bone in space is consistent with the already cited finding of Schneider in bed-rested normal subjects.

Several pharmacological regimens have been studied for their possible protective effect. Earlier Whedon and Shorr (1957c) had shown, in paralytic polio, that administration of testosterone proprionate provided partial protection against calcium and nitrogen losses and that estradiol benzoate protected against calcium losses. The same investigators who performed the exercise countermeasure studies in bed-rested subjects (Schneider and McDonald, 1984) also evaluated several pharmacologic and nutritional interventions. Salmon calcitonin (100 MRC units daily) and phosphate supplements were ineffective in preventing the negative calcium balance during bed rest. Oral calcium (1.2 g/d) and phosphorus (1.3 g/d) supplements held calcium in balance for 12 weeks of bed rest, but thereafter gradually increasing fecal calcium shifted the balance negatively by more than 100 mg/d. Disodium etidronate in low dose was ineffective, but in a higher dose (20 mg/kg/d) reduced the negative calcium balance during bed rest to 30 mg/ d and reduced urinary hydroxyproline to 10 mg below the control ambulatory level. The most promising regimen explicitly tested to date was administration of the bisphosphonate, clodronate, for 3 weeks prior to bed rest as well as throughout the bed-rest phase; it prevented calcium loss during 17 weeks of bed rest. Most likely the newer, third-generation bisphosphonates would be at least as effective.

Significance of Calcium Losses in Weightlessness and Immobilization

The increases in urinary calcium of astronauts in space flight were strikingly similar in pattern to those observed in immobile bed rest and nearly as great in degree. The negative shift in calcium balance also indicated slightly greater loss from immobilization, -280 mg/d vs. -184 mg/d for the six astronauts of the first two Skylab flights. In studies of ordinary (unimmobilized) bed rest, calcium losses have been about the same as those noted in the space studies. The total calcium loss rate generated by the 2nd month in space amounted to approximately 5.5 g/month or about 0.4% of total body calcium per month.

Although this rate seems small in relation to the whole skeleton, the general similarity to bed rest calcium losses (particularly in the failure to show any tendency toward abatement in 3 months' time) suggests that mineral loss in weightlessness will continue for a very long time, presumably many months. After 6 months of weightless flight, the calcium loss could amount to about 2.5% of total body calcium. This is slightly more than the amount of loss which, in studies of paralytic poliomyelitis, resulted in X-ray-visible rarefaction in the distal tibiae (Whedon and Shorr, 1957a). Assuming that such excess excretion would continue in weightlessness, the calcium loss rate of 0.4%/month observed in Skylab takes on potentially serious significance in view of the fact that the losses from inactivity are predominantly in the weight-bearing bones of the lower extremities, and with the realization that flights to Mars and back (for example) will take 1.5 or more years. A loss of 5% of total body calcium in 1 year could be as much as 15% or more in the lower extremities, putting them clearly at risk for fracture.

Immobilization for any medical or surgical reason will also result in bone loss, just as occurs in weightlessness. We have already noted that the bed-rest studies showed that bone loss began approximately concurrently with immobilization (e.g., Hulley *et al.*, 1971). Krolner and Toft (1983) found losses from the lumbar spine averaging 0.9%/week in patients bed rested for intervertebral disc disease for 11 to 61 d. Recovery was slow, but nearly complete by 4 months. Young *et al.* (1983), investigating immobilization in monkeys, also found extensive bone loss, but recovery was slow and potentially inadequate. Similarly, in recent bed-rest studies, in subjects who spent 17 weeks in bed and then were followed for 6 months after reambulation, bone loss was not completely recovered (LeBlanc *et al.*, 1990).

Recovery might be a serious potential problem in mature humans for two reasons. First, typical adult calcium intakes are barely adequate to sustain bone mass, and are generally not sufficient to repair skeletal mass deficits. Rarely do physicians pay attention to the need for calcium supplementation in patients recovering otherwise successfully from illnesses involving prolonged bed rest. Second, lost trabecular structure can probably not be replaced, and thickening of remaining trabeculae would not be predicted to exhibit the same mechanical functionality as the original, more connected structure.

Possible Mechanisms of Bone Loss

With respect to the pathogenesis of bone loss in immobilization or weight-lessness, the evidence is mixed. The rapid onset of hypercalciuria and slight elevation in serum calcium in both situations clearly indicate unbalanced resorption of bone as the predominant early process. All workers have found suppression of plasma PTH and calcitriol, suggestive of resorptive hyper-calciuria. Stewart *et al.* (1982), for example, came to this conclusion in 14 patients with spinal cord injury. In the Skylab flights urinary hydroxyproline excretion increased, along with the increases in urinary calcium, suggesting increased resorption of bone. Leuken *et al.* (1989) found increases in urinary hydroxyproline in bed-rested, normal subjects, and Minaire *et al.* (1974) also found elevated hydroxyproline excretion in patients with spinal cord injury. Thus the evidence points toward, not only resorptive excess, but an absolute increase in resorption as well.

On the other hand, histomorphometric studies, entirely in rats, either flown on one of the Cosmos missions or in simulated weightlessness on Earth, have shown mainly a profound early suppression of new bone for-mation (Morey and Baylink, 1978, Wronski and Morey, 1983; Jee *et al.*, 1983). Most had little or no evidence of increased osteoclastic resorption, although Vico *et al.* (1987) did find increased osteoclast numbers in the bone of pregnant rats flown on one of the Cosmos missions. Young *et al.* (1983), on histologic grounds, also concluded that resorption was increased in a simulated weightlessness model in monkeys. The mode of development of decreased bone in weightlessness is undoubtedly complex, and is probably different in different species. The rat, for example, does not remodel bone as do primates and humans.

It is likely also that what one finds is partly dependent on when one measures the system, relative to the onset of weightlessness or immobiliza-tion. Thus Heaney (1962), using calcium tracer kinetics, found clear evi-dence of elevations in both formation and resorption, but with resorption greater than formation, in polio patients studied 3 to 12 months after onset of paralysis. Chantraine *et al.* (1979) also found elevated values for bone formation (as well as resorption) by calcium kinetics in patients with spinal cord injury. However, most studies have also found that, after the disuse atrophy has developed, bone remodeling drops to normal or subnormal levels.

The high values reported for formation in the kinetics studies might seem paradoxical, but these findings probably reflect the general coupling of formation and resorption found in most osseous conditions. At its earliest phases the bone loss process clearly involves osteoblastic suppression with probable increases in osteoclastic resorption. As the process advances, re-sorption increases further, which inevitably pulls formation with it; hence, the late finding of increased formation.

In any case, it seems abundantly clear that bone loss is mediated mainly by local mechanisms. To begin with, the lost bone is confined to the unloaded skeletal members, an unlikely outcome if the change were systemically mediated. The bone loss during bed rest and in the weightlessness of space flight is mainly in the lower extremities. LeBlanc *et al.* (1990) even found a small *increase* in bone mass in the skulls of normal subjects bedrested for 17 weeks. This probably represents what Parfitt (1980) has termed a decrease in the remodeling space, rather than true bony increase. It would be produced in this instance by a pan-skeletal depression of homeostatically mediated resorption, caused by a relative surplus of calcium released from the resorption of unloaded skeletal regions.

It has not been possible to attribute the local bone loss to measured changes in systemic hormones. Zero gravity, with its psychological and physiological stresses, would be expected to evoke increased secretion of adrenal glucocorticoids, and indeed such was observed in the Skylab personnel (Whedon, 1979). However, Halloran *et al.* (1988) found that adrenalectomized rats lost at least as much bone from unloaded hindquarters as did sham-operated controls, indicating both that the bone loss was not mediated by a nonspecific stress response and that glucocorticoids are not necessary for the production of disuse atrophy. Finally, by clamping calcitriol at normal values, Halloran *et al.* (1986) have also ruled out any role for the decreased calcitriol levels also known to occur during unloading.

Summary

Bone is a mechanical organ, the mass density of which is dynamically adjusted to match the level of current loading. Among its other functions the bone-remodeling apparatus revises bone density and architecture so that ordinary physical activity produces deformations on the order of 1000 microstrain. Decreased loading, whether from paralysis, weightlessness, or simple inactivity, inevitably results in bone loss. The effects on bone of decreased loading have been observed in a series of studies of bed rest in normal human subjects, in patients with paralytic disease, and in astronauts in the weightlessness of space.

In bed-rested normal subjects, depending upon the degree of restriction of activity, bone loss is reflected in urinary calcium, which may be doubled by 4 to 5 weeks and remain elevated for weeks to months, and by fecal calcium which also gradually increases, suggestive of impaired intestinal calcium absorption. Recovery of lost bone mass on resumption of ambulation is gradual and may be incomplete.

In paralytic diseases, such as anterior poliomyelitis, the pattern of calcium loss is similar to that in immobilized normal individuals, but the degree is often greater and in some instances is associated with hypercalcemia. Ra-

diographically detectable bone rarefaction develops in the ends of the long
bones of the lower extremities as early as 2 months after onset of paralysis.
Sizeable losses of nitrogen and phosphorus occur during the first few months,
associated with progressive loss of muscle mass.

In weightlessness, metabolic studies of the Skylab astronauts revealed a
pattern of urinary calcium loss similar to that observed in bed rest, gradually
increasing to a plateau, accompanied by an increase in urinary hydroxyproline; there was also gradually increasing fecal calcium, continuing for the
duration of the flights, the longest being 89 d. Significant decreases in the
density of the os calcis occurred in the three astronauts with the greatest
measured losses of calcium. In Soviet space flights of 75 to 184 d the mean
decrease in cosmonaut os calcis density was 1.35%/month; in flights of 187
and 211 days vertebral density losses were variable and small. In the Cosmos
series of space flights, observations of growing rats by American and Soviet
investigators have shown decreased trabecular bone mass in both fore and
hind limbs; histomorphometric measurements indicated decreased bone formation.

The principal features of mineral losses from the skeleton in all of the
conditions of decreased load conditions are that they are not only significant
in amount but persistent in pattern, at least over the several months of
observation available thus far. In weightlessness, human losses of 0.4% of
total body calcium per month might put lower extremities at risk for fracture
in as soon as 1 year because of the greater differential loss in this particular
area of the skeleton. Studies to date suggest that recovery is slow and
potentially incomplete.

Pharmacologic countermeasures, such as the bisphosphonates, seem the
best means for reducing bone loss in situations where the condition of
unloading is temporary. Exercise countermeasures, at least those devised
and implemented to date, have generally been ineffective.

Bone loss from decreased loading is a local process, not directly mediated
by systemic hormones. It comes about by remodeling in which resorption
exceeds formation. Early in the process formation appears to be depressed,
at least in rats. Resorption is generally elevated and becomes more so as
the process advances. Factors that interfere with resorption will slow the
process, but may not prevent its ultimate development.

Increased Loading

Although the emphasis of this chapter has been on the effects of unloading,
our treatment of this topic would be incomplete if we were not to point out
that the effects of changed loading are bidirectional. Not only can bone lost
from inactivity be replaced (or nearly so) by resumption of normal loading,

but even normally active individuals, with normal skeletons, can increase bone mass if they increase their level of physical activity (Dalsky *et al.*, 1988). However, evidence derived from female runners (Drinkwater, 1990) shows that it is difficult for normally active individuals to increase bone mass by more than a few percentage points, despite exposure to relatively intense activity. This is also despite the fact that there is a great deal of bone that can be lost by physical inactivity. Part of the reason for this apparent asymmetry is undoubtedly that the stimulus Drinkwater used was simply for the runners to do more of what they were already doing. Nevertheless, there should be no doubt that increased activity results in an increase in bone mass and strength, without any change in chemical composition. This has been convincingly shown, for example, in rats and pigs (Saville and Whyte, 1969; Woo *et al.*, 1981; Saville and Smith, 1966; Smith and Saville, 1966; Raab *et al.*, 1990) as well as in humans (Simkin *et al.*, 1987; Huddleston *et al.*, 1980; Jones *et al.*, 1977; Nilsson and Westlin, 1971; Montoye *et al.*, 1980; Pocock *et al.*, 1989, 1986; Sinaki *et al.*, 1986; Lane *et al.*, 1986; Block *et al.*, 1986; Chow *et al.*, 1986).

Acknowledgment

The authors gratefully acknowledge the assistance of Diane Raab, Ph.D., in the preparation of this chapter, and particularly her help with the extensive literature of this field.

References

Barengolts, E. I., Rosol, T. J., Botsis, J., and Kukreja, S. C. (1990). Comparison of the effects of progesterone, estrogen, and medroxyprogesterone on established bone loss in ovariectomized aged rats (abstract). *J. Bone Miner. Res.*, **5** (suppl.): 246.

Beaupré, G. S., Orr, T. E., and Carter, D. R. (1990). An approach for time-dependent bone modeling and remodeling—theoretical development. *J. Orthop. Res.*, **8**: 651–661.

Birkhead, N. E., Blizzard, J. J., Daly, J. W., Haupt, G. J., Issekutz, B., Jr., Myers, R. N., and Rodahl, K. (1963). AMRL-TDR-63–37.

Biryukov, Y. N. and Krasnykh, I. G. (1970). Changes in optical density of bone tissue and calcium metabolism in the cosmonauts, A. G. Nikolayev and V. I. Sevastyanov. *Kosm. Biol. Med.*, **4**:42.

Block, J. E., Genant, H. K., and Black, D. (1986). Greater vertebral bone mineral mass in exercising young men. *West. J. Med.*, **145**: 39–42.

Bloomfield, S. A., Mysiw, W. J., and Jackson, R. D. (1990). Changes in regional bone mineral density with immobilization due to spinal cord injury (abstract). *Med. Sci. Sports Exerc.*, **22** (suppl.): 76.

Chantraine, A., Heynen, G., and Franchimont, P. (1979). Bone metabolism, parathyroid hormone, and calcitonin in paraplegia. *Calcif. Tissue Int.*, **27**: 199–204.

Chow, R. K., Harrison, J. E., Brown, C. F., and Hajek, V. (1986). Physical fitness effect on bone mass in postmenopausal women. *Arch. Phys. Med. Rehab.*, **67**: 231–234.

Currey, J. (1984). *The Mechanical Adaptations of Bones*. Princeton University Press, Princeton, NJ.

Cuthbertson, D. P. (1929). The influence of prolonged muscular rest on metabolism. *Biochem. J.*, **23**: 1328.

Dalsky, G. P., Stocke, K. S., *et al.* (1988). Weight-bearing exercise training and lumbar bone mineral content in postmenopausal women. *Ann. Intern. Med.*, **108**: 824–828.

Deitrick, J. E., Whedon, G. D., and Shorr, E. (1948). Effects of immobilization upon various metabolic and physiologic functions of normal men. *Am. J. Med.*, **4**: 3–36.

Donaldson, C. L., Hulley, S. B., Vogel, J. M., Hattner, R. S., Boyers, J. H., and McMillan, D. E. (1970). Effect of prolonged bed rest on bone mineral. *Metabolism*, **19**: 1071–1084.

Drinkwater, B. L. (1990). Physical exercise and bone health. *JAMWA*, **45**: 91–97.

El Haj, A. J., Minter, S. L., Rawlinson, S. C. F., Suswillo, R., and Lanyon, L. E. (1990). Cellular responses to mechanical loading *in vitro. J. Bone Miner. Res.*, **5**: 923–932.

Flocks, R. H. (1945). Calcium phosphate renal lithiasis. *J. Iowa Med. Soc.*, **35**: 321.

Halloran, B. P., Bikle, D. D., Cone, C. M., and Morey-Holton, E. (1988). Glucocorticoids and inhibition of bone formation induced by skeletal unloading. *Am. J. Physiol.*, **255**: E875–879.

Halloran, B. P., Bikle, D. D., Wronski, T. J., Globus, R. K., Levens, J. M., and Morey-Holton, E. (1986). The role of 1,25-dihydroxyvitamin D in the inhibition of bone formation induced by skeletal unloading. *Endocrinology*, **118**: 948–954.

Hantman, D. A., Vogel, J. M., Donaldson, C. L., Friedman, R. J., Goldsmith, R. S., and Hulley, S. B. (1973). Attempts to prevent disuse osteoporosis by treatment with calcitonin, longitudinal compression and supplementary calcium and phosphate. *J. Clin. Endocrinol. Metab.*, **36**: 845–858.

Heaney, R. P. (1962). Radiocalcium metabolism in human disuse osteoporosis. *Am. J. Med.*, **33**: 188–200.

Huddleston, A. L., Rockwell, D., *et al.* (1980). Bone mass in lifetime tennis athletes. *JAMA*, **244**: 1107–1109.

Hulley, S. B., Vogel, J. M., Donaldson, C. L., Bayers, J. H., Friedman, R. J., and Rosen, S. N. (1971). The effect of supplemental oral phosphate on the bone mineral changes during prolonged bed rest. *J. Clin. Invest.*, **50**: 2506–2518.

Jee, W. S. S., Wronski, T. J., Morey, E. R., and Kimmel, D. B. (1983). Effects of space flight on trabecular bone in rats. *Am. J. Physiol.: Regul. Integ. Compar. Physiol.*, **244(13)**: 310–314.

Jones, H. H., Priest, J. D., Hayes, W. C., *et al.* (1977). Humeral hypertrophy to response to exercise. *J. Bone Jt. Surg.*, **59A**: 204–208.

Keys, A. (1945). Deconditioning and reconditioning in convalescence. *S. Clin. N. Am.*, **25**: 442.

Kiratli, B. J., Agre, J. C., and Smith, E. L. (1989). Effects of chronic immobilization (paralysis) on vertebral and femoral bone mineral density (abstract). *J. Bone Miner. Res.*, **4** (suppl.): 173.

Krølner, B. and Toft, B. (1983). Vertebral bone loss: an unheeded side effect of therapeutic bed rest. *Clin. Sci.*, **64**: 537–540.

Lane, N. E., Bloch, D. A., Jones, H. H., *et al.* (1986). Long-distance running, bone density, and osteoarthritis. *JAMA*, **255**: 1147–1151.

Lockwood, D., Vogel, J. M., Schneider, V. S., and Hulley, S. F. (1975). Effects of diphosphonate EHDP on bone mineral metabolism loss during prolonged bed rest. *J. Clin. Endocrinol. Metab.*, **41**: 533–541.

LeBlanc, A. D., Schneider, V. S., Evans, H. J., Engelbretson, D. A., and Krebs, J. M. (1990). Bone mineral loss and recovery after 17 weeks of bed rest. *J. Bone Miner. Res.*, **5**: 843–850.

Lueken, S., Arnaud, S., Taylor, A. K., Lau, K. H. W., Perkel, V., and Baylink, D. J. (1989). Bed rest causes an acute and progressive increase in skeletal resorption in normal men: indirect evidence that this is mediated by osteocalcin (abstract). *J. Bone Miner. Res.*, **4** (suppl.): 308.

Lutwak, L., Whedon, G. D., LaChance, P. A., Reid, J. M., and Lipscomb, H. S. (1969). Mineral, electrolyte and nitrogen balance studies of the Gemini-VII fourteen-day orbital space flight. *J. Clin. Endocrinol. Metab.*, **29**: 1140–1156.

Minaire, P., Meunier, P., Edouard, C., Bernard, J., Courpron, P., and Bourret, J. (1974). Quantitative histological data on disuse osteoporosis. *Calcif. Tissue Res.*, **17**: 57–73.

Montoye, H. J., Smith, E. L., and Fardon, D. F. (1980). Bone mineral in senior tennis players. *Scand. J. Sports Sci.*, **2**: 26–32.

Morey, E. R. and Baylink, D. J. (1978). Inhibition of bone formation during space flight. *Science*, **201**: 1138–1141.

Nilsson, B. E. and Westlin, N. E. (1971). Bone density in athletes. *Clin. Orthop. Relat. Res.*, **77**: 179–182.

O'Connor, J. A., Lanyon, L. E., and MacFie, H. (1982). The influence of strain rate on adaptive bone remodelling. *J. Biomech.*, **15**: 767–781.

Oganov, V. and Cann, C. (1989). Determination of Spine Mineral and Muscle Density using Computerized Tomography. Aerospace Medical Association Annual Meeting, Washington, D.C.

Parfitt, A. M. (1980). Morphologic basis of bone mineral measurements: transient and steady state effects of treatment in osteoporosis. *Miner. Electrolyte Metab.*, **4**: 273–287.

Pead, M. J., Skerry, T. M., and Lanyon, L. E. (1988a). Direct transformation from quiescence to bone formation in the adult periosteum following a single brief period of bone loading. *J. Bone Miner. Res.*, **3**: 647–655.

Pead, M. J., Suswillo, R., et al. (1988b). Increased ^{3}H-uridine levels in osteocytes following a single short period of dynamic loading *in vivo*. *Calcif. Tissue Int.*, **43**: 92–96.

Pocock, N., Eisman, J., Gwinn, T., et al. (1989). Muscle strength, physical fitness, and weight but not age predict femoral neck bone mass. *J. Bone Miner. Res.*, **4**: 441–448.

Pocock, N., Eisman, J., Yeates, M. G., et al. (1986). Physical fitness is a major determinant of femoral neck and lumbar spine bone mineral density. *J. Clin. Invest.*, **78**: 618–621.

Raab, D. M., Smith, E. L., Crenshaw, T. D., and Thomas, D. P. (1990). Bone mechanical properties after exercise training in young and old rats. *J. Appl. Physiol.*, **68**: 130–134.

Roberts, W. E., Mozary, P. G., and Morey, E. R. (1981). Suppression of osteoblast differentiation during weightlessness. *Physiologist* **24** (suppl.): 75–76.

Rubin, C. T. and Lanyon, L. E. (1982). Limb mechanics as a function of speed and gait: a study of functional strains in the radius and tibia of horse and dog. *J. Exp. Biol.*, **101**: 187–211.

Rubin, C. T. and Lanyon, L. E. (1984). Regulation of bone formation by applied dynamic loads. *J. Bone Jt. Surg.*, **66A**: 397–402.

Rubin, C. T. and Lanyon, L. E. (1985). Regulation of bone mass by mechanical strain magnitude. *Calcif. Tissue Int.*, **37**: 411–417.

Saville, P. D. and Smith, R. (1966). Bone density, breaking force and leg muscle mass as functions of weight in bipedal rats. *Am. J. Phys. Anthrop.*, **25**: 35–40.

Saville, P. D. and Whyte, M. P. (1969). Muscle and bone hypertrophy. *Clin. Orthop. Relat. Res.*, **65**: 81–88.

Schneider, V. S. (1981). Modification of Calcium Balance and Bone Mineral Loss during Prolonged Bed Rest. Vol. I–III, NASA Terminal Report, #T-66D.

Schneider, V. S. and McDonald, J. (1984). Skeletal homeostasis and countermeasures to prevent disuse osteoporosis. *Calcif. Tissue Int.*, **36** (suppl.): 151–154.

Simkin, A., Ayalon, J., and Leichter, I. (1987). Increased trabecular bone density due to bone-loading exercises in postmenopausal osteoporotic women. *Calcif. Tissue Int.*, **40**: 59–63.

Simmons, D. J., Russell, J. E., Winter, F., Baron, R., Vignery, A., Tran, V. T., Rosenberg, G. D., and Walker, W. (1980). Bone growth in the mandible during space flight. *Physiologist,* **24** (suppl.): 87–90.

Sinaki, M., McPhee, M. C., Hodgson, S. F., *et al.* (1986). Relationship between bone mineral density of spine and strength of back extensors in healthy postmenopausal women. *Mayo Clin. Proc.,* **61**: 116–122.

Skerry, T. M., Bitensky, L., *et al.* (1988). Loading-related reorientation of bone proteoglycan *in vivo.* Strain memory in bone tissue. *J. Orthop. Res.,* **6**: 547–551.

Skerry, T. M., Bitensky, L., *et al.* (1989). Early strain-related changes in enzyme activity in osteocytes following bone loading *in vivo. J. Bone Miner. Res.,* **4**: 783–788.

Smith, E. L. and Gilligan, C. (1989). Mechanical forces and bone. *Bone Miner. Res.,* **6**: 139–173.

Smith, R. E. and Saville, P. D. (1966). Bone breaking stress as a function of weight bearing in bipedal rats. *Am. J. Phys. Anthrop.,* **25**: 159–164.

Stewart, A. F., Adler, M., Byers, C. M., Segre, G. V., and Broadus, A. E. (1982). Calcium homeostasis in immobilization: an example of resorptive hypercalciuria. *N. Engl. J. Med.,* **306**: 1136–1140.

Stubakov, G. P., Kaseykin, V. S., Koslovskiy, A. P., and Korolev, V. V. (1984). Evaluation of changes in human axial skeletal bone structures during long-term space flights. *Kosm. Biol. Aviakosmicheskaya Med.,* **18**: 33–37.

Thornton, W. D. and Rummel, J. A. (1977). Muscular deconditioning and its prevention in space flight. In: *Biomedical Results from Skylab.* Johnston, R. S. and Dietlein, L. R., Eds., NASA, 191–197.

Turner, C. H. (1991). Homeostatic control of bone structure: an application of feedback theory. *Bone,* **12**: 203–217.

Vico, L., Chappard, D., Alexandre, C., Palle, S., Minaire, P., Riffat, G., Novikov, V. E., and Bakulin, A. V. (1987). Effects of weightlessness on bone mass and osteoclast number in pregnant rats after a five-day spaceflight (Cosmos 1514). *Bone,* **8**: 95–103.

Vogel, J. M. and Anderson, J. T. (1972). Rectilinear transmission scanning of irregular bones for quantification of mineral content. *J. Nuclear Med.,* **13**: 13–18.

Vogel, J. M. and Whittle, M. W. (1976). Bone mineral content changes in the Skylab astronauts. *Am. J. Roentgenol. Radium Ther. Nuclear Med.,* **126**: 1296–1297.

Whedon, G. D. (1984). Disuse osteoporosis: physiological aspects. *Calcif. Tissue Int.,* **36** (suppl.): 146–150.

Whedon, G. D., Deitrick, J. E., and Shorr, E. (1949). Modification of the effects of immobilization upon metabolic and physiologic functions of normal men by the use of an oscillating bed. *Am. J. Med.,* **6**: 684–711.

Whedon, G. D., Leach, C. S., and Rambaut, P. (1979). Metabolic and endocrine hormone studies in manned space flights. In: *Molecular Endocrinology,* Mac Intyre, I. and Szelke, M., Eds., Elsevier/North-Holland Biomedical Press, Amsterdam, 229–250.

Whedon, G. D., Lutwak, L., Reid, J., Rambaut, P. C., Whittle, M. W., Smith, M. C., and Leach, C. (1974). Mineral and nitrogen metabolic studies on Skylab orbital space flights. *Trans. Assoc. Am. Physicians,* **87**: 95–108.

Whedon, G. D. and Shorr, E. (1957a). Metabolic studies in paralytic acute anterior poliomyelitis. II. Alterations in calcium and phosphorus metabolism. *J. Clin. Invest.,* **36**: 966–981.

Whedon, G. D. and Shorr, E. (1957b). Metabolic studies in paralytic acute anterior poliomyelitis. III. Metabolic and circulatory effects of the slowly oscillating bed. *J. Clin. Invest.,* **36**: 982–994.

Whedon, G. D. and Shorr, E. (1957c). Metabolic studies in paralytic acute anterior poliomyelitis. IV. Effects of testosterone proprionate and estradiol benzoate on calcium, phosphorus, nitrogen, creatine, and electrolyte metabolism. *J. Clin. Invest.,* **36**: 995–1018.

Woo, S. L.-Y., Kuei, S. C., Amiel, D., *et al.* (1981). The effect of prolonged physical training on the properties of long bone: a study of Wolff's law. *J. Bone Jt. Surg.*, **63A**: 780–787.

Wolff, J. (1892). *The Law of Bone Transformation*. Royal Academy of Berlin.

Wronski, T. J. and Morey, E. R. (1983). Effect of space flight on periosteal bone formation in rats. *Am J. Physiol: Regul. Integ. Compar. Physiol.*, **244(13)**: 305–309.

Yagodovsky, V. S., Tristanidi, L. A., and Gorokohova, G. P. (1976). Space flight effects on skeletal bones of rats (light and electron microscopic examinations). *Aviat. Space Environ. Med.*, **47**: 734–738.

Young, D. R., Niklowitz, W. J., and Steele, C. R. (1983). Tibial changes in experimental disuse osteoporosis in the monkey. *Calcif. Tissue Int.*, **35**: 304–308.

4

Adaptation of Bone Growth to Miniaturization of Body Size

JAMES HANKEN

Department of Environmental, Population, and Organismic Biology
University of Colorado
Boulder, Colorado

Introduction

One of the most evolutionarily plastic vertebrate features is adult body size. A predominant trend towards size increase is seen in so many lineages that it has been embodied as an evolutionary "law" — Cope's rule (Cope, 1885; Stanley, 1973). However, the opposite trend — evolutionary decrease in body size — is also widely known, and in certain respects has been of greater evolutionary significance than has size increase (Gould, 1977). Indeed, extreme body size decrease, or miniaturization, is regarded as a key factor in the evolution of the derived bauplans that define several major taxa, including the earliest reptiles (Carroll, 1969, 1970), as well as snakes (Rieppel, 1988), lizards (Carroll, 1970, 1977), and recent amphibians (Bolt, 1977, 1979; Carroll and Holmes, 1980; Milner, 1988). Moreover, miniaturization is extremely common. Among South American freshwater fishes, for example, miniaturization has independently evolved at least 34 times and is represented by no less than 85 species of adult standard length less than 26 mm (Weitzman and Vari, 1988).

As is typical of size change generally (Schmidt-Nielsen, 1984), miniaturization has structural and functional consequences for a variety of organ systems (e.g., vascular system — Villalobos *et al*.,, 1988; brain and visual system — Roth *et al*.,, 1988, 1990). Nowhere, however, are the consequences more pervasive and profound than in the skeleton. This chapter addresses these consequences for the skeleton and especially for bone because of its predominance in the adult. In doing so, I hope to provide insights into how and to what extent patterns and processes of bone growth are modified in the evolution of body size decrease.

The chapter is organized into three parts. First, I briefly review models for evolutionary decrease in body size. These models depict the range of potential effects on the skeleton and how patterns of bone growth may be perturbed. They also reveal the difficulty in inferring the developmental mechanisms underlying changes in body size and adult skeletal morphology solely from adult stages. Second, I illustrate the consequences for the vertebrate skeleton that typically accompany size change and discuss them in terms of patterns and processes of bone growth. These consequences encompass four broad categories: reduction, hyperossification, increased variability, and morphological novelty. I conclude with a brief discussion of the evolutionary implications of altered patterns of bone growth and associated effects on the adult skeleton.

In this review, I draw examples exclusively from fishes, amphibians, and reptiles. This bias reflects in part my personal greater familiarity with these taxa, especially amphibians. However, it is also justified by the simple fact that, in absolute terms, miniaturization of body size is more extreme in representatives of each of these taxa than in birds and mammals. This no doubt is related to the endothermic metabolism of the latter two groups, which, as a consequence of surface area-volume relations, dictates a larger minimum adult body size for them. Thus, fishes, amphibians, and reptiles may provide more appropriate and effective models than do birds and mammals for illustrating both the consequences of miniaturization for the skeleton and the ways in which patterns and processes of bone growth are altered to effect these changes. This is not to say, however, that evolutionary decrease in body size for birds and mammals is of little consequence for the skeleton or of little interest from the standpoint of skeletal growth, as illustrated by recent studies by Bertram (1989) and Biewener (1982, 1989a, b). (See also Chapter 1.)

Mechanisms of Body Size Decrease

Understanding the morphological and functional consequences of miniaturization for the skeleton is facilitated by an appreciation of the various

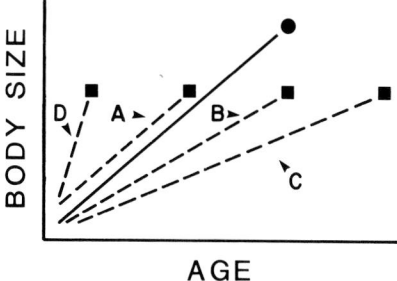

Fig. 1. Hypothetical mechanisms for evolutionary decrease in adult body size. The solid line depicts the ancestral ontogenetic trajectory relating body size to age. Reduced adult size in a descendant may result from (A) precocious cessation of growth (i.e., decrease in offset age) or (B) decrease in overall growth rate. Extending the growth period (i.e., increase in offset age) may also lead to size decrease if it is accompanied by a sufficiently low growth rate (C). Similarly, even an increase in growth rate may lead to size decrease if growth is terminated early enough (D). ●, adult ancestor; ■, adult descendant.

developmental pathways by which evolutionary decrease in body size may occur. The model of Alberch *et al.*, (1979), which relates ontogenetic and phylogenetic changes in organismal size and shape to alterations in the relative rate or timing of discrete developmental events, i.e., to heterochrony, is particularly helpful (see also Fink, 1982). In light of the model, miniaturization emerges as only one of a number of potential evolutionary results of heterochrony, but one that may follow from any of a series of distinct developmental perturbations.

Miniaturization typically involves changes in two distinct developmental parameters: the age at which overall growth stops, or offset age, and growth rate. These parameters may change in a variety of ways, either alone or in combination, to effect size decrease (Fig. 1). If the ancestral rates of organ and tissue differentiation, morphogenesis, and growth with respect to body size are retained in the smaller descendant, the effect will be to produce a pedomorphic adult morphology which resembles juvenile stages of the ancestor more closely than it does the adult (Fig. 2A). If, however, the rates of differentiation, morphogenesis, and growth relative to body size also change, the adult morphology of the descendant could, depending on the nature of the change, resemble the adult ancestor, albeit at a smaller size ("proportional dwarfism", Gould, 1971; Fig. 2B), or could even exceed that of the ancestor ("peramorphosis", Alberch *et al.*, 1979; Fig. 2C).

Several important rules follow from this model. First, the consequences of body size reduction for adult morphology may be quite variable, according to how size decrease has been achieved. Moreover, it is impossible to predict the consequences of size reduction for adult morphology from knowledge of

James Hanken

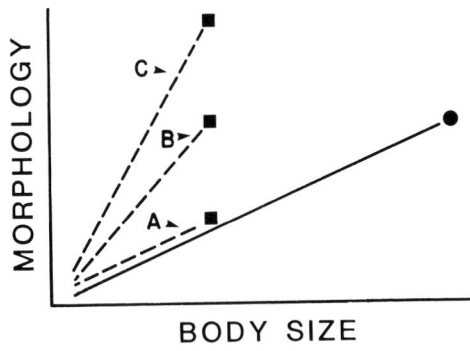

Fig. 2. Potential effects of adult body size decrease on organ and tissue morphology. If ancestral ontogenetic rates of organ and tissue differentiation, morphogenesis, and growth with respect to body size (solid line) are retained, the adult morphology of the descendant will be pedomorphic (A). If, however, differentiation, morphogenesis, and growth occur at a faster rate in the descendant, the ancestral adult morphology could be retained, albeit at a smaller body size ("proportional dwarfism"; Gould, 1971) (B). If the rates of differentiation, morphogenesis, and growth are elevated even more, then the ontogenetic trajectory may go beyond that of the ancestor ("peramorphosis"; Alberch *et al.*, 1979) (C). ●, adult ancestor; ■, adult descendant.

a single developmental parameter. Indeed, the same change in one parameter (e.g., offset age, growth rate) may produce a different adult size or morphology, depending on whether, and in what ways, other parameters are affected. Second, and conversely, similar changes in adult morphology may be brought about by fundamentally dissimilar developmental pathways. For example, evolution of pedomorphosis, as described above, may involve shortening, prolongation, or no change in the growth *period*; similarly, it may involve an increase, a decrease, or no change in the growth *rate* (Fig. 1). Finally, and following from rules 1 and 2, it is impossible to reliably infer the specific developmental changes that led either to decreased body size or to a derived adult morphology from adult stages alone. Addressing this problem requires knowledge of rates of differentiation, morphogenesis, and growth throughout ontogeny in both the descendant and putative ancestral forms — information that is rarely available in most real situations (Fig. 3). Consequently, much more is known about the effects of miniaturization on adult morphology than about the developmental mechanisms underlying them.

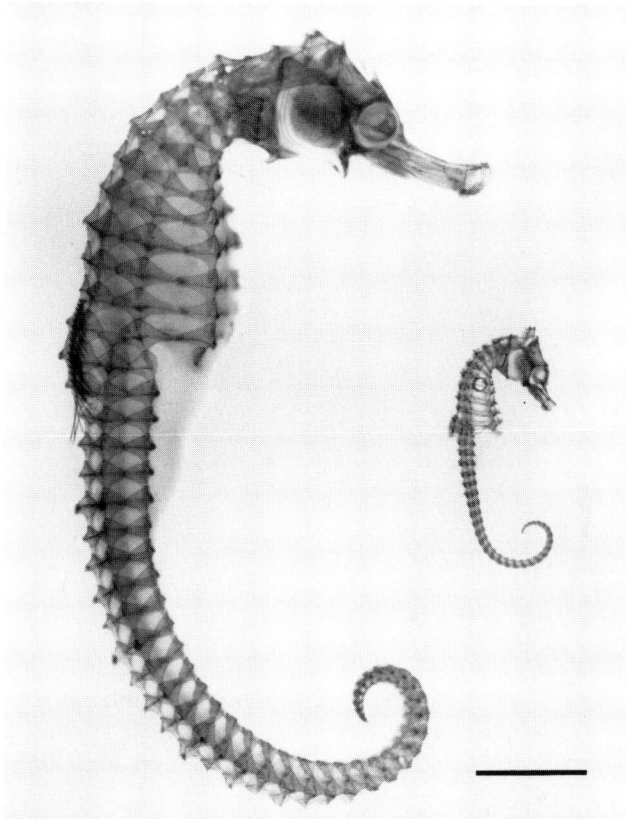

Fig. 3. Adult skeletons of the dwarf seahorse, *Hippocampus zosterae* (right) and the golden seahorse, *H. kuda*. Resolution of mechanisms underlying miniaturization and its consequences for bone growth requires knowledge of rates of differentiation, morphogenesis, and growth throughout ontogeny in both the dwarfed and putative ancestral taxa, in addition to adult morphology. Such information is largely unavailable for these fishes. Recently, Azzarello (1989) described ossification of the pterygoid series in the skull of *H. zosterae*. Scale bar equals 1 cm.

Consequences for the Skeleton

Reduction

As described above, the adult skeletal morphology of a miniaturized taxon may in theory be equally, more, or less developed than that of the ancestor. The most prevalent outcome of size decrease is reduced ossification (e.g., Fink, 1981) (Table 1). A wide range of skeletal components may be affected, including the skull, vertebrae, girdles, limbs, and/or fins. Reduced ossification may take many forms, ranging from subtle changes in the degree of

Table 1.
Incidence of Four Derived Skeletal Features (reduced ossification, R; hyperossification, H; increased variability, V; and morphological novelty, N) in a Variety of Miniaturized Taxa

Taxon	Adult Size[a]	Features	Structures Affected	Citation[b]
Osteichthyes				
Elachocharax mitopterus	12–14	R	Skull, vertebrae, scales	1
Hyphessobrycon elachys	14–20	R	Skull	2
Nannostomus anduzei	11–16	R	Laterosensory canals, pelvic and caudal fins	3
Paracheirodon spp.	17–22	R	Skull, laterosensory canals, pectoral girdle	4, 5
Priocharax ariel, P. pygmaeus	11–17	R	Skull, pectoral girdle, and fins	6
Scopaeocharax spp., *Tyttocharax* spp.	12–25	N	Caudal fin	7
Xenurobrycon macropus	12–20	H	Caudal fin	7
X. polyancistrus	11–14	R	Anal fin	8
Xenurobryconin spp.	12–25	R, N	Laterosensory canals, scales, pectoral and pelvic girdles, fins	7
Ceratostethus bicornis	17–27	R, N	Skull, priaprium	9
Manacopus falcifer	17–27	R, N	Pelvic girdle and fins, priaprium	10
Neostethus siamensis	<40	N	Lower jaw	9, 11
Phallostethus dunckeri, *Phenacostethus* spp.	17	R, N	Skull, pectoral girdle, pelvic girdle and fins, priaprium	12, 13
Oryzias latipes	16–25	R, N	Skull	14

Sundasalanx praecox, S. microps	15–18	R, N	Skull and hyobranchial skeleton, pectoral and pelvic girdles and fins, scales	15
Danionella translucida	10–12	R, N	Skull and hyobranchial skeleton, Weberian apparatus, pelvic girdle, pectoral, pelvic and caudal fins, scales	16
Tyson belos	19	R	Skull, pectoral girdle, pectoral and caudal fins, scales	17
Schindleria praematura, S. pietschmanni	15–20	R	Pelvic fins	18
Amphibia				
Idiocranium russeli	74–113 (total)	R, H, N	Skull, vertebrae	19
Lineatriton lineola	40–55	H	Hyolaryngeal skeleton, mesopodials	20–23
Parvimolge townsendi	23	H	Hyolaryngeal skeleton, mesopodials	20–22, 24
Thorius spp.	14–31	R, H, V, N	Skull and hyolaryngeal skeleton, limbs (epiphyses, phalanges, mesopodials), vertebrae	21, 22, 24–30
Atopophrynus syntomopus	19	R	Skull, sternum, pectoral girdle, limbs (digits, phalanges)	31
Brachycephalus ephippium, B. nototerega, Psyllophryne didactyla	9–16	R, H, N	Skull, digits	32, 33

Table 1 (continued).
Incidence of Four Derived Skeletal Features (reduced ossification, R; hyperossification, H; increased variability, V; and morphological novelty, N) in a Variety of Miniaturized Taxa

Taxon	Adult Size[a]	Features	Structures Affected	Citation[b]
Didynamipus sjoestedti	19	R, N	Skull, sternum, pectoral girdle, limbs (digits, phalanges), vertebrae	34
Mertensophryne micranotis	24	R	Phalanges	34
Phyllonastes heyeri, Phrynopus bagrecito	13–19	R, N	Skull, sternum, pectoral girdle	35
Pseudhymenochirus merlini	40	R, H, N	Skull, hyolaryngeal skeleton, sternum, pectoral girdle, phalanges	36
Sminthillus limbatus	8	N	Pectoral girdle	37
Spea bombifrons	38–64	R, H	Skull, vertebrae	38, 39
Uperoleia spp.	16–35	R, H, V	Skull, sternum, pectoral girdle, sacrum, vertebrae	40–49
Reptilia				
Acontias spp., Acontophiops lineatus, Anniella pulchra, Aprasia repens, Dibamus novaeguineae, Pletholax spp., Typhlosaurus spp.	4–15 (skull)	R, H, N	Skull	50–54
Anolis bimaculatus	110	R	Skull, limbs, pectoral and pelvic girdles	55
Chamaelinorops barbouri	41	H, N	Vertebrae	56

[a] Sizes are only approximate: some denote sample averages, others are maximum recorded values. All represent standard (snout-vent) length, in millimeters, except as otherwise indicated.

[b] Citations: 1 — Weitzman, 1986; 2 — Weitzman, 1985; 3 — Fernandez and Weitzman, 1987; 4 — Weitzman and Fink, 1983; 5 — Weitzman and Vari, 1988; 6 — Weitzman and Vari, 1987; 7 — Weitzman and Fink, 1985; 8 — Weitzman, 1987; 9 — Roberts, 1971; 10 — Parenti, 1986b; 11 — Parenti, 1986a; 12 — Parenti, 1984; 13 — Parenti 1986c; 14 — Parenti, 1987; 15 — Roberts, 1981; 16 — Roberts, 1986; 17 — Springer, 1983; 18 — Watson et al., 1984; 19 — Wake, 1986; 20 — Rabb, 1955; 21 — Uzzell, 1961; 22 — Wake and Elias, 1983; 23 — Wake and Lynch, 1976; 24 — Wake, 1966; 25 — Hanken, 1982; 26 — Hanken, 1983a; 27 — Hanken, 1984; 28 — Hanken, 1985; 29 — Lombard and Wake, 1977; 30 — Wake, 1970; 31 — Lynch and Ruiz-Carranza, 1982; 32 — Trueb and Alberch, 1984; 33 — Trueb and Alberch, 1985; 34 — Grandison, 1981; 35 — Lynch, 1986; 36 — Cannatella and Trueb, 1988; 37 — Griffiths, 1959; 38 — Wiens, 1989; 39 — Stebbins, 1966; 40 — Davies, 1989; 41 — Davies and Littlejohn, 1986; 42 — Davies and McDonald, 1985; 43 — Davies et al., 1986; 44 — Davies et al., 1987; 45 — Stephenson, 1965; 46 — Tyler and Davies, 1984; 47 — Tyler et al., 1980; 48 — Tyler et al., 1981a; 49 — Tyler et al., 1981b; 50 — Rieppel, 1981; 51 — Rieppel, 1982; 52 — Rieppel, 1984a; 53 — Rieppel, 1984b; 54 — Rieppel, 1984c; 55 — Pregill, 1986; 56 — Forsgaard, 1983.

mineralization to the outright absence of one or more bones due to the failure of a cartilaginous precursor to ossify. Typically, it is interpreted as the result of precocious truncation of the ancestral pattern of skeletal ontogeny, i.e., pedomorphosis, because the adult skeletal morphology often resembles, in overall degree of ossification as well as gross size and shape, juvenile stages of a presumed ancestral ontogeny (e.g., Hanken, 1984; Rieppel, 1984a; Wake, 1986).

While pedomorphosis may be the most parsimonious interpretation of skeletal reduction in adults, it must be emphasized that such an interpretation remains only a hypothesis in the absence of corroborating ontogenetic data; as discussed above, developmental mechanisms responsible for skeletal reduction cannot be inferred solely from adult morphology. This is underscored by documented instances in which reduced adult ossification results not simply from precocious cessation of skeletal growth, but from secondary reduction, and sometimes complete loss, of structures that are well developed in juvenile stages. For example, in females of the unusual Philippine phallostethid fish *Manacopus falcifer*, the entire pelvic girdle and several fin rays, which are well developed in subadults, are absent in adults (Parenti, 1986b). Consequently, in instances of the limited development or absence of a bone from an adult stage, it simply is not possible, in the absence of ontogenetic data, to resolve whether this has resulted from precocious cessation of an ancestral developmental program (i.e., decrease in offset age), from change in rates of bone differentiation, morphogenesis, and growth, or even from secondary reduction from a more developed juvenile condition.

One of the important reasons for distinguishing among these alternate routes to skeletal reduction concerns their implications for bone growth. In cases of pedomorphosis, the ancestral patterns and processes of bone growth seemingly are largely conserved, notwithstanding changes in timing and rate (but see discussion below). In cases of secondary reduction, however, ancestral patterns of bone growth have undergone more fundamental alterations, primarily with respect to greater emphasis on processes of bone resorption.

The variability in reduction that frequently accompanies miniaturization, as well as the difficulties in interpreting the reduction from the standpoint of mechanisms of bone growth, are well illustrated by some especially speciose dwarfed taxa. Here, closely related members of a monophyletic group frequently display a gradient of reduction, of all the skeleton or of individual bones, from modest to extreme. It is tempting to envision that such a "morphocline" represents the actual phylogenetic sequence by which size decrease and skeletal reduction occurred, via a series of truncation events at smaller and smaller sizes. This interpretation, however, is not always supported by additional evidence. For example, body size and degree of

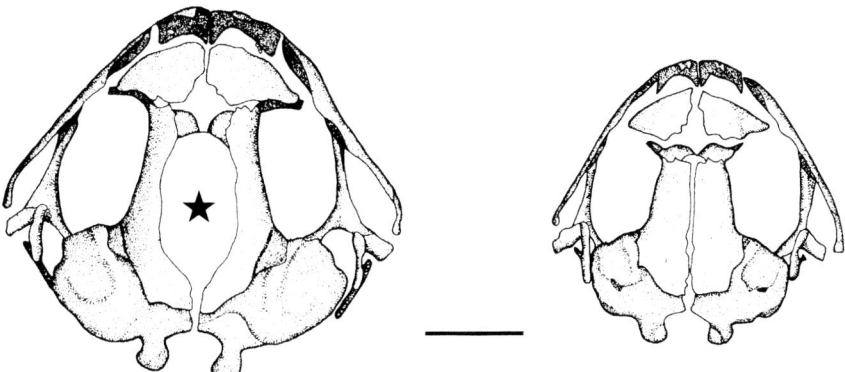

Fig. 4. Adult skulls of the miniaturized Australian frogs of the genus *Uperoleia* (dorsal views). Ossification is more complete in *U. minima* (right) than in the much larger *U. russelli* (left). Note, for example, the extensive frontoparietal fontanelle in *U. russelli* (star); these bones nearly meet in *U. minima*. Reproduced with permission from Tyler *et al.* (1981). Scale bar equals 2 mm.

skeletal reduction may not be well correlated. (If the graded array of reduced morphologies depicts the phylogenetic sequence, reduction should be minimal in the largest species and more pronounced with each successive decrease in adult body size.) Consequently, it often is impossible to resolve whether the existing array of forms represents a single graded phylogenetic sequence, or a series of reduced morphologies that independently evolved from a fully developed ancestral form. Moreover, in the absence of ontogenetic data, it is not even appropriate to accept the hypothesis of pedomorphosis as an explanation of reduced adult ossification, as opposed to secondary reduction (see earlier discussion).

An excellent example is *Uperoleia*, a genus of at least 23 species of tiny frogs endemic to Australia and New Guinea, whose osteology has been extensively studied by Davies and colleagues (Davies, 1989; Davies and Littlejohn, 1986; Davies and McDonald, 1985; Davies *et al.*,, 1986, 1987; Tyler and Davies, 1984; Tyler *et al.*,, 1980, 1981a, b). Adult body size in the genus ranges from 16 mm standard length (snout to vent; SL) in *U. minima* to 35 mm SL in *U. russelli*. The skeleton, especially the skull and vertebrae, is generally reduced relative to that of larger frogs. However, there is extensive interspecific variation in the degree of reduction, ranging from moderate to extreme. This is well illustrated by the frontoparietals, paired bones of the cranial roof (Fig. 4). In some species, the frontoparietals are well developed, abutting or even fusing in the dorsal midline and enclosing at most a small opening, or fontanelle, between them. In other species, they are little more than longitudinal splints of bone confined to the lateral margins of the skull roof and enclosing a broad, gaping fontanelle.

Table 2.
Cranial Variation in Frogs of the Australian Genus *Uperoleia*

Species	Exposure of Frontoparietal Fontanelle	Maxillary Teeth	Degree of Ossification	Size Class
U. variegata	Minimal or none	Absent	Well	Small
U. minima	Minimal or none	Absent	Moderate	Very small
U. rugosa	Minimal or none	Absent	Well	Small
U. aspera	Minimal or none	Absent	Moderate	Moderate
U. martini	Minimal or none	Present	Moderately well	Large
U. fusca	Minimal or none	Present	Well	Moderate
U. lithomoda	Slight	Absent	Moderate	Small
U. micromeles	Slight	Vestigial	Well	Large
U. crassa	Moderate	Absent	Moderate	Large
U. russelli	Extensive	Absent	Well	Large
U. arenicola	Extensive	Absent	Poor	Small
U. borealis	Extensive	Absent	Poor	Moderate
U. talpa	Extensive	Absent	Very poor	Large

Thirteen of the 23 known species are ordered according to relative exposure of the frontoparietal fontanelle in adults, which is a measure of the degree of reduced ossification of these bones. "Degree of ossification" applies to the skull overall. The four size classes encompass the full range of adult body size in these frogs, from the smallest species, *U. minima* (16 mm SL) to the largest, *U. russelli* (35 mm SL).

Data are taken from Davies, 1989; Davies and Littlejohn, 1986; Davies and McDonald, 1985; Davies et al., 1986, 1987; Tyler and Davies, 1984; Tyler et al., 1980, 1981a.

Other species show intermediate configurations. Together, all the species define a nearly continuous gradient in adult frontoparietal morphology (Table 2).

Does the gradient in frontoparietal morphology in *Uperoleia* correspond either with evolutionary decrease in body size or with the phylogenetic sequence of skeletal reduction? In both cases, the answer is no (Table 2). First, adult frontoparietal morphology (or inversely, size of the fontanelle) and body size are poorly correlated. Species showing minimal exposure of the fontanelle include the smallest known species in the genus, *U. minima*, as well as both moderately sized (*U. aspera*) and large species (*U. martini*). Conversely, extensive exposure of the fontanelle is found in small (*U. arenicola*), moderate (*U. borealis*), and large (*U. russelli*) species. Second, based on comparisons to putative sister taxa (*Pseudophryne*) and other outgroups (*Crinia*), in which the frontoparietals are extremely reduced (and the fontanelle correspondingly large), the more extensive development of the frontoparietal in many species of *Uperoleia* represents an *increase* in ossification over the ancestral condition for the genus. In other words, whereas extreme reduction apparently is the ancestral character state of the frontoparietal in *Uperoleia*, many species evince a reversal of this character state toward the more complete ossification characteristic of larger, more typical frogs.

Variable development of the frontoparietal in *Uperoleia* can also be used to test the hypothesis of simple truncation of the ancestral program of bone growth as a mechanism of achieving reduced ossification in adults. If the hypothesis were true, the degree of frontoparietal development should closely correspond with the degree of ossification elsewhere in the skeleton, especially in the skull. If the hypothesis were false, there likely would be little correspondence between the degree of ossification of the frontoparietals and other bones. The latter alternative prevails (Table 2). While in some species (e.g., *U. variegata*) well-developed frontoparietals are associated with a high degree of cranial ossification overall; in other species (e.g., *U. minima*) well-developed frontoparietals are found in skulls that are otherwise only moderately ossified. Similarly, species with extremely reduced frontoparietals include those with very poorly (*U. talpa*), poorly (*U. arenicola*), or well (*U. russelli*)-ossified skulls. In other words, the hypothesis of a simple truncation of the ancestral program of bone growth cannot account for the diversity in adult cranial morphology in *Uperoleia*. At the very least, there has been dissociation of the patterns of growth of individual bones, such that their development has been truncated both independently and to differing degrees.

Thus, in *Uperoleia*, the characteristically reduced ossification in adults is the result of a complex interplay between evolutionary change in body size and patterns of bone growth and morphological and developmental integration. Similar adult skeletal configurations have likely evolved repeatedly and independently, and in at least some instances represent reversals from the otherwise pervasive trend towards skeletal reduction.

Hyperossification

A second characteristic feature of the skeletons of many miniaturized taxa is hyperossification, which is bone growth or some other form of calcification (usually involving cartilage) in excess of that found in the ancestor. In terms of the developmental mechanisms and their effects on the skeleton reviewed earlier, hyperossification may be considered an example of peramorphosis (Alberch *et al.*, 1979; Fig. 2). Obviously, hyperossification stands in stark contrast to the reduced ossification that is otherwise so typical of dwarfed forms. That miniaturization can affect patterns and processes of bone growth and calcification in such a way that it may have opposite effects on the adult skeleton is remarkable. Even more surprising is the observation that hyperossification frequently occurs in groups that also show extensive skeletal reduction (e.g., *Thorius* — Hanken, 1982; *Brachycephalus* — Trueb and Alberch, 1984, 1985; Fig. 5). Extreme reduction involving one portion of the skeleton is commonly associated with excessive ossification of another

92 James Hanken

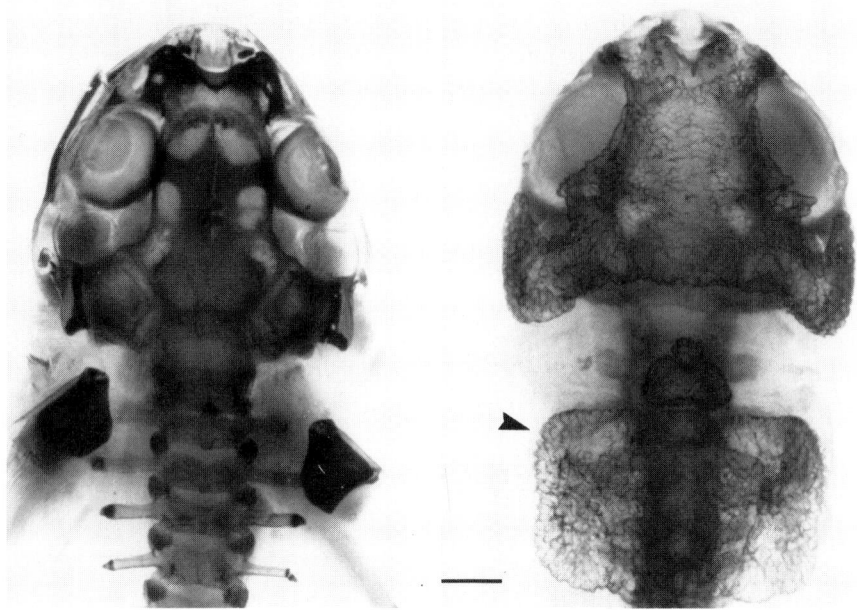

Fig. 5. Adult skulls and anterior vertebrae of two species of dwarf frogs (dorsal views). Left: *Geobatrachus walkeri* (Leptodactylidae; MCZ 20252); right: *Brachycephalus ephippium* (Brachycephalidae; MCZ 15659; pectoral girdle and forelimbs removed). *Brachycephalus* provides an outstanding example of hyperossification. Note, for example, the extensive fusion among cranial bones, which form virtually a single element dorsally; the novel dorsal shield lying above the presacral vertebrae and transverse processes (arrow); and the generally encrusted nature of the bone tissue itself. All of these features are absent in *Geobatrachus*, which displays a more generalized adult osteology for anurans, including abundant cartilage (darker areas). Scale bar equals 1 mm.

portion. Indeed, reduced ossification and hyperossification are often present within the same functional unit, such as the skull. To date, most examples of hyperossification ascribable to miniaturization come from amphibians (Table 1). It is not clear, however, if this reflects a greater liability of a derived pattern of bone growth in this class or if it is simply a consequence of the greater attention paid to this phenomenon (and miniaturization generally) in amphibians in recent years (e.g., Hanken, 1983a, 1984, 1985; Trueb and Alberch, 1985).

A number of explanations have been offered for hyperossification in miniaturized forms. These range from viewing hyperossification as a maladaptive consequence of the physiological mechanisms responsible for size decrease (e.g., "hormonal imbalance associated with dwarfing", Trueb and Alberch [1984]), to a variety of functional or adaptive explanations in which the excessive mineralization is seen to confer some physical or mechanical advantage or benefit (e.g., Forsgaard, 1983; Rieppel, 1984a). Frequently, increased calcification is interpreted as compensating for the mechanical weakening that is presumed to result from decreased body size in general and from reduction in the number and/or size of bones in particular (e.g., Wake, 1986; Lombard and Wake, 1977; Uzzell, 1961.) In such cases, reduced ossification and hyperossification would be functionally linked and part of the same phenomenon of skeletal growth and adaptation.

While mechanical explanations for hyperossification may be plausible in some instances, to my knowledge none has ever been tested by functional analysis, at least not among the groups considered here; they remain speculative. Moreover, alternative and frequently less-obvious explanations for the same phenomenon are rarely considered, even though they may provide, in at least some cases, a more parsimonious and consistent explanation for the data.

An excellent example comes from Mexican salamanders of the genera *Thorius*, *Parvimolge*, and *Lineatriton*. Miniaturization has evolved independently and via different routes in these three taxa, resulting in both convergent and dissimilar morphologies (Wake, 1966; Wake and Elias, 1983). One of the features they share is calcification of mesopodial elements, which typically remain cartilaginous in adults of larger, related taxa (Hanken, 1982; Rabb, 1955; Uzzell, 1961; Wake, 1966; Wake and Elias, 1983). This phenomenon was first analyzed in a meaningful way by Uzzell, who offered a mechanical explanation in proposing that hyperossification "may compensate for the paedomorphic and presumably weak condition of the adult foot of these genera; the absence of calcified mesopodials in other weak-limbed plethodontid genera may reflect different kinds of locomotion in those forms" (1961, p. 83). This was subsequently challenged by Wake (1966), who pointed out that Uzzell's postulated distribution of mechanical forces in the limb did not agree with that inferred from patterns of mesopodial fusion and digital loss. Wake, however, did not offer an alternative explanation for the excess calcification. Later, Hanken (1982) documented that mesopodial calcification, at least in *Thorius*, was actually only one manifestation of a broader pattern of hyperossification involving the entire limb skeleton, which in turn was part of an overall mechanism of skeletal growth regulation that conferred determinate growth in these salamanders. In *Thorius*, onset of limb hyperossification is not strictly associated with a particular body size, as might be expected if it were a primarily mechanical phenomenon. Instead, it coincides with sexual maturity, which occurs at widely different body sizes in different species.

Where does this leave the mechanical explanation for limb hyperossification in the remaining two genera, *Parvimolge* and *Lineatriton*? At present, phylogenetic analyses cannot resolve whether mesopodial calcification in these genera is homologous to that in *Thorius* or if it evolved independently

(Wake and Elias, 1983). Thus, what holds for *Thorius* may not, indeed need not, apply to them. Results from *Thorius*, however, indicate that a mechanical explanation for hyperossification is not the only plausible one. To further underscore the difficulties that may accompany efforts to account for derived patterns of bone growth such as hyperossification, it should be pointed out that hyperossification may have different explanations, even within the same skeleton. Thus, whereas in *Thorius* mechanical factors do not adequately explain mesopodial calcification, they do provide a much more satisfactory and realistic explanation for calcification in the hyolaryngeal skeleton (Lombard and Wake, 1977).

Finally, it is important to remember that, while hyperossification is observed in many miniaturized taxa, it may not in every instance primarily result from phylogenetic decrease in body size. As with reduced ossification, the evolution of hyperossification must be analyzed in a rigorous phylogenetic context in order to distinguish those instances that accompanied body size decrease from those that did not. For example, in the small pipid frog *Pseudhymenochirus merlini*, some examples of cranial hyperossification (coalescence of frontoparietals, fusion of tympanic annulus) cannot be attributed to size decrease, as they also are characteristic of larger, more-primitive species (Cannatella and Trueb, 1988). However, other examples of hyperossification within the same skull (ossification of ceratohyals, prootic-squamosal fusion) are unique to *Pseudhymenochirus* and are therefore more appropriately interpreted as correlates of size decrease.

Increased Variability

The third feature associated with miniaturization is increased intraspecific variability of the adult skeleton. This includes variation among or within individuals in the size, shape, or even presence/absence of individual bones. Increased variability is the most difficult feature to document and, therefore, to defend, as characteristic of dwarfed taxa, simply because of the paucity of studies that assay skeletal variation in natural populations of vertebrates, miniaturized or not. Nevertheless, extensive skeletal variability has been observed in several dwarfed forms (Table 1), providing further insights into how ancestral patterns and processes of bone growth have been affected by size change. Marshall and Corruccini (1978) provide numerous additional examples of increased variability in tooth dimensions accompanying dwarfism in fossil mammals.

The observed variation is basically of two kinds with respect to bone growth. The first variation involves typically late-forming elements, whose development is precociously truncated as part of the common pattern of reduced ossification via pedomorphosis described above. While a common level of development may be attained by many individuals in a species,

Table 3.

Skeletal Variation in Five Species of the Diminutive Mexican
Salamander Genus *Thorius*

Species	Absent	Septomaxilla Present, Small	Present, Large	Right-Left Asymmetry	Distal Carpal 1-2 + Distal Carpal 3 Fused	Right-Left Asymmetry
T. pennatulus	62	3	35	25	51	26
T. macdougalli	97	3	—	5	15	20
T. minutissimus	86	8	6	28	17	28
T. schmidti	89	3	8	11	11	22
T. narisovalis	85	—	15	—	8	5

Values denote frequencies (%) observed in approximately 20 specimens per species,
which are arranged in order of increasing adult body size. Intraspecific variation overall
is much more extensive than that represented by these two characters from the skull
and limb skeleton, respectively. For example, seven different carpal fusion combinations
are each variable in at least one species, and right-left asymmetry of overall carpal or
tarsal pattern ranges as high as 68% in some species.

Data are from Hanken (1982, 1984).

remaining individuals develop to substantially greater or lesser degrees. In
other words, variation in the stage at which the ancestral pattern of bone
growth is truncated leads directly to variation in adult morphology. The
magnitude of variation is larger than in nonminiaturized species, in which
individuals typically complete the ontogenetic sequence, resulting in the
bone(s) in question being fully formed in most individuals. Variation of this
kind is most conspicuous in cases in which truncation of the ancestral
program of skeletal ontogeny leads to the failure of a bone to form in some
but not all individuals. Even when present, the bone may be very poorly
developed (e.g., septomaxilla in *Thorius* — Table 3). If this involves paired
bones, there may even be right-left asymmetry in terms of presence or
absence. In such cases, the mean extent to which the species completes the
ancestral ontogeny can be thought of as lying precisely atop the developmental threshold (*sensu* Falconer, 1981) for the bone in question. Individuals
for which the combination of prevailing genetic and environmental factors
fails to exceed the threshold will lack the bone; those in which the combination exceeds the threshold will have it.

An interesting consequence of this kind of variation for phylogenetic
analysis is seen in speciose taxa. Because the skeleton often is a primary
source of morphological characters for taxonomic and phylogenetic studies,
extensive intraspecific variation may obscure interspecific differences in adult
morphology, even when such differences exist. Consequently, the systematics
of many groups of miniaturized vertebrates has been difficult to resolve

using morphology alone, and researchers often have to resort to nonskeletal features or molecular techniques to discern phylogenetic relationships (e.g., *Thorius* — Hanken, 1983b, 1984).

The second kind of variation involves features that form early in development and whose variability reflects a fundamental alteration of skeletal patterning. Hence, unlike the first kind of variation, it cannot be readily linked to alterations in the patterns or processes of bone growth at later stages. One example is the extensive variability in mesopodial arrangement and phalangeal number in *Thorius* (Hanken, 1982, 1985; Table 3). The primary reason for excluding bone growth as a factor in accounting for this variation is very simply that mesopodial and phalangeal patterns are established during early stages of chondrogenesis, well before bone has formed. Moreover, there is no evidence that the observed skeletal patterns change once ossification begins (Hanken, unpublished data). This does not mean, however, that the variation is unrelated to evolutionary change in body size. Indeed, smaller body size, acting through decreased cell number or absolute size of limb primordia during embryonic development, may well underlie many of the documented evolutionary changes in skeletal patterning (Alberch and Gale, 1983, 1985; Hanken, 1985; Wake and Larson, 1987). Alternatively, increased skeletal variability in dwarfed taxa may simply reflect relaxed selection pressures on the morphology of certain structures when built at a much smaller size (Gould, 1977; Hanken, 1984). In other words, excessive variation may follow as a by-product of size decrease and have nothing directly to do with the particular developmental mechanism by which miniaturization is achieved.

Morphological Novelty

The final feature prevalent in the skeletons of miniaturized vertebrates is morphological novelty. Novel morphologies are observed in virtually all regions of the skeleton, although the skull, distal portions of the limbs, and the limb girdles are affected most frequently (Table 1). There are three categories of novelties that differ in the extent to which the novel features can be regarded as specific adaptations that permit or allow size decrease.

The first category includes novel skeletal arrangements that represent virtually inevitable consequences of adult body size decrease. Unlike features that apparently solve problems posed by body size reduction (see below), these novel arrangements seem to represent little more than side effects of miniaturization. Such changes frequently occur, for example, when conservative allometric growth relations are extrapolated to tiny adult body sizes, resulting in substantial change in the relative proportions among skeletal and nonskeletal components. In such cases, a novel shape or disposition of a cartilage or bone may simply represent a mechanical consequence of the altered physical positioning of these components brought on by the change in relative sizes — a packaging effect. While novelties of this kind may appropriately be viewed as by-products of changes primarily affecting other tissues, they nevertheless often entail a substantial and fundamental change in structure and/or function. In this way, they may represent an important source of morphological variation for subsequent adaptation and diversification (Hanken, 1985).

In salamanders of the genus *Thorius*, for example, extrapolation of the negatively allometric relationship between brain, eye, and inner ear size relative to body size (a characteristic of vertebrates generally) to their tiny adult head size has resulted in predominance of these organs and a substantial shift in their relative positions (Hanken, 1983a). This, in turn, has effected a dramatic change in braincase shape and a reorientation of the jaw suspension in the tiny skull, which barely exceeds 3 mm in total length in some species. If such changes in cranial morphology are a consequence of size decrease acting in concert with evolutionarily conservative allometric growth patterns, then similar scaling effects dictated by the brain and sense organs should accompany cranial miniaturization in other groups. Indeed, this is the case, in groups as divergent as Recent amphibians (Carroll and Holmes, 1980; Milner, 1988) and squamate reptiles (Carroll, 1969, 1970; Rieppel, 1981, 1984c). Interestingly, while morphological novelty is observed in each of these cases, the particular novel structure or arrangement often differs, reflecting fundamental differences in the "initial conditions" of cranial structure among these groups before miniaturization.

The second category of morphological novelty comprises changes in the skeleton that may be interpreted as specific adaptations that permit size decrease: in other words, structures that maintain or confer skeletal function at reduced body size. In some cases this involves little more than enhanced deposition of bone, which may compensate for the mechanical weakening that presumably follows as a result of the reduction or even loss of other portions of the skeleton (see above section on reduced ossification). In the miniaturized caecilian *Idiocranium russeli*, for example, extensive ossification of the mesethmoid region of the skull may compensate for reduction of other cranial bones, and thereby maintain rigidity and strength necessary for use of the head in burrowing by this fossorial species (Wake, 1986).

In other instances, the anatomical changes are more extensive, involving functional systems that comprise both skeletal and nonskeletal components. For example, novel configurations of the braincase (closure) and upper temporal arcade (reduction or loss) have evolved repeatedly in the skulls of miniaturized fossorial lizards (Rieppel, 1981, 1984a, b, c; Table 1). In the extremely derived skull of *Dibamus novaeguineae*, there is in addition a novel dorsal enlargement of the coronoid process on the lower jaw (Fig. 6). These

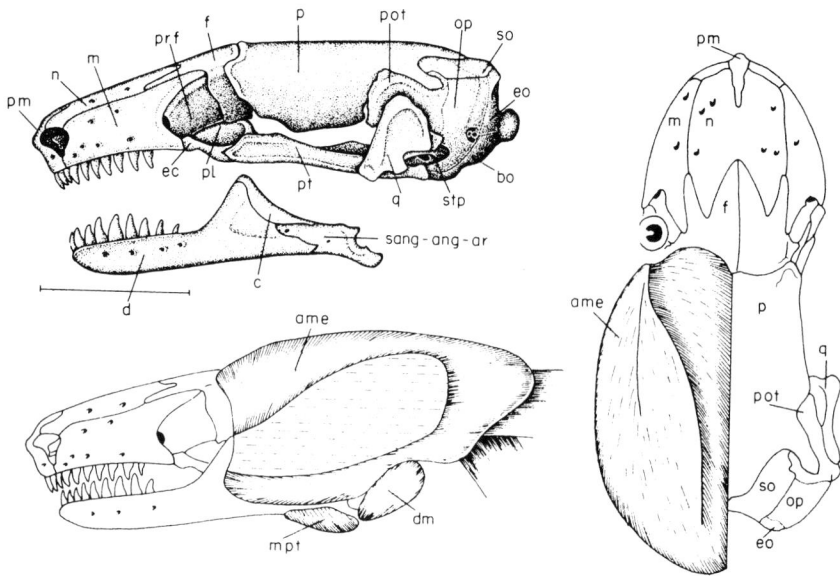

Fig. 6. Skull and superficial jaw adductor musculature of the miniaturized, fossorial lizard, *Dibamus novaeguineae* (Dibamidae) in lateral (left) and dorsal (right) views. Novel features include a closed lateral braincase wall formed by a descending process of the parietal (p) and an anterior process of the prootic (pot); absence of the postorbitofrontal and squamosal, i.e., the upper temporal arcade; and a dorsally expanded coronoid process (c) on the lower jaw. Additional abbreviations: ame, m. adductor mandibulae externus; ang, angular; ar, articular; bo, basioccipital; d, dentary; dm, depressor mandibulae; ec, ectopterygoid; eo, exoccipital; f, frontal; m, maxilla; mpt, m. pterygoideus; n, nasal; op, opisthotic; pl, palatine; pm, premaxilla; prf, prefrontal; pt, pterygoid; q, quadrate; sang, surangular; so, supraoccipital; stp, stapes. Reproduced with permission from Rieppel (1984c). Scale bar equals 2 mm.

changes are associated with — and, indeed, permit — posterodorsal expansion of the jaw adductor musculature that maintains an effective fiber length, which is important in assuring an adequate gape and enhancing mechanical advantage for feeding. Without these modifications, it is unlikely that miniaturization could have proceeded to the tiny adult skull sizes attained in some genera. Interestingly, however, not all small lizards show these modifications — only those that are also fossorial. Thus, evolutionary and developmental responses by the skeleton to size decrease have been mediated by skull function as well as habitus and life history.

The third category of morphological novelty contains a series of functionally diverse, unique specializations that are the most difficult to explain in the context of miniaturization. Unlike the examples discussed above, they are not readily interpreted either as primary, functionally mandated changes that facilitate or permit size decrease or as incidental, yet sometimes inevitable, consequences of miniaturization. Instead, if their evolution is causally linked to size decrease, it most likely is a result of their relation to other features of the organism that are more directly affected by size change, such as reproductive mode or clutch size (Miller, 1979). A bizarre yet wonderful example is the priaprium, or subcephalic copulatory organ, of male fishes in the teleost family Phallostethidae (Parenti, 1984, 1986c; Roberts, 1971). Males use this structure to hold onto the female during head-to-head courtship, which leads to internal fertilization of her eggs. The skeletal morphology of the priaprium, which is unique to these tiny fishes among all teleosts, is so odd that resolving homologies between it and skeletal structures in other fishes — indeed, whether it is homologous to skeletal structures in other fishes — has been a vexing problem since it was first described more than 75 years ago (Parenti, 1986b). In fact, this question was only adequately resolved recently following careful comparative and ontogenetic analyses by Parenti (1986b), who demonstrated that the priaprium is derived from pelvic fin structures, particularly the rays and girdle.

Each of these examples of morphological novelty involves modification of the ancestral patterns of bone growth. In some instances, the modifications may represent little more than a labile morphogenetic response of osteogenic tissues to changes primarily involving adjacent, nonskeletal tissues, especially nervous and sensory components and musculature, which are known to exert a predominant influence on skeletal pattern formation and growth generally (reviewed by Hanken, 1983a; Moss, 1968, 1972). Such an explanation likely applies to novel arrangements that seemingly are incidental consequences of size decrease (first category, above) as well as those that primarily comprise increased mineralization in areas of high mechanical stress (e.g., the hyolaryngeal skeleton of small bolitoglossine salamanders [Lombard and Wake, 1977]). Other instances, however, such as the novel configuration of the braincase in miniaturized burrowing reptiles (Rieppel, 1981, 1984a, b, c) and the priaprium of phallostethid fishes (Parenti, 1984, 1986c; Roberts, 1971), are not readily explained by this model. Instead, they likely denote a more fundamental alteration to the developmental processes underlying skeletal pattern formation and growth. Thus, just as the novel skeletal configurations in miniaturized vertebrates are diverse, so too are the ways in which bone growth has been modified to effect these evolutionary changes. Together, these examples document the significant potential for evolutionary change that resides within general patterns and processes of bone growth and which can be evoked with relatively little perturbation.

Concluding Remarks

Four distinct features of skeletal morphology are associated with miniaturization of adult body size in vertebrates: reduced ossification, hyperossification, increased variability, and morphological novelty. None of these features is an inevitable consequence of size decrease, nor is size reduction a prerequisite for the evolutionary appearance of any one of them. Nevertheless, the high frequency with which dwarfed taxa display them (Table 1) is evidence of the significant effect that miniaturization may have on skeletal development, and especially bone growth. It is thus surprising how frequently body size *per se* is ignored in considerations of the derived features of the skeleton in dwarfed forms. One likely explanation is the frequent difficulty of evaluating a specific instance of reduced ossification, morphological novelty, etc., in the context of size decrease vs. plausible alternatives such as retention of an ancestral trait.

The adult skeleton of dwarfed forms is the product of both phylogenetic and ontogenetic constraints and functional modification mediated by natural selection (Hanken, 1983a, 1984; Trueb and Alberch, 1985). The main difficulty, of course, is to partition the effects of these often-conflicting influences. This can be especially difficult when the consequences of small size for the skeleton are not especially important in terms of natural selection, whose primary target may lie elsewhere. As the evolutionary changes that accompany size decrease are mediated in large part by patterns and processes of bone growth, greater knowledge of these phenomena likely will aid our understanding of how miniaturization itself is achieved.

Acknowledgments

Patricia van Buskirk, University of Colorado, and Linda Trueb, The University of Kansas, provided specimens used to prepare Figs. 3 and 5, respectively. Margaret Davies and Olivier Rieppel generously granted permission to reproduce their published illustrations.

References

Alberch, P. and Gale, E. A. (1983). Size dependence during the development of the amphibian foot. Colchicine-induced digital loss and reduction. *J. Embryol. Exp. Morphol.*, **76**: 177–197.

Alberch, P. and Gale, E. A. (1985). A developmental analysis of an evolutionary trend: digital reduction in amphibians. *Evolution*, **39**: 8–23.

Alberch, P., Gould, S. J., Oster, G. F., and Wake, D. B. (1979). Size and shape in ontogeny and phylogeny. *Paleobiology*, **5**: 296–317.

Azzarello, M. Y. (1989). The pterygoid series in *Hippocampus zosterae* and *Syngnathus scovelli* (Pisces: Syngnathidae). *Copeia*, **1989**: 621–628.

Bertram, J. E. A. (1989). Size transitions in terrestrial mammals: the interesting case of dwarf elephants. *Am. Zool.*, **29**: 182A.

Biewener, A. A. (1982). Bone strength in small mammals and bipedal birds: do safety factors change with body size? *J. Exp. Biol.*, **98**: 289–301.

Biewener, A. A. (1989a). Mammalian terrestrial locomotion and size. BioScience, **39**: 776–783.

Biewener, A. A. (1989b). Scaling body support in mammals: limb posture and muscle mechanics. *Science*, **245**: 45–48.

Bolt, J. R. (1977). Dissorophoid relationships and ontogeny, and the origin of the Lissamphibia. *J. Paleontol.*, **51**: 235–249.

Bolt, J. R. (1979). *Amphibamus grandiceps* as a juvenile dissorophid: evidence and implications. In: *Mazon Creek Fossils*. Nitecki, M. H., Ed., Academic Press, New York, 529–563.

Cannatella, D. C., and Trueb, L. (1988). Evolution of pipoid frogs: morphology and phylogenetic relationships of *Pseudhymenochirus*. *J. Herpetol.*, **22**: 439–456.

Carroll, R. L. (1969). Problems of the origin of reptiles. *Biol. Rev.*, **44**: 393–432.

Carroll, R. L. (1970). Quantitative aspects of the amphibian-reptilian transition. *Forma Functio*, **3**: 165–178.

Carroll, R. L. (1977). The origin of lizards. In: *Problems in Vertebrate Evolution*, Linnean Society Symposium Series, No. 4. Andres, S. M., Miles, R. S., and Walker, A. D., Eds., Academic Press, New York, 359–396.

Carroll, R. L. and Holmes, R. (1980). The skull and jaw musculature as guides to the ancestry of salamanders. *Zool. J. Linn. Soc.*, **68**: 1–40.

Cope, E. D. (1885). On the evolution of the vertebrates. *Am. Nat.* **19**: 140–148, 234–247, 341–353.

Davies, M. (1989). Ontogeny of bone and the role of heterochrony in the myobatrachine genera *Uperoleia, Crinia,* and *Pseudophryne* (Anura: Leptodactylidae: Myobatrachinae). *J. Morphol.*, **200**: 269–300.

Davies, M. and Littlejohn, M. J. (1986). Frogs of the genus *Uperoleia* Gray (Anura: Leptodactylidae) in south-eastern Australia. *Trans. R. Soc. S. Aust.*, **109**: 111–143.

Davies, M. and McDonald, K. R. (1985). A redefinition of *Uperoleia rugosa* (Andersson) (Anura: Leptodactylidae). *Trans. R. Soc. S. Aust.*, **109**: 37–42.

Davies, M., McDonald, K. R., and Corben, C. (1986). The genus *Uperoleia* Gray (Anura: Leptodactylidae) in Queensland, Australia. *Proc. R. Soc. Vict.*, **98**: 147–188.

Davies, M., Watson, G. F., and Miller, A. (1987). New records of *Uperoleia* (Anura: Leptodactylidae) from Western Australia with supplementary osteological data on *Uperoleia micromeles*. *Trans. Roy. Soc. South Aust.*, **111**: 201–202.

Falconer, D. S. (1981). Introduction to Quantitative Genetics, 2nd ed., Longman Group, London.

Fernandez, J. M. and Weitzman, S. H. (1987). A new species of *Nannostomus* (Teleostei: Lebiasinidae) from near Puerto Ayacucho, Rio Orinoco drainage, Venezuela. *Proc. Biol. Soc. Wash.*, **100**: 164–172.

Fink, W. L. (1981). Ontogeny and phylogeny of tooth attachment modes in actinopterygian fishes. *J. Morphol.*, **167**: 167–184.

Fink, W. L. (1982). The conceptual relationships between ontogeny and phylogeny. *Paleobiology*, **8**: 254–264.

Forsgaard, K. (1983). The axial skeleton of *Chamaelinorops*. In: *Advances in Herpetology and Evolutionary Biology*. Rhodin, A. G. J. and Miyata, K., Eds., Museum of Comparative Zoology, Cambridge, 284–295.

Gould, S. J. (1971). Geometric scaling in allometric growth: a contribution to the problem of scaling in the evolution of size. *Am. Nat.*, **105**: 113–136.

Gould, S. J. (1977). *Ontogeny and Phylogeny.* Harvard University Press, Cambridge.

Grandison, A. G. (1981). Morphology and phylogenetic position of the West African *Didynamipus sjoestedti* Anderson, 1903 (Anura, Bufonidae). *Ital. J. Zool.*, **40**: 187–215.

Griffiths, I. (1959). The phylogeny of *Sminthillus limbatus* and the status of the Brachycephalidae (Amphibia: Salientia). *Proc. Zool. Soc. London*, **132**: 457–491.

Hanken, J. (1982). Appendicular skeletal morphology in minute salamanders, genus *Thorius* (Amphibia: Plethodontidae): growth regulation, adult size determination, and natural variation. *J. Morphol.*, **174**: 57–77.

Hanken, J. (1983a). Miniaturization and its effects on cranial morphology in plethodontid salamanders, genus *Thorius* (Amphibia, Plethodontidae). II. The fate of the brain and sense organs and their role in skull morphogenesis and evolution. *J. Morphol.*, **177**: 255–268.

Hanken, J. (1983b). Genetic variation in a dwarfed lineage, the Mexican salamander genus *Thorius* (Amphibia: Plethodontidae): taxonomic, ecologic, and evolutionary implications. *Copeia*, **1983**: 1051–1073.

Hanken, J. (1984). Miniaturization and its effects on cranial morphology in plethodontid salamanders, genus *Thorius* (Amphibia: Plethodontidae). I. Osteological variation. *.Biol. J. Linn. Soc.*, **23**: 55–75.

Hanken, J. (1985). Morphological novelty in the limb skeleton accompanies miniaturization in salamanders. *Science*, **229**: 871–874.

Lombard, R. E. and Wake, D. B. (1977). Tongue evolution in the lungless salamanders, family Plethodontidae. II. Function and evolutionary diversity. *J. Morphol.*, **153**: 39–80.

Lynch, J. D. (1986). New species of minute leptodactylid frogs from the Andes of Ecuador and Peru. *J. Herpetol.*, **20**: 423–431.

Lynch, J. D. and Ruiz-Carranza, P. M. (1982). A new genus and species of poison-dart frog (Amphibia: Dendrobatidae) from the Andes of northern Colombia. *Proc. Biol. Soc. Wash.*, **95**: 557–562.

Marshall, L. G. and Corruccini, R. S. (1978). Variability, evolutionary rates, and allometry in dwarfing lineages. *Paleobiology*, **4**: 101–119.

Miller, P. J. (1979). Adaptiveness and implications of small size in teleosts. *Symp. Zool. Soc. London*, **44**: 263–306.

Milner, A. R. (1988). The relationships and origin of living amphibians. In: *The Phylogeny and Classification of the Tetrapods*, Vol. 1, Benton, M. J., Ed., Systematics Association Special Volume, No. 35A. Clarendon Press, Oxford, 59–102.

Moss, M. L. (1968). A theoretical analysis of the functional matrix. *Acta Biotheor.*, **18**: 195–203.

Moss, M. L. (1972). The regulation of skeletal growth. In: *Regulation of Organ and Tissue Growth*. Goss, R., Ed., Academic Press, New York, 127–142.

Parenti, L. R. (1984). On the relationships of phallostethid fishes (Atherinomorpha), with notes on the anatomy of *Phallostethus dunckeri* Regan, 1913. *Am. Mus. Nov.*, No. **2779**: 1–12.

Parenti, L. R. (1986a). The phylogenetic significance of bone types in euteleost fishes. *Zool. J. Linn. Soc.*, **87**: 37–51.

Parenti, L. R. (1986b). Homology of pelvic fin structures in female phallostethid fishes (Atherinomorpha, Phallostethidae). *Copeia*, **1986**: 305–310.

Parenti, L. R. (1986c). Bilateral asymmetry in phallostethid fishes (Atherinomorpha) with description of a new species from sarawak. *Aoc. Calif. Acad. Sci.*, **44**: 225–236.

Parenti, L. R. (1986c). Bilateral asymmetry in phallostethid fishes (Atherinomorpha) with description of a new species from Sarawak. *Proc. Calif. Acad. Sci.*, **44**: 225–236.

Pregill, G. (1986). Body size of insular lizards: a pattern of Holocene dwarfism. *Evolution*, **40**: 997–1008.

Rabb, G. B. (1955). A new salamander of the genus *Parvimolge* from Mexico. *Breviora*, **42**: 1–9.

Rieppel, O. (1981). The skull and the jaw adductor musculature in some burrowing scincomorph lizards of the genera *Acontias*, *Typhlosaurus* and *Feylinia*. *J. Zool.*, **195**: 493–528.

Rieppel, O. (1982). The phylogenetic relationships of the genus *Acontophiops* Sternfeld (Sauria: Scincidae), with a note on mosaic evolution. *Ann. Transvaal Mus.*, **33**: 241–257.

Rieppel, O. (1984a). The upper temporal arcade of lizards: an ontogenetic problem. *Rev. Suisse Zool.*, **91**: 475–482.

Rieppel, O. (1984b). The cranial morphology of the fossorial lizard genus *Dibamus* with a consideration of its phylogenetic relationships. *J. Zool.*, **204**: 289–327.

Rieppel, O. (1984c). Miniaturization of the lizard skull: its functional and evolutionary implications. *Symp. Zool. Soc. London*, **52**: 503–520.

Rieppel, O. (1988). A review of the origin of snakes. In: *Evolutionary Biology*, Vol. 22, Hecht, M. K., Wallace, B., and Prance, G. T., Eds., Plenum Press, New York, 37–130.

Roberts, T. R. (1971). Osteology of the Malaysian phallostethid fish (*Ceratostethus bicornis*), with a discussion of the evolution of remarkable structural novelties in its jaws and external genitalia. *Bull. Mus. Comp. Zool.*, **142**: 393–418.

Roberts, T. R. (1981). Sundasalangidae, a new family of minute freshwater salmoniform fishes from southeast Asia. *Proc. Calif. Acad. Sci.*, **42:** 295–302.

Roberts, T. R. (1986). *Danionella translucida*, a new genus and species of cyprinid fish from Burma, one of the smallest living vertebrates. *Env. Biol. Fishes*, **16**: 231–241.

Roth, G., Rottluff, B., Grunwald, W., Hanken, J., and Linke, R. (1990). Miniaturization in plethodontid salamanders (Caudata: Plethodontidae) and its consequences for the brain and visual system. *Biol. J. Linn. Soc.* **40**: 165–190.

Roth, G., Rottluff, B., and Linke, R. (1988). Miniaturization, genome size and the origin of functional constraints in the visual system of salamanders. *Naturwissenschaften*, **75**: 297–304.

Schmidt-Nielsen, K. (1984). *Scaling: Why is Animal Size so Important?* Cambridge University Press, Cambridge.

Springer, V. G. (1983). *Tyson belos*, new genus and species of western Pacific fish (Gobiidae, Xenisthminae), with discussions of gobioid osteology and classification. *Smithsonian Contrib. Zool.*, no. **390**: 1–40.

Stanley, S. M. (1973). An explanation for Cope's rule. *Evolution*, **27**: 1–26.

Stebbins, R. C. (1966). *A Field Guide to Western Reptiles and Amphibians*. Houghton Mifflin, Boston.

Stephenson, N. G. (1965). Heterochronous changes among Australian leptodactylid frogs. *Proc. Zool. Soc. London*, **144**: 339–350.

Trueb, L. and Alberch, P. (1984). Hyperossification in dwarf frogs of the family Brachycephalidae. *Am. Zool.*, **24**: 64A.

Trueb, L. and Alberch, P. (1985). Miniaturization and the anuran skull: a case study of heterochrony. In: *Functional Morphology of Vertebrates*. Duncker, H. R. and Fleischer, G., Eds., Gustav Fisher Verlag, Stuttgart, 113–121.

Tyler, M. J. and Davies, M. (1984). *Uperoleia* Gray (Anura: Leptodactylidae) in New Guinea. *Trans. R. Soc. S. Aust.*, **108**: 123–125.

Tyler, M. J., Davies, M., and Martin, A. A. (1980). Australian frogs of the leptodactylid genus *Uperoleia* Gray. *Aust. J. Zool. Suppl. Ser.*, no. **79**: 1–64.

Tyler, M. J., Davies, M., and Martin, A. A., (1981a). New and rediscovered species of frogs from the Derby-Broome area of Western Australia. *Rec. West. Aust. Mus.*, **9**: 147–172.

Tyler, M. J., Davies, M., and Martin, A. A. (1981b). Frog fauna of the northern territory: new distributional records and the description of a new species. *Trans. R. Soc. South Aust.*, **105**: 149–154.

Uzzell, T. M. J. (1961). Calcified hyoid and mesopodial elements of plethodontid salamanders. *Copeia*, **1961**: 78–86.

Villalobos, M., Leon, P., Sessions, S. K., and Kezer, J. (1988). Enucleated erythrocytes in plethodontid salamanders. *Herpetologica*, **44**: 243–250.

Wake, D. B. (1966). Comparative osteology and evolution of the lungless salamanders, family Plethodontidae. *Mem. South. Calif. Acad. Sci.*, **4**: 1–111.

Wake, D. B. and Elias, P. (1983). New genera and a new species of Central American sala-
    manders, with a review of the tropical genera (Amphibia, Plethodontidae). *Contrib. Sci.
    Los Angeles Co. Mus.*, **345**: 1–19.
Wake, D. B. and Larson, A. (1987). Multidimensional analysis of an evolving lineage. *Science*,
    238: 42–48.
Wake, D. B. and Lynch, J. F. (1976). The distribution, ecology, and evolutionary history of
    plethodontid salamanders in tropical America. *Nat. Hist. Mus. Los Angeles Co. Sci. Bull.* **25**:
    1–65.
Wake, M. H. (1986). The morphology of *Idiocranium russeli* (Amphibia: Gymnophiona), with
    comments on miniaturization through heterochrony. *J. Morphol.*, **189**: 1–16.
Watson, W., Stevens, E. G., and Matarese, A. C. (1984). Schindlerioidei: development and
    relationships. In: *Ontogeny and Systematics of Fishes*. Moser, H. G., Ed., Allen Press, Law-
    rence, KS, 552–554.
Weitzman, M. (1985). *Hyphessobrycon elachys*, a new miniature characid from eastern Paraguay
    (Pisces: Characiforms). *Proc. Biol. Soc. Wash.*, **98**: 799–808.
Weitzman, S. H. (1986). A new species of *Elachocharax* (Teleostei: Characidae) from the Rio
    Negro region of Venezuela and Brazil. *Proc. Biol. Soc. Wash.*, **99**: 739–747.
Weitzman, S. H. (1987). A new species of *Xenurobrycon* (Teleostei: Characidae) from the Rio
    Mamore basin of Bolivia. *Proc. Biol. Soc. Wash.*, **100**: 112–120.
Weitzman, S. H. and Fink, S. V. (1985). Xenurobryconin phylogeny and putative pheromone
    pumps in glandulocaudine fishes (Teleostei: Characidae). *Smithson. Contrib. Zool.*, no. **421**:
    1–121.
Weitzman, S. H. and Fink, S. V. (1983). Relationships of the neon tetras, a group of South
    American freshwater fishes (Teleostei, Characidae) with comments on the phylogeny of
    the New World characiforms. *Bull. Mus. Comp. Zool. Harvard Univ.*, **150**: 339–365.
Weitzman, S. H. and Vari, R. P. (1987). Two new species and a new genus of miniature
    characid fishes (Teleostei: Characiformes) from northern South America. *Proc. Biol. Soc.
    Wash.*, **100**: 640–652.
Weitzman, S. H. and Vari, R. P. (1988). Miniaturization in South American freshwater fishes;
    an overview and discussion. *Proc. Biol. Soc. Wash.*, **101**: 444–465.
Wiens, J. J. (1989). Ontogeny of the skeleton of *Spea bombifrons* (Anura: Pelobatidae). *J. Morphol.*,
    202: 29–51.

5

Domestication and Bone Growth

R. K. WAYNE
Department of Biology
University of California at Los Angeles
Los Angeles, California

AND

C. B. RUFF
Department of Cell Biology and Anatomy
The Johns Hopkins School of Medicine
Baltimore, Maryland

Introduction

Many domestic mammals have changed dramatically in morphology and behavior relative to their wild progenitors (see Zeuner, 1963; Epstein, 1971; Clutton-Brock, 1987). Such changes led Darwin (1859) to use artificial selection as a metaphor to explain long-term changes among discrete species. Darwin emphasized the analogy between artificial and natural selection and the potential for either, given the appropriate time period, to completely remodel the phenotype of an organism. However, this view of selection as omnipotent has recently been challenged (Gould and Lewontin, 1978; Lauder, 1981; Gould and Vrba, 1982; Albrech, 1982, 1985; Kauffmann, 1983). Morphologic change in nature often follows regular rules that are an expression of the underlying complexity of genetic and developmental systems. Selection for larger or smaller individuals may cause a change in body size that often carries with it coordinated changes in the proportions of body structures. For instance, simple decreases in growth rates will often produce adults of smaller size which have juvenile proportions (neoteny). Such morphologic characteristics may not reflect selection for juvenile characteristics as much as selection for small size. Therefore, the study of domestic animals may provide insights into both the potential of selection and the associated developmental constraints on morphologic change.

In this chapter, we outline a quantitative approach to the study of morphologic change in bone length and width. We exemplify the approach using data from the domestic dog, but the methods can be applied to any domestic mammal. Morphologic variability within the domestic dog is interpreted within a developmental context. We also examine the potential causes of morphologic change in domestic mammals including the effect of selection, developmental constraints, and varying levels of exercise and nutrition on morphology.

Methodology

Measurements

Twenty-one measurements were made on the cranium and dentition of museum specimens from 202 domestic dogs and 3 to 10 individuals from each of 27 wild canid species (Fig. 1, top; Wayne, 1986a). Sixteen measurements were also made on the limb bones of museum specimens from 118 domestic dogs and 1 to 21 individuals from each of 27 wild canid species (Fig. 1, bottom; Wayne, 1986b). These measurements were chosen to reflect differences in length and width of anatomical structures and also to reflect differences in diet and locomotion (Hildebrand, 1954, 1974; Crusafont-Pairo

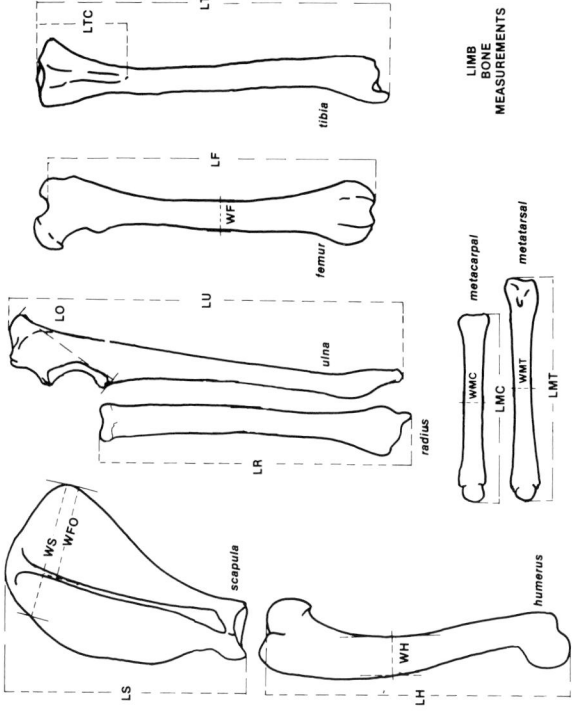

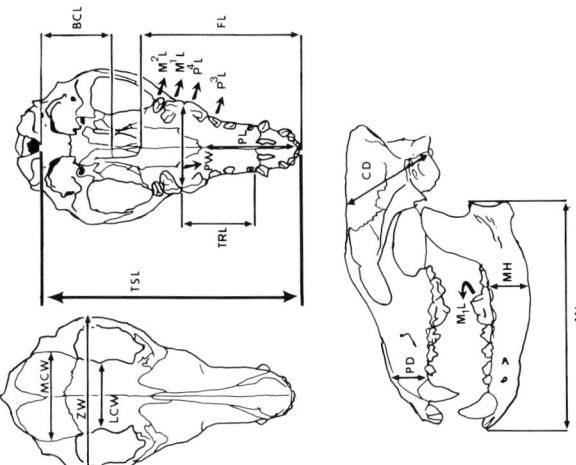

Fig. 1. Diagram of 21 cranial and dental measurements (left) and 16 limb bone measurements (right) made on domestic dogs and wild canids. Mandible width is not figured and is defined as medial-lateral width at posterior end of P⁴. All dental measurements are maximum lengths and widths of teeth. Abbreviations: Left — total skull length (TSL), face length (FL), palatal length (PL), basicranial length (BCL), upper premolar tooth row length (TRL), mandible length (ML), palatal width (PW), maximum cranial width (MCW), zygomatic width (ZW), least cranial width (LCW), cranial depth (CD), premaxilla depth (PD), mandible width (MW), mandible height (MH), P³ length (P³L), P⁴ length (P⁴L), M¹ length (M¹L), M² length (M²L), M¹ width (M¹W), M² width (M²W), M₁ length (M₁L). Right — femur length (LF), metacarpal length (LMT), radius length (LR), ulna length (LU), humerus length (LH), metatarsal length (LMT), olecranon length (LO), tibia crest length (LTC), tibia length (LT), metacarpal width (WMC), humerus width (WH), femur width (WF), metatarsal width (WMT), femoral end width (WFE), scapula length (LS), scapula width (WS), width infraspinous fossa (WFO).

and Truyols-Santonja, 1956; Taylor, 1970; Gonyea, 1976; Radinsky, 1981a, b; Van Valkenburgh, 1985, 1989). Although the precise homologous anatomical landmarks may not be present for some measurements on other domestic species, a set of analogous measurements can be constructed for any domestic mammal.

A subset of these measurements was also taken from monthly or bimonthly radiographs of a growing puppy from the Lhasa Apso, Cocker Spaniel, Labrador Retriever, and the Great Dane. Radiographs were taken from age 3 weeks to 10 months of age. These breeds were chosen because they span a wide range of body size and conformation.

Allometric Analysis

Anatomical structures often change in a regular fashion with a change in overall size (Huxley, 1932; Gould, 1966). This change can be expressed as the ratio of two dimensions, for instance, width vs. length. If the ratio remains the same over a wide range of sizes (e.g., the effect of photographic enlargement), such change is considered isometric; otherwise the change is allometric. The relation between two variables may be expressed simply as $y = a + bx$ where x and y are base ten or natural logarithms of two variables and a is the y-intercept and b is the slope of the regression line. If the slope of the regression line is one, the change is isometric. The slope will be less than one if the y-axis variable decreases in relative size with an increase in size of the x variable (negative allometry) and more than one if the reverse situation exists (positive allometry). The study of the bivariate or allometric scaling of two variables has been undertaken in a wide diversity of taxa and for a great variety of measurements (Huxley, 1932; Gould, 1966; Cock, 1966). Results of these studies suggest that many measurements have a relatively fixed relationship to each other and to body size. Such invariant allometric relationships have led to the development of biomechanical models relating form to function (e.g., Brody, 1945; Klieber, 1961; Taylor, 1970; Schmidt-Knielsen, 1984).

In this study, our principal interest concerns the pattern of allometric scaling in the dentition, cranium, mandible, and limb skeleton. We compare allometric scaling in the domestic dog to that observed among a similar body size array of wild canids. In this way, we hope to identify allometric scaling patterns that are unique to the domestic dog. We also examine scaling among differently aged juvenile dogs of several breeds in hopes of understanding the relationship of developmental alterations to morphologic variability among adults.

In an allometric analysis, change in each variable must be viewed relative to another variable. In many studies, body mass is used as the constant reference variable because many features are expected to scale as a function of body mass due to metabolic considerations (Brody, 1945; Klieber, 1961;

Schmidt-Knielsen, 1984). We have chosen total skull length (Fig. 1, top) as our index variable for cranial and dental measurements because differences in the scaling of measurements are readily interpreted as changes in the skull outline and because differences in the scaling of the dentition and cranium may reflect dietary differences when viewed relative to skull length (Radinsky, 1981a, b; Jaslow, 1987; Van Valkenburgh and Ruff, 1987; Van Valkenburgh, 1989). Similarly, we have chosen femur length for our index variable for the limb skeleton analysis because differences in locomotion appear as scaling differences when femur length is used as the standard of comparison (e.g., McMahon, 1975). However, as seen in Fig. 2, both total skull length and femur length are well correlated with body weight. The slope of total skull length vs. body size is 0.32 which is near the isometric expectation of 0.33 for linear dimensions vs. body mass estimates. The slope of femur length vs. body mass is 0.43 which indicates positive allometry. Therefore, allometric patterns of limb measurements to femur length as presented in this paper should not be taken as representative of the relationship of linear measurements to body mass. Least-squares regression was used to calculate allometric coefficients (a and b of the equation $y = a + bx$ where $x =$ base ten logarithm of the index variable and $y =$ base ten logarithm of the dependent variable, $a =$ y-intercept, $b =$ slope). Other regression techniques such as reduced major axes (Ricker, 1973) can also be used but the results are very similar so long as the correlation among variables is high (see discussion in Siem and Saether, 1983; Smith, 1984). We chose least-squares regression because correlation coefficients among variables are high and because statistical analyses of slope and intercept differences are well defined (Zar, 1983).

Specific growth rates were calculated from data on developing dogs from four breeds. The specific growth rate (SGR) is estimated as $SGR = [\ln(s_2) - \ln(s_1)]/(t_2 - t_1)$ where s_1 and s_2 are the sizes of the same measurement at age t_1 and t_2 (Brody, 1945; Laird, 1965). The units for SGR are expressed as a rate per unit size (cm/d/cm) or by letting the size units cancel out as a fractional increase per day (day^{-1}). Two properties of SGR make it a desirable measure of growth. First, because SGR is the proportional increment of growth with an increase in age, animals of different sizes can be compared on an equivalent basis. Second, because the ratio of SGR of two measurements at any point in time equals their allometric slope (see below), SGR data are useful in explaining patterns of allometric scaling (Wayne, 1986c).

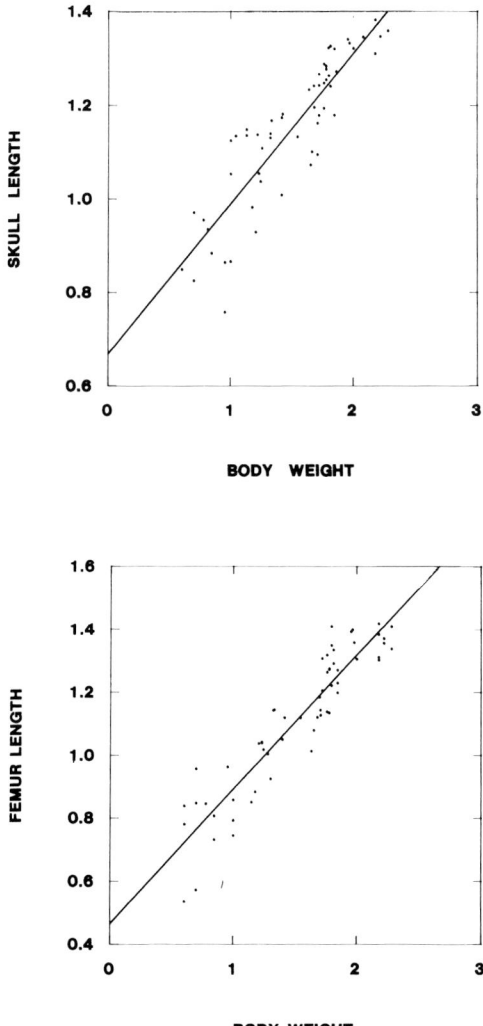

Fig. 2. Log/log plots of avearge total skull length and femur length of dog breeds plotted against their average total body weight (Hubbard, 1964). Top regression line: slope = 0.321, intercept = 0.668, r = 0.884, number of breeds = 58. Bottom regression line: slope = 0.427, intercept = 0.464, r = 0.922, number of breeds = 61.

Allometry among Adults from Different Dog Breeds and Wild Canid Species

Cranial and Dental Measurements

Domestic dogs differ from wild canids principally in the scaling of measurements of cranial width and depth and dental length and width (Table 1). These variables always have smaller slopes and larger intercepts in the domestic dog than in the wild canids. In contrast, the allometric slopes and intercepts of skull length variables are very similar in dogs and wild canids (Table 1). The consequences of these allometric differences can be visualized in bivariate plots (Fig. 3). As a result of the decreased slope and increased intercept of domestic dog cranial width allometry relative to that of wild canids, regression lines of the two groups cross only among canids of large skull length (Fig. 3b and c). Therefore, all large domestic dogs have similar skull proportions to their wolf-like ancestors, whereas all small domestic dogs have relatively wider crania than wild canids of equivalent skull size. Similarly, with the exception of M_2 length, all small domestic dogs have relatively longer teeth than wild canids of similar skull size (Fig. 3d). In contrast, measurements of skull length, such as face length, are proportioned similarly in domestic dogs and their wild counterparts (Fig. 3a).

In the domestic dog, measurements of skull length tend to be isometric (slope equals one) while those of skull width and depth and dental length and width are negatively allometric (slopes less than one, Table 1). As a result, the proportion of face length to skull length is similar in both small and large dogs (e.g., 0.75 in a Chihuahua, 0.78 in a Great Dane). In contrast, measurements of relative cranial width and depth and dental length and width change dramatically with skull size such that smaller dogs always have relatively wider crania and larger teeth than do bigger dogs. For example, the ratio of cranial width to total skull length in the Chihuahua is 0.59, while in the Great Dane it is 0.31.

A final observation concerns differences in variability among cranial and dental measurements. The standard error about the regression line is clearly less for measurements of skull length than for other variables (Table 1) . In addition, the standard error of the regressions for dog breeds are almost always greater than those for wild canids (Table 1). This increased scatter is also evident in scatter plots of cranial width and dental length and width; domestic dogs show considerably more scatter about the regression line than the wild canids. The same increase in morphologic variability has been observed in other domestic mammals vs. their wild progenitors (Clutton-Brock, 1963; Herre, 1963).

In conclusion, there are dramatic scaling differences between wild canids and domestic dogs. Except for measurements of skull length, small domestic

Table 1.
Standard Errors of the Regression, Slope (b) and Intercept (a) for the Regression of the Log of the Indicated Variable on the Log of Total Skull Length

Dependent Variable	Wild Canids			Adult Domestic Dogs			Developing Domestic Dogs		
	SE	b	a	SE	b	a	SE	b	a
Cranial Length									
FL	0.012	1.04	−0.32	0.014	1.00	−0.25	0.017	0.94	−0.17
PL	0.021	1.02	−0.47	0.027	0.97	−0.40	0.011	0.95	−0.38
BCL[a]	0.021	0.83	−0.26	0.034	0.88	−0.33	0.031	1.05	−0.48
TRL	0.034	1.02	−0.55	0.041	0.96	−0.48	—	—	—
ML[b]	0.012	1.06	−0.16	0.022	0.96	−0.03	0.017	1.04	−0.11
Cranial Width and Depth									
PW[a,b]	0.033	1.10	−0.61	0.060	0.57	0.09	0.029	0.69	−0.08
MCW[a,b]	0.027	0.60	0.01	0.026	0.24	0.47	0.025	0.38	0.35
ZW[a,b]	0.028	1.03	−0.26	0.050	0.59	0.30	0.030	0.81	0.00
LCW[a,b]	0.050	0.76	−0.41	0.059	0.19	0.34	0.013	0.11	0.61
CD[b]	0.031	0.85	−0.22	0.037	0.52	0.24	0.023	0.47	0.25
PD[b]	0.046	1.24	−1.13	0.065	0.94	−0.70	0.041	0.86	−0.67
MW[b]	0.041	1.29	−1.60	0.064	0.78	−0.93	0.041	0.73	−0.83
MH[a,b]	0.047	1.39	−1.42	0.052	1.16	−1.08	0.069	0.95	−0.78

Dental Length and Width

P^3L[b]	0.042	1.09	−1.29	0.050	0.67	−0.77	—	—	—	—
P^4L[b]	0.041	1.15	−1.18	0.035	0.58	−0.49	—	—	—	—
M^1L[b]	0.062	0.84	−1.00	0.054	0.64	−0.74	—	—	—	—
M^2L[b]	0.072	0.54	−0.86	0.082	0.72	−1.07	—	—	—	—
M^1W[b]	0.032	0.97	−0.96	0.038	0.67	−0.60	—	—	—	—
M^2W	0.048	0.74	−0.86	0.037	0.68	−0.82	—	—	—	—
M_1L[b]	0.042	1.17	−1.15	0.032	0.62	−0.46	—	—	—	—

[a] Regression lines of adult domestic dogs and developing domestic dogs are significantly different ($p < 0.05$).

[b] Regression lines of wild canids and adult domestic dogs are significantly different ($p < 0.05$).

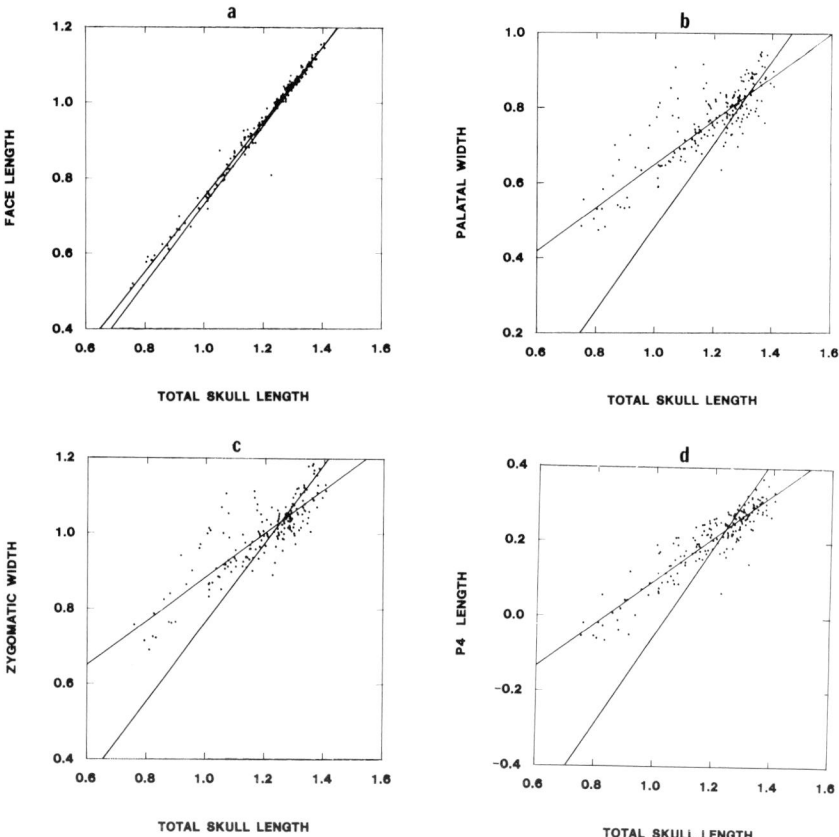

Fig. 3. Log/log plots of face length (a), palatal width (b), zygomatic width (c), and P4 length (d) against total skull length for domestic dogs and wild species. Individual values (points) are plotted for the domestic dog only. The domestic dog line is always above that of the wild canids. See Table 1 for regression statistics.

dogs tend to have wider crania and larger teeth relative to their skull length than the wild canids. Moreover, because most measurements of skull width and dental length and width show strong negative allometry, large dogs differ from small dogs in the proportions of skull and dental measurements.

Limb Bone Measurements

The scaling of limb bone measurements in domestic dogs and wild canids is much more similar than the scaling of cranial measurements (Table 2). For two limb bone measurements, allometric regressions are not significantly different between domestic dogs and wild canids (Table 2). Scaling similarities are apparent in allometric plots of limb bone lengths such as humerus length vs. femur length (Fig. 4a). In this plot, domestic dogs and wild canids have similarly sized humeri over the measured range of femur lengths.

The greatest dissimilarity between regression lines of domestic dogs and wild canids appears with measurements of metacarpal length, olecranon length, scapula length, and long bone width (Table 2, Fig. 4c and d). With the latter three measurements, slopes are always smaller and the intercepts greater in the domestic dog than in wild canids (Table 2). The reverse is true of metatarsal length (Fig. 4b). As with skull measurements, allometric regression lines generally cross at large size and thus small dogs have slightly shorter metatarsals, longer olecrana and scapulas than small wild canids of equivalent femur length, whereas large dogs are similar in proportion to equivalently sized wild canids (Fig. 4). Similarly, limb bones of all but the largest dogs are wide relative to wild canids of equivalent femur size (Table 2, Fig. 4d). However, limb bone width is increased by the same proportion in all limb bones as indicated by the similarity of regressions of width of one long bone relative to another (Table 2).

For most limb bone length measurements, the slope of the allometric regression is near one, indicating isometric or no change in proportion with increased limb bone length (Table 2). Thus, small and large dogs are closely scaled versions of one another with respect to femur length. In the domestic dog, the measurements that depart most significantly from isometry include olecranon, metapodial, and scapula length and width, and measurements of limb bone width. All these variables show negative scaling; thus, small dogs have proportionately greater values on these measurements.

In conclusion, allometry of limb bone length in domestic dogs and wild canids is very similar. There are subtle differences in some measurements, but the general coincidence of many regression lines contrasts strongly with the differences observed in the cranial and dental analysis. As before, where scaling differences between the two groups are evident, only large domestic dogs and wild canids overlap in size and proportion. These large wild canids (the gray wolf and its relatives) are the species most closely related to domestic dogs. Moreover, morphologic differences in limb bone scaling between large and small dogs are evident in only a few measurements of limb bone length and are most apparent in measurements of limb bone width.

Ontogenetic Allometry in the Domestic Dog

Cranial Allometry

Data on cranial allometry were obtained from measurements of four domestic dog puppies from different breeds and from Becker (1923, see Wayne, 1986a). Allometry of juvenile domestic dogs of various ages and sizes shows some similarity to that of adults of different sizes. Regression

Table 2.
Standard Errors of the Regression, Slope (b) and Intercept (a) for the Regression of the Log of the Indicated Variable on the Log of Femur Length

Dependent Variable	Wild Canids			Adult Domestic Dogs			Developing Domestic Dogs		
	SE	b	a	SE	b	a	SE	b	a
Long Bone Length									
LR[a]	0.029	1.08	−0.12	0.023	1.04	−0.07	0.012	1.00	−0.07
LU[b]	0.030	1.05	−0.02	0.017	1.02	0.02	0.024	0.98	0.04
LH	0.016	0.95	0.03	0.014	0.95	0.02	0.018	0.95	0.01
LT[a,b]	0.026	0.95	0.09	0.020	1.01	0.09	0.023	1.06	−0.11
LTC[a]	0.037	0.98	−0.61	0.060	1.03	−0.63	—	—	—
LO[a]	0.052	0.99	−0.62	0.045	0.83	−0.36	0.030	0.93	−0.31
LMC[a]	0.030	1.04	−0.45	0.032	0.90	−0.29	0.023	0.93	−0.27
LMT[a]	0.037	0.89	−0.21	0.207	0.93	−0.29	0.037	0.83	0.30
Long Bone Width									
WMC[a]	0.103	1.00	−1.50	0.120	0.85	−1.18	—	—	—
WH[a]	0.056	0.96	−1.10	0.088	0.85	−0.89	0.871	0.82	−0.77
WMT[a]	0.060	0.91	−1.32	0.075	0.76	−1.05	—	—	—
WF[a]	0.043	0.88	−1.00	0.074	0.76	−0.78	0.420	0.76	−0.73
WFE[a]	0.036	0.92	−0.59	0.066	0.89	−0.50	—	—	—

Relative Width

WMC:WMT	0.081	1.08	−0.02	0.108	1.08	−0.01	—	—	—
WH:WF	0.040	1.07	−0.02	0.050	1.09	−0.01	0.381	1.07	0.02
WMC:WH	0.098	1.00	−0.30	0.108	0.92	−0.29	—	—	—
WMT:WF	0.055	1.00	−0.28	0.057	0.95	−0.26	—	—	—

Scapula Length and Width

LS[a,b]	0.03	1.06	−0.21	0.037	0.87	0.08	0.029	0.92	−0.09
WS[b]	0.04	0.89	−0.23	0.067	0.84	−0.17	0.053	0.93	−0.23
WFO[a]	0.04	0.94	−0.48	0.070	0.82	−0.33	—	—	—

[a] Regression lines of wild canids and adult domestic dogs are significantly different ($p < 0.05$).
[b] Regression lines of adult domestic dogs and developing domestic dogs are significantly different ($p < 0.05$).

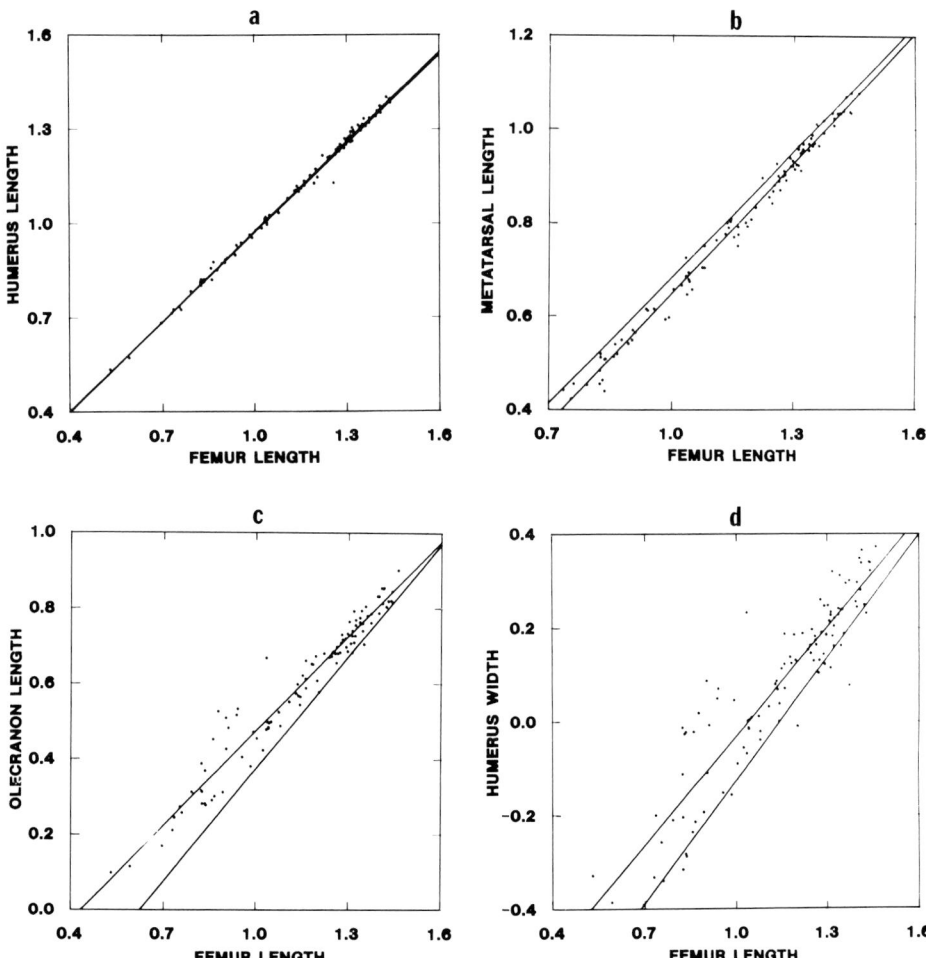

Fig. 4. Log/log plots of humerus length (a), metatarsal length (b), olecranon length (c), humerus width (d) against femur length for domestic dogs and wild species. Individuals values (points) are plotted for the domestic dog only. The domestic dog line is always above that of the wild canids except for b, where it is below that of the wild canid regression line. See Table 2 for regression statistics.

coefficients of several measurements are not significantly different between the two groups (Table 1, e.g., FL, PL, CD, PD). In those measurements that do show allometric scaling differences between juvenile and adult domestic dogs, adults from small breeds (less than 15 cm total skull length, approximately 1.2 in Fig. 5, top) are positioned above or very near to the ontogenetic regression line. As a result, adults from small dog breeds have

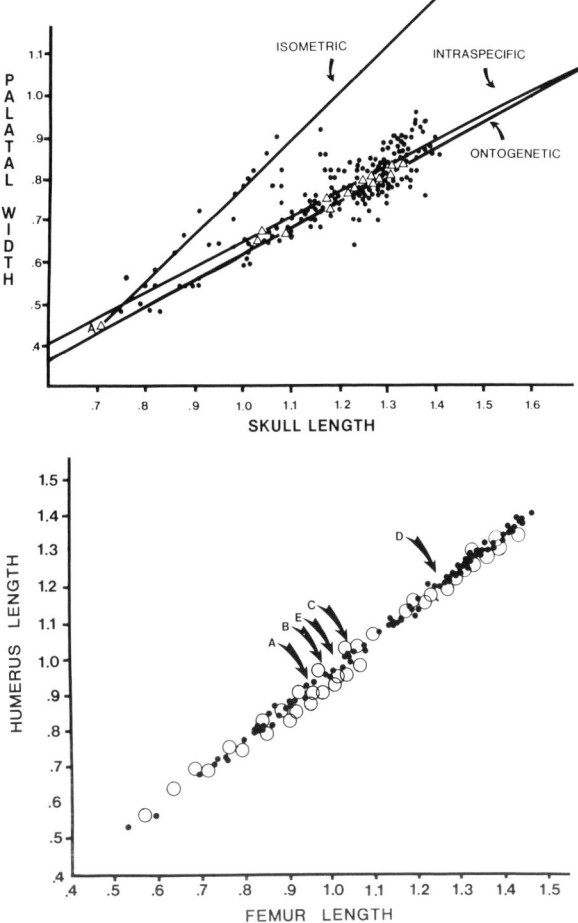

Fig. 5. Top — log/log plots of palatal width against total skull length for juvenile German Shepherds (triangles; Becker, 1923) and adult domestic dogs (solid circles). Since the isometric line indicates an extension of neonate proportions (denoted by point "A") into large size, many domestic dogs have neonate proportions as adults. Ontogenetic and adult domestic dog ("intraspecific") regression lines are shown. Measurements in centimeters. See Table 1 for regression statistics. Bottom — log/log plot of humerus length against femur length for juvenile dogs from four breeds (circles) and adult domestic dogs (dots). A is the normal 250-day-old juvenile of the Lhasa Apso. B, C, D, and E represent the morphology that results if the specific growth rate of a Lhasa Apso neonate is increased according to Fig. 6.

skull proportions like those of juvenile dogs of the same or smaller skull size, that is, all small breeds are to some extent juvenilized, i.e., paedomorphic (see Gould, 1977). In the extreme, some adults have the same proportions as a neonate German shepherd (points along isometric line, Fig. 5, top).

Large breeds tend to fall to either side of the ontogenetic line and are thus either juvenilized or hypermorphic (equivalent in proportion to a dog that exceeded the ancestral ontogeny).

Finally, the ontogenetic scaling of skull length variables is nearly isometric and has smaller standard errors than cranial width and depth measurements (Table 1). The ontogenetic scaling of cranial width and depth measurements is negatively allometric (slopes less than one). Therefore, the pattern of allometric scaling among adults of different sizes and among juveniles of different ages is similar in the domestic dog.

Limb Bone Allometry

Limb bone growth allometry, based on measurements of four individuals from different dog breeds, shows a close similarity to allometry among adults from different breeds (Table 2). The allometric scaling of most measurements does not differ statistically between the two groups and those that do differ are very close in slope and intercept (Table 2). As seen in Fig. 5 (bottom), some adult domestic dogs are identical in size and proportion to juvenile domestic dogs from a large breed. Thus, as with cranial measurements, many small dog breeds share more proportional similarity with juvenile domestic dogs than with adults from larger breeds. However, because many measurements are not strongly allometric (slopes near one, Table 2), adults and juveniles differ to a lesser extent in scaling of limb bone measurements than in scaling of cranial width and depth measurements. The most strongly allometric measurements are those of long bone width; puppies have proportionately wider bones than older juveniles or adults.

Relationship of Growth Rates to Ontogenetic Allometry

The morphological differences in cranial and limb morphology among dog breeds could conceivably be due to differences in size and shape evident at birth, in post-natal growth, and/or in time of growth onset and cessation. The extent to which breeds differ at birth is unclear; preliminary data suggest that, although differences in adult limb bone proportions may be evident at birth, the large part of breed differences appear to be acquired through differences in post-natal growth rates and the timing of growth onset and cessation (Wayne, 1986c). Growth rate changes that would produce the similarity of ontogenetic and adult allometry observed in the domestic dog are outlined in Fig. 6 for growth in humerus and femur length. In general, ontogenetic and adult allometry will always be similar if the specific growth rate curves for each measurement are changed by the same

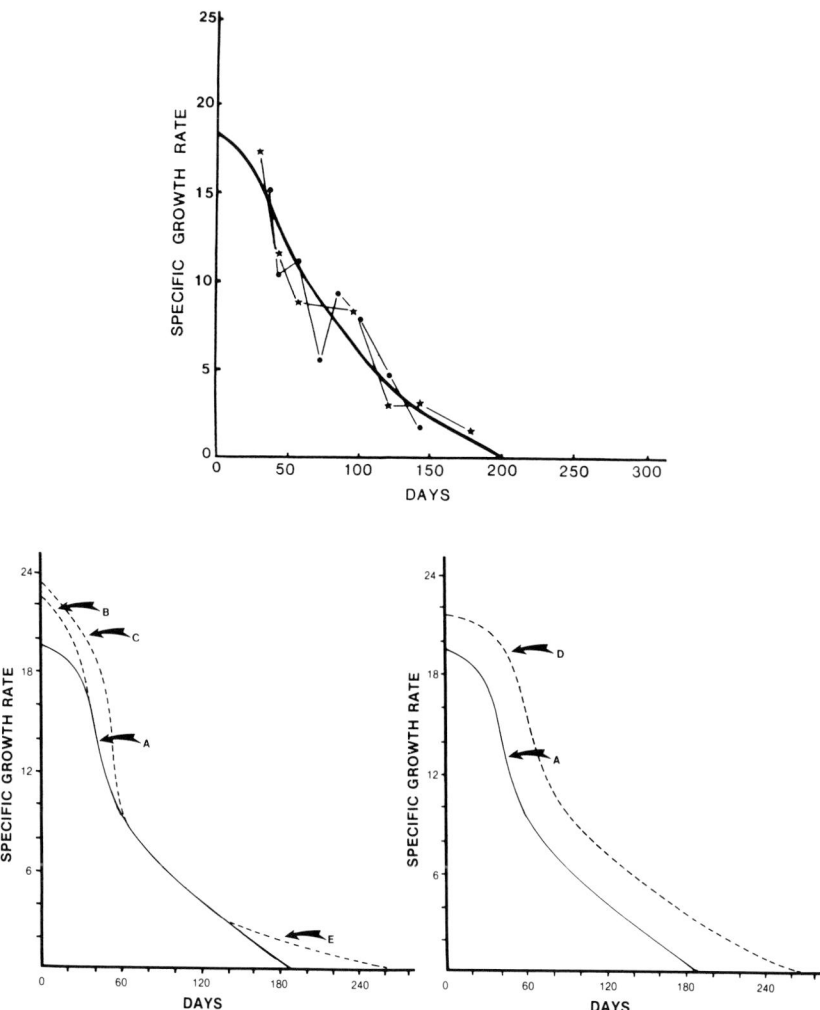

Fig. 6. Top — specific growth rates of femur length (solid circles) and humerus length (stars) vs. time for the Lhasa Apso. Composite growth rate curve fitted empirically with flexible rule and shown as solid line. Specific growth rate in units of 1/day times 1000. Bottom — hypothetical growth rate changes superimposed on the composite humerus and femur Lhasa Apso growth rate curve. A is the normal composite growth rate curve taken from the top figure. B represents a growth rate increase over the perinatal period (0 to 25 d). C represents a growth rate increase over the entire period of rapid growth (0 to 60 d). D represents an increase only in the initial specific growth rate and E represents a growth rate increase late in ontogeny. Specific growth rate in units of 1/day times 1000.

proportion. Such an alteration maintains the same ratio of specific growth rates, and consequently the same allometric slope at corresponding points in development (see Fig. 5 and 6; A, B, C, D, and E). As long as the relationship among growth curves remains the same, and the size at birth and the length of the growth period is similar among breeds, ontogenetic and adult allometry will resemble one another.

Although a proportional change in growth rates may explain the coincidence of ontogenetic and adult regression lines, it cannot account for breeds positioned above the ontogenetic regression line in Fig. 5 (top). For these breeds, in addition to an overall decrease in growth rate, the relative growth rates of measurements must change. Our limited data on cranial growth suggest that in the Lhasa Apso growth rates of zygomatic width are similar to those of the Great Dane but growth rates of total skull length are lower (Fig. 7). As a result, the ontogenetic regression line of zygomatic width vs. total skull length for the Lhasa Apso will have a larger slope than that of the Great Dane and, thus, assuming the two breeds have similar cranial morphology at birth, the adult Lhasa Apso will have a proportionately wider skull than that of an adult or juvenile Great Dane.

Because ontogenetic and adult limb bone allometry corresponds closely in domestic dogs, differences in growth rates among limb bones in large and small dogs seem less prevalent than with cranial allometry. Instead, simple proportional changes in the overall growth rates of limb bones are all that is required to produce the array of skeletal proportions exhibited by the domestic dog. However, our data on development of limb bones in four different dog breeds, from age 50 to 250 d, suggest growth rates are identical over this time span (Fig. 8). Apparently, differences in adult size and proportion between large and small dogs are determined by 50 d of age because after that time limb bone growth rate is similar in all limb bones (Wayne, 1986c). Therefore, differences in limb bone growth rates must exist before or soon after birth.

A final observation concerns differences in the scaling of limb bones. Because the ratio of specific growth rates for two measurements equals their allometric slope, ontogenetic allometry should directly reflect differences in limb bone growth rates. For instance, growth rates of femur and humerus length in the Lhasa Apso are given in Fig. 6 (top). The two growth curves correspond; hence their allometric scaling is nearly isometric (slope equals one, Table 2). Growth rates of metatarsal and femur length do not correspond (Fig. 9). The metatarsal specific growth rate is at first greater than the femur growth rate but crosses the femur growth rate curve at approximately 85 d. Thereafter, the specific growth rate is lower than that of the femur. This pattern of relative growth is similar in the other breeds studied: the metapodials grow faster than the femur for the first 75 to 100 d of growth and slower thereafter. As a result, the ontogenetic slope of the two measurements (LMT vs. LF) is at first greater than one and then less than one.

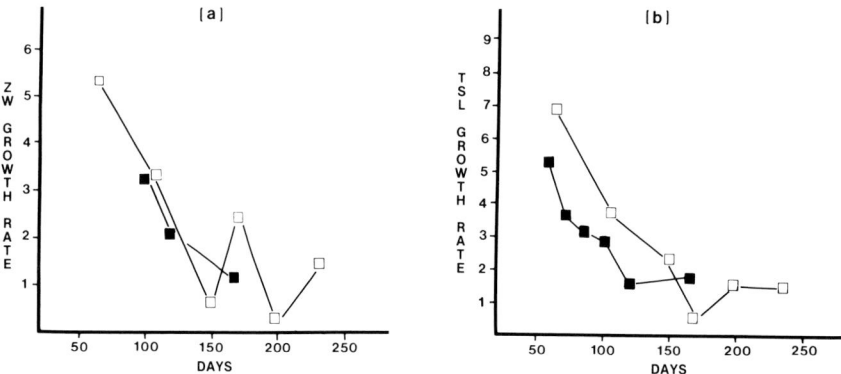

Fig. 7. Specific growth rate of zygomatic width (A) and total skull length (B) against time for the Great Dane (open squares) and the Lhasa Apso, (solid squares). Specific growth rate in units of 1/day times 1000.

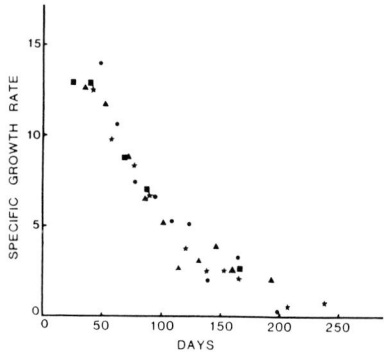

Fig. 8. Specific growth rate of radius length vs. time for growing domestic dogs. Great Dane (solid circles), Labrador Retriever (stars), Cocker Spaniel (triangles), Lhasa Apso (solid squares). Specific growth rate in units of 1/day times 1000.

Thus, puppies have relatively large metatarsals that decrease in proportion to femur length after approximately 100 d of age. The overall ontogenetic slope is less than one (Table 2). In general, the ontogenetic scaling of limb bones is unlikely to be isometric if specific growth rate curves cross or are offset.

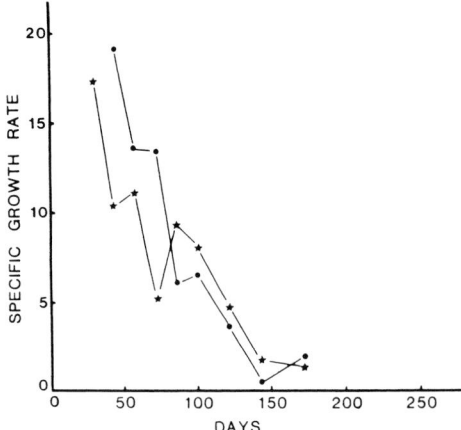

Fig. 9. Specific growth rates of metatarsal length (solid circles) and femur length (stars) vs. time for the Lhasa Apso. Specific growth rate in units of 1/day times 1000.

In conclusion, the cranium and limb bones show different patterns of allometric growth with respect to adult allometry. Cranial allometry of juveniles and adults is similar but many breeds show a highly juvenilized morphology which may result from both proportionate and disproportionate changes in post-natal growth rates. Limb bone growth rates are more uniform and less variable; hence, ontogenetic and adult allometries are nearly identical. Apparently, differences in adult limb bone size and proportion stem from inequities in perinatal or fetal specific growth rates.

The Role of Selection, Environment, and Development on Morphology

Directional Selection

To a varying extent, all small domestic dog breeds have skull proportions resembling that of juveniles of larger breeds. Both juvenile morphology and behavior may provide the appearance of docility and helplessness that increases the desirability and success of a breed (see Gould, 1979; Coppinger and Coppinger, 1982). However, selection for ferocity and aggressiveness are also characteristics desired by some dog breeders. It is odd then that all mid- and small-sized breeds measured in this study are juvenilized. None shows morphologic similarity with smaller fox-sized wild canids, all of which, have relatively narrow skulls.

Such uniformity in the direction of morphologic change under domestication is even more apparent with measurements of limb length. Allometric scaling is nearly identical between juveniles and adult domestic dogs and is similar between the latter and the wild canids. This uniformity in scaling over three allometric levels seems unlikely to stem from a similarity of artificial and natural selection. The limb morphology of wild canids probably reflects adaptations for locomotion and prey capture (Howells, 1944; Smith and Savage, 1956; Taylor, 1970; Hildebrand, 1952; 1974; Van Valkenburgh, 1985; 1987). Although some large working or hunting breeds may have been selected for similar behaviors, such selection would seem unimportant in the development of most toy, miniature, or mid-sized breeds as these are not required to hunt regularly or to catch and dismember prey. Despite the obscure origin of most breeds, they have clearly originated in numerous places, under various conditions and at various times. In fact, with the exception of walking, the locomotor requirements of different breeds would seem as varied as the breeds themselves. Nevertheless, small dogs are proportioned like larger more wolf-like breeds. In conclusion, directional selection may be an important force in the evolution of some specific breeds, but it does not explain the pervasive morphologic trends observed among small- and mid-sized breeds.

Environmental Effects

The domestic environment often involves a change in nutrition or exercise that can potentially alter bone size and proportion as well as bone microstructure over the lifetime of an individual. Two major environmental effects on skeletal structure which could vary among domestic mammals are diet and mechanical loading. The effects of these variables may be interrelated because an increase in nutritional plane may lead to greater body size which in turn could increase the mechanical loading on skeletal elements (see Hammond and Appleton, 1932). Experimental studies have shown that changes in mechanical stimuli primarily affect bone volume and proportion rather than mechanical properties (e.g., Woo et al., 1981; see review by Meade, 1989), while dietary alterations in young growing animals may affect tissue quality, i.e., material strength and stiffness (Ferretti et al., 1985). Only a few investigators have carried out comparisons between domestic animals and their wild counterparts and none of these has distinguished clearly between exercise and dietary influences on bone proportions or material properties.

In an early study of wild-captured but zoo-reared adult lions, Hollister (1917) reported significant changes in cranial shape of adult lions when compared to their wild counterparts. Specifically, the crania of zoo-reared lions were relatively shorter and broader with a more circular zygomatic arch cross-section. These changes in morphology were attributed to reduced muscle development, particularly of the masseter, due to an absence of killing behavior in zoo lions. Similar morphologic differences between wild and captive-reared wolves were also claimed to exist. Thus, because small domestic dogs have relatively wider crania they may also have a weaker bite (see Radinsky, 1981a, b).

Hammond and Appleton (1932), in a study of the effects of domestication on bone growth and morphology of the sheep hindlimb, reported that the most highly improved breeds had wider long bones with more oval cross-sections than "semiwild" breeds. They considered the increase in body mass as due to increased nutrition to be a possible explanation for this result. A more in-depth study was undertaken by Palsson and Verdes (1952) on the effects of different planes of nutrition on the growth of lambs. They found, as had others, that the timing of nutritional changes was critical in determining the specific effects on the skeleton. The greatest effect occurred during the most rapid growth of a particular skeletal element. For example, because long bone width continues growth at a high rate after growth in length has slowed, animals that are fed an abundance of food late in post-natal growth will have relatively wider bones than those underfed during the same period. Palsson and Verges also note that the effects of different nutritional planes could vary between species due to the species differences in the timing of maximum growth.

It is important to note, however, that in these studies no attempt was made beyond measurements of bone length and width to further understand the underlying mechanical processes causing the change. For example, Hammond and Appleton (1932) observed that "domestic animals,... though actually heavier, lead a less active life and the internal stresses on bones are presumably lessened: the bones are indeed less able to withstand stress in spite of greater thickness". This implies that the long bones of the more domesticated breeds, while externally wider, have thinner cortices and reduced bone material strength than less thoroughly domesticated semiwild breeds. Clearly, comparisons of relevant bone dimensions and microstructure need to be made in wild and domestic mammals under different nutritional and exercise regimes if we are to understand how these variables influence bone morphology.

Developmental Constraints

The close similarity of cranial and limb bone allometry in adults and in juvenile dogs suggests a causal relationship between post-natal development and the generation of diverse adult morphologies (e.g., breeds). Measurements which are strongly allometric in developing domestic dogs are also those measurements which show the most dramatic shape differences among adults. Dog puppies have wide, rounded crania, and broad palates. The average, large adult domestic dog has a long, narrow rostrum and a tapered cranium. To some extent, many dog breeds represent morphological snapshots between these developmental endpoints. In general, the morphologic diversity seen among domestic breeds of mammals may be dependent upon the morphological discrepancy between neonate and adult. For instance, the cat has been domesticated for as long as 9500 years (Clutton-Brock, 1981), yet there is minimal variability in size or shape among cat breeds. Such morphologic similarity among adults may reflect the lack of proportional variability between neonate and adult cats; kittens look relatively similar to adult cats (Wayne, 1986a). Because ontogenetic growth in the domestic cat cranium is nearly isometric, simple changes in overall growth rate will not result in differences in proportion among adults as they would in the domestic dog.

The near identity of adult and juvenile limb bone allometry in domestic dogs suggests even more strongly that the diversity in limb proportions among adult dog breeds is largely determined by the magnitude of ontogenetic scaling. The extent and direction of breed evolution and the observed differences between domestic dogs and wild canids are seemingly reflected in the development of a single dog. It would appear that, despite the great diversity of the domestic dog, morphologic variability among dogs is limited in ways predictable from an analysis of ontogeny. Given this, how might development be changed such that small domestic dogs acquire cranial and limb proportions more similar to small wild canids? In the cranium, changes in the relationship of specific growth rates can result in adults with relatively wider skulls (e.g., Fig. 7). Changes in relative growth rate might also produce small adults with long narrow skulls more similar to small wild canids if total skull length growth was increased relative to zygomatic width instead of being decreased. However, neonate domestic dogs have very wide skulls and are already half the size of an adult small wild canid such as a kit fox. Thus, a dramatic departure in the relative growth rate of total skull length would be needed to produce a small narrow-skulled dog similar to a kit fox. This suggests that small domestic dogs differ from small wild canids because puppies of small dogs cannot grow out of their distinctive neonate morphology. Similarly, because post-natal limb bone growth rates are so constant among dogs, the limb proportions of neonates may limit morphologic diversity among adults.

One conceivable way to alter cranial and limb bone morphology further would be to change gestation time. If fetal growth of cranial or limb bone dimensions is allometric (slopes different from one), then domestic dogs born at different times will have different cranial and limb proportions. In fact, small wild canids all have gestation times of approximately 50 to 53 d, whereas all domestic dogs have gestations times of approximately 60 to 63 d,

(Wayne, 1986c). Thus, smaller dogs might be more similar in proportion to small wild canids if they were born earlier (see Wayne, 1986c). In the domestic dog, the apparent lack of variability in gestation time may act as a fundamental constraint on the morphologic diversity of dog breeds.

Other Domestic Mammals

Our results suggest that in other domestic mammals, especially those in which the conditions of evolution were similar to the domestic dog (e.g., other pet species), morphologic characters whose ontogenetic scaling departs significantly from isometry (e.g., zygomatic width, olecranon length) would be predicted to show between-breed differences in proportion. For instance, the domestic pig shows considerable change in skull proportions with growth. Piglets are born with broad crania and short faces and adults have narrow crania and long faces. For example, the ratio of palate length to width changes from 3:1 at 1 month to 5:1 at 6 months of age (Epstein, 1971, p.365). This ontogenetic change is mirrored among adults from different pig breeds which, among domestic mammals, appear to be second only to domestic dogs in morphologic diversity (Epstein, 1971).

In contrast, the isometric scaling among juvenile cats is reflected in the lack of cranial diversity among adult domestic cats. The domestic horse provides a better example because adults from different breeds vary in size almost as much as the domestic dog but are considerably less variable than domestic dogs in cranial shape (Zeuner, 1963; Epstein, 1971). As with dogs, the lack of skull shape diversity among adults reflects that among an age series of juvenile horses (Hilzheimer, 1935; Hammond, 1935; Robb, 1935; Epstein, 1971; Radinsky, 1984; Devillars et al., 1984).

Conclusions

(1) The scaling of cranial and dental measurements in the domestic dog differs from that among wild canids. Small domestic dogs generally have wider and deeper skulls than wild canids of equivalent skull size. Overlap in size and proportion is apparent only among large domestic dogs and their close relatives, the wolf-like canids.

(2) The scaling of limb bone measurements is similar between domestic dogs and wild canids. Minor differences in scaling are apparent between small domestic dogs and small wild canids in measurements of olecranon length, metapodial length, scapula length, and long bone width.

(3) Ontogenetic allometry is similar to allometry among adults. Hence, all small adult dogs have proportions similar to that of juveniles of large domestic dogs and are thus puppy-like. Simple alterations in absolute and relative specific growth rates can account for much of the variation in adult morphology.

(4) Given that gestation time is constant, the morphologic diversity among adults from different breeds appears to be limited by that expressed during post-natal development.

(5) Skeletal morphology of domestic mammals may be altered over the life time of an individual due to differences in exercise and nutritional regime. The differences observed among domestic breeds however reflects both selection for specific physical attributes and the developmental association of these attributes and other morphologic features.

Acknowledgments

We are grateful for the assistance of the mammalogy curators and staff of the following museums: the National Museum of Natural History, The Field Museum of Chicago, and the American Museum of Natural History. We thank Blaire Van Valkenburgh and Derek Girman for discussion and critical review of the manuscript.

References

Alberch, P. (1983). Developmental constraints in the evolutionary process. In: *Evolution and Development*. Bonner, J. T., Ed., Springer-Verlag, Berlin, 313–332.

Alberch, P. (1985). Developmental constraints: why St. Bernards often have an extra digit and poodles never do. *Am. Nat.,* **126**: 430–433.

Brody, S. (1945). *Bioenergetics and Growth*. Reinhold, New York.

Clutton-Brock, J. (1963). The origins of the dog. In: *Science in Archaeology*. Brothwell, D., Higgs, E., and Clark, C., Eds., Thames and Hudson, Bristol, 269–274.

Clutton-Brock, J. (1987). *A Natural History of Domesticated Mammals*. Cambridge University Press, Cambridge.

Cock, A. G. (1966). Genetical aspects of metrical growth and form in animals. *Q. Rev. Biol.,* **41**: 131–190.

Coppinger, L. and Coppinger, R. (1982). Livestock-guarding dogs that wear sheep's clothing. *Smithsonian*. April: 65–73.

Crusafont-Pairo, M. and Truyols-Santonja, J. (1956). A biometric study of the evolution of Fissiped carnivores. *Evolution,* **10**: 314–322.

Darwin, C. (1859). *On the Origin of Species*. Facsimile of the first edition, Harvard University Press, Cambridge.

Devillers, Ch., Mahe, J., Ambroise, D., Bauchot, R., and Chatelain, E. (1984). Allometric studies on the skull of living and fossil Equidae (Mammalia: Perissodactyla). *J. Vert. Paleontol.*, **4**: 471–480.

Epstein, H. (1971). *The Origins of the Domestic Animals of Africa.* Vol. 1, Africana, New York.

Ferretti, J. L., Tessaro, R. D., Audisio, E. O., and Galassi, C. D. (1985). Long term effects of high and low CA intakes and lack of parathyroid function on rat femur biomechanics. *Calcif. Tissue Int.*, **37**: 608–612.

Gonyea, W. S. (1976). Adaptive differences in the body proportions of large Felids. *Acta Anat.*, **96**: 81–96.

Gould, S. J. (1966). Allometry and size in ontogeny and phylogeny. *Biol. Rev. Cambridge Phil. Soc.*, **41**: 587–640.

Gould, S. J. (1979). Mickey Mouse meets Konrad Lorenz. *Nat. Hist.*, **88**: 30–37.

Gould, S. J. and Lewontin, R. C. (1978). The Spandrels of San Marco and the Panglossiam paradigm: a critique of the adaptationist programme. *Proc. R. Soc. London*, **205**: 581–598.

Gould, S. J. and Vrba, E. S. (1982). Exadaptation — A missing term in the science of form. *Paleobiology*, **8**: 4–15.

Hammond, J. (1935). The inheritance of productivity in farm livestock. I. *Meat Emp. J. Exp. Agric.*, **3**: 1–18.

Hammond, J. and Appleton, A. B. (1932). Studies of the leg in mutton. In: *Growth and Development of the Mutton Qualities in Sheep.* Hammond, J., Ed., Oliver and Tweed, London, 351–581.

Herre, W. (1963). The science and history of domestic animals. In: *Science in Archaeology.* Brothwell, D., Higgs, E., and Clark, C., Eds., Thames and Hudson, Bristol, 269–274.

Hildebrand, M. (1952). An analysis of body proportions in the Canidae. *Am. J. Anat.*, **90**: 217–256.

Hildebrand, M. (1974). *Analysis of Vertebrate Structure.* John Wiley & Sons, New York.

Hilzheimer, M. (1935). On the evolution of the horse. *Antiquity*, **9**(34).

Hollister, N. (1917). Some effects of environment and habit on captive lions. *Proc. U.S. Natl. Mus.*, **53**: 177–193.

Howells, H. H. (1944). *Speed in Animals. Their Specialization for Running and Leaping.* University of Chicago Press, Chicago.

Hubbard, C. L. B. (1964). *The Observer's Book of Dogs.* Frederick Warne and Co., London.

Huxley, J. S. (1932). *Problems of Relative Growth.* Dover, New York.

Jaslow, C. R. (1987). Morphology and digestive efficiency of red foxes (*Vulpes vulpes*) and gray foxes (*Urocyon cinereoagenteus*). *Can. J. Zool.*, **65**: 72–79.

Jungers, W. L. (1985). Body size and scaling of limb proportions in primates. In: *Size and Scaling in Primate Biology.* Jungers, W. L., Ed., Plenum Press, New York, 345–382.

Kauffmann, S. A. (1983). Developmental constraints: internal factors in evolution. In: *Development and Evolution.* Goodwin, B. C., Holder, N., Wylie, C. C., Eds., Cambridge University Press, Cambridge, 332–386.

Klieber, M. (1961). *The Fire of Life. An Introduction to Animal Energetics.* John Wiley & Sons, New York.

Lauder, G. V. (1981). Form and function: structural analysis in evolutionary morphology. *Paleobiology*, **7**: 430–455.

McMahon, T. A. (1975). Allometry and biomechanics: limb bones of adult ungulates. *Am. Nat.*, **109**: 547–563.

Meade, J. B. (1989). The adaptation of bone to mechanical stress: experimentation and current concepts. In: *Bone Mechanics.* Cowin, S. C., Ed., CRC Press, Boca Raton, FL, 211–251.

Palsson, H. and Verges, J. B. (1952). Effects of the plane of nutrition on the growth and development of carcass quality in lambs. I. *J. Agric. Sci.*, **42**: 1–92.

Radinsky, L. B. (1981a). Evolution of skull shape in carnivores. I. Representative modern carnivores. *Biol. J. Linn. Soc.*, **15**: 369–388.

Radinsky, L. B. (1981b). Evolution of skull shape in carnivores: additional modern carnivores. *Biol. J. Linn. Soc.*, **16**: 337–355.

Radinsky, L. B. (1984). Ontogeny and phylogeny in horse skull evolution. *Evolution*, **38**: 1–15.

Robb, R. C. (1935). A study of mutation in evolution. II: Ontogeny in the equine skull. *J. Genet.*, **31**: 47–52.

Schmidt-Nielsen, K. (1984). *Scaling: Why is Animal Size so Important?* Cambridge University Press, Cambridge.

Seim, E. and Saether, B. E. (1983). On rethinking allometry: which regression model to use? *J. Theor. Biol.*, **104**: 161–168.

Smith, R. J. (1984). Allometric scaling in comparative biology: problems of concept and method. *Am. J. Physiol.*, **245**: R152–R160.

Smith, J. M. and Savage, R. J. G. (1956). Some locomotory adaptations in mammals. *J. Linn. Soc. Zool.*, **42**: 603–622.

Taylor, M. E. (1970). Locomotion in some east African viverrids. *J. Mammal.*, **51**: 42–51.

Van Valkenburgh, B. (1985). Locomotor diversity within past and present guilds of large predatory mammals. *Paleobiology*, **11**: 406–428.

Van Valkenburgh, B. (1987). Skeletal indicators of locomotor behavior in living and extinct carnivores. *J. Vert. Paleo.*, **7**: 162–182.

Van Valkenburgh, B. (1988). Incidence of tooth breakage among large predatory mammals. *Am. Nat.*, **131**: 291–302.

Van Valkenburgh, B. Carnivore dental adaptations and diet: a study of trophic diversity in guilds. In: *Carnivore Behavior, Ecology and Evolution.* Gittleman, J. L., Ed., Cornell University Press, Cornell, NY, in press.

Van Valkenburgh, B. and Ruff, C. B. (1987). Canine tooth strength and killing behavior in large carnivores. *J. Zool.*, **212**: 379–397.

Wayne, R. K. (1986a). Cranial morphology of domestic and wild canids: the influence of development on morphologic change. *Evolution*, **40**:243–261.

Wayne, R. K. (1986b). Limb morphology of domestic and wild canids: the influence of development on morphologic change. *J. Morphol.*, **187**: 301–319.

Wayne, R. K. (1986c). Developmental contraints on limb growth in domestic and some wild canids. *J. Zool.*, **210A**: 381–399.

Woo, S. L., Kuei, S. C., Amiel, D., Gomez, M. A., Hayes, W. C., White, F. C., and Akeson, W. H. (1981). The effect of prolonged physical training on the properties of long bones: a study of Wolff's Law. *J. Bone Jt. Surg.*, **63A**: 78–87.

Zar, B. (1984). *Biostatistical Analysis.* John Wiley & Sons, New York.

Zeuner, F. E. (1963). *A History of Domesticated Animals.* Harper and Row, London.

6

Bone Growth and Primate Evolution

BRIAN T. SHEA
Department of Cell, Molecular and Structural Biology
Department of Anthropology
Northwestern University
Chicago, Illinois

Introduction
Background
Bone growth and adaptation
Bone growth and phylogenetic reconstruction
Bone growth and the evolution of growth patterns
Allometry and heterochrony
Control of bone growth — evolutionary implications
References

Introduction

This chapter presents a brief overview of how knowledge of bone growth may contribute to our understanding of various aspects of primate evolution. Bone growth is defined here broadly, and includes both early development and ossification as well as later morphogenesis, or ontogenetic changes in form and size. A variety of topics of interest to evolutionary biologists will be considered below, but all are based upon a single premise, which I hope will capture the commitment especially of students and young researchers. This is simply a claim that more is generally better, and that ontogenetic data invariably yield more information than the traditional static adult data that are normally collected. (The exception to this is if collection of growth data prevents collection of other data due to time constraints, etc. — then the issue becomes debatable.) Furthermore, certain key issues in evolutionary biology require the special information provided by studies of growth and development. These include the issues of homology determination in systematics, size correction in studies of adaptation and/or systematics, heterochrony and evolutionary mechanisms, and developmental constraints and directionality in evolutionary transformations. Since the evolutionary sequences and adaptations which we reconstruct from adult specimens found in statigraphic series and museum drawers are connected by a chain of ontogenies, growth mechanisms and patterns must be analyzed in detail in

8827-9/93/$0.00 + $.50

order to fully understand evolutionary mechanisms and patterns. I will try to illustrate this through a discussion of bone growth and the evolution of our own Order, the Primates. Fig. 1 presents one of many possible systematic arrangements of genera within the primates. It is included here as a reference for those not intimately familiar with the taxa and basic phylogenetic relationships discussed below.

Background

The need for an understanding of the causes and consequences of bone growth in primates was seen very clearly in the early 1800s, when the comparative anatomist Geoffroy Saint-Hilaire had to correct his previous error of placing the differently shaped skulls of juvenile and adult orangutans into two distinct genera (Gould, 1977). Subsequent work did much to document the sometimes dramatic changes in bone size and proportions which are observed during ontogeny. Among primatologists involved in these endeavors, the work of A. H. Schultz stands out in its breadth and detail. Schultz's research, much of which is summarized and cited in his 1969 book, *The Life of Primates*, was focused on documenting the age changes and variability in the morphology of various primates, and interpreting these patterns of variability and divergence in light of adult adaptive specializations and phylogenetic relationships. The rich body of Schultz's empirical work will continue to provide his successors with a valuable research resource.

Somewhat surprisingly, Schultz's concentration on growth and form almost studiously avoided a major theoretical current developing in other areas of evolutionary biology in the 1920s and later. This current focused on relative growth rates and the integration of growth patterns (as opposed to the more traditional foci on growth-in-time), and emerged from the important general theoretical and empirical writings of Thompson (1917), Huxley (1932), and DeBeer (1930), among others. Hyman Lumer's 1939 publication on relative growth of the limbs in anthropoid apes represents one of the first applications of growth allometric analyses to the primate skeleton. Lumer's theoretical orientation toward growth allometry was combined with Schultz's primate expertise in subsequent studies of limb and tail growth in macaques (Lumer and Schultz, 1941) and spider (*Ateles geoffroyi*) vs. cebus (*Cebus capucinus*) monkeys (Lumer and Schultz, 1947). Giles' (1956) work on cranial growth allometry in the great apes was another important application of this growth perspective to problems in primate evolution, a fact I well recognize since my own early work is an extension of Giles' research in many ways.

Even in this body of early research on primate bone growth and morphology we can perceive two overlapping but somewhat distinct areas of emphasis. The relationships between these two broad orientations are the subject of rekindled debates in evolutionary biology at present, reflecting the resurgent interest in development and evolution, emerging in large part from Gould's 1977 book, *Ontogeny and Phylogeny*. In the recent program for research proposed by Wake and Larson (1987), these two overlapping emphases are described as *structuralist* and *Darwinian* approaches. Basically, the first is concerned with developmental integration and the constraints and directionality which may be imposed on evolutionary change, while the second is focused on adaptive evolutionary transformations arising from selection for improved performance in particular ecological contexts. Both of these frameworks require detailed reconstruction of phylogenetic relationships, and thus systematic theory plays a central role in structuralist or Darwinian undertakings (Lauder, 1981). That these broad areas of evolutionary theory and change are not independent should be obvious; indeed, the developmental relationships which may come to direct and constrain patterns of change are in all likelihood normally the result of both internal and external selection (e.g., Reidl, 1975; Buss, 1987). Nevertheless, workers generally concentrate on one realm or the other, and our subsequent discussion will also be organized along these lines.

Bone Growth and Adaptation

Changes in bone form or composition during ontogeny can and should be as much the object of analyses of adaptation by evolutionary morphologists as are interspecific adult differences. However, relatively few studies of form/function interrelationships have focused on bone growth, as opposed to static adult comparisons, and this is particularly true for investigations of primate morphology. That such work can reveal much about the function of bones and related structures is nicely illustrated by Carrier's (1983) study of changes in postcranial skeletal dimensions, mechanical properties of bone, and contractile properties of muscle during ontogeny in jack rabbits.

The framework for assessing evolutionary adaptations proposed by Arnold (1983) can easily be extended to the realm of ontogenetic transformations, as I discuss in more detail in Shea (1990). In this framework, heritable ontogenetic transformations within and between species would be mapped onto gradients of performance and fitness variation to assess adaptation. At present, there are no examples of which I am aware in primatology that have rigorously applied such an approach to adult morphological variation, let alone ontogenetic trajectories. Hopefully, this will be an area of major work in the next several decades, for comparative ontogenetic analyses offer a wonderful opportunity to integrate the evolutionary themes of development, constraint, function, selection, and fitness (Shea, 1990).

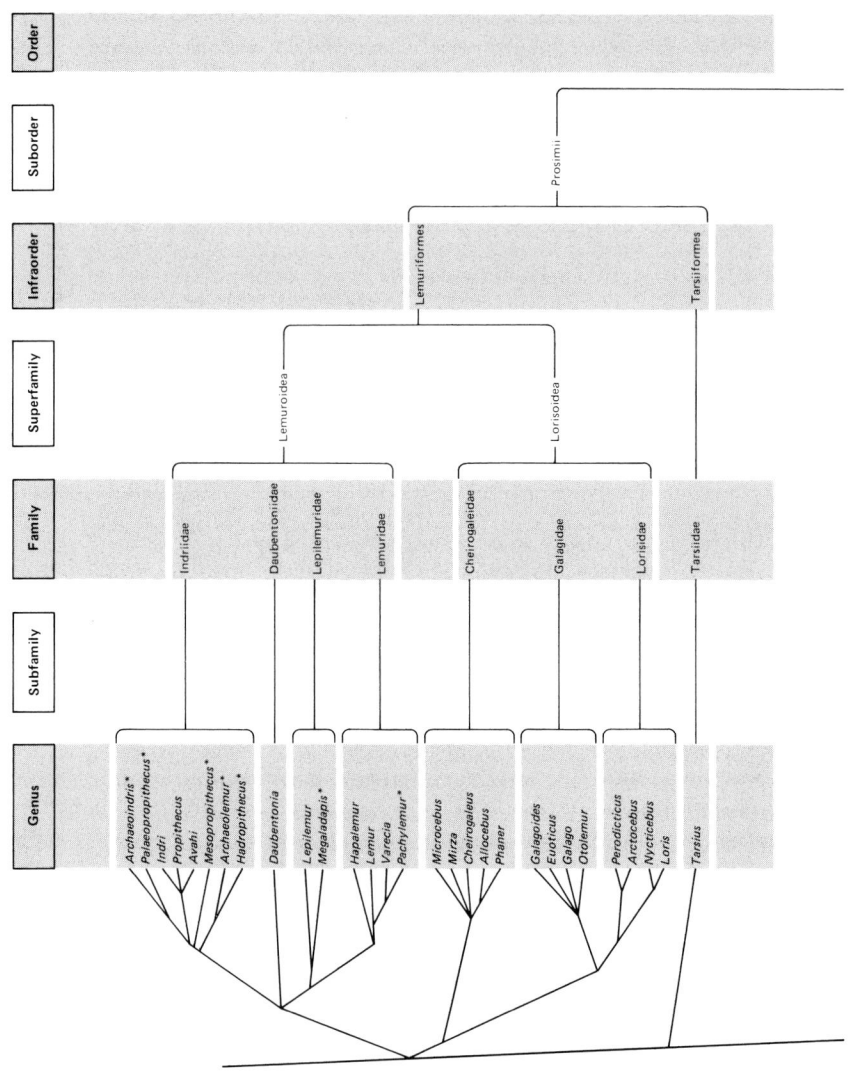

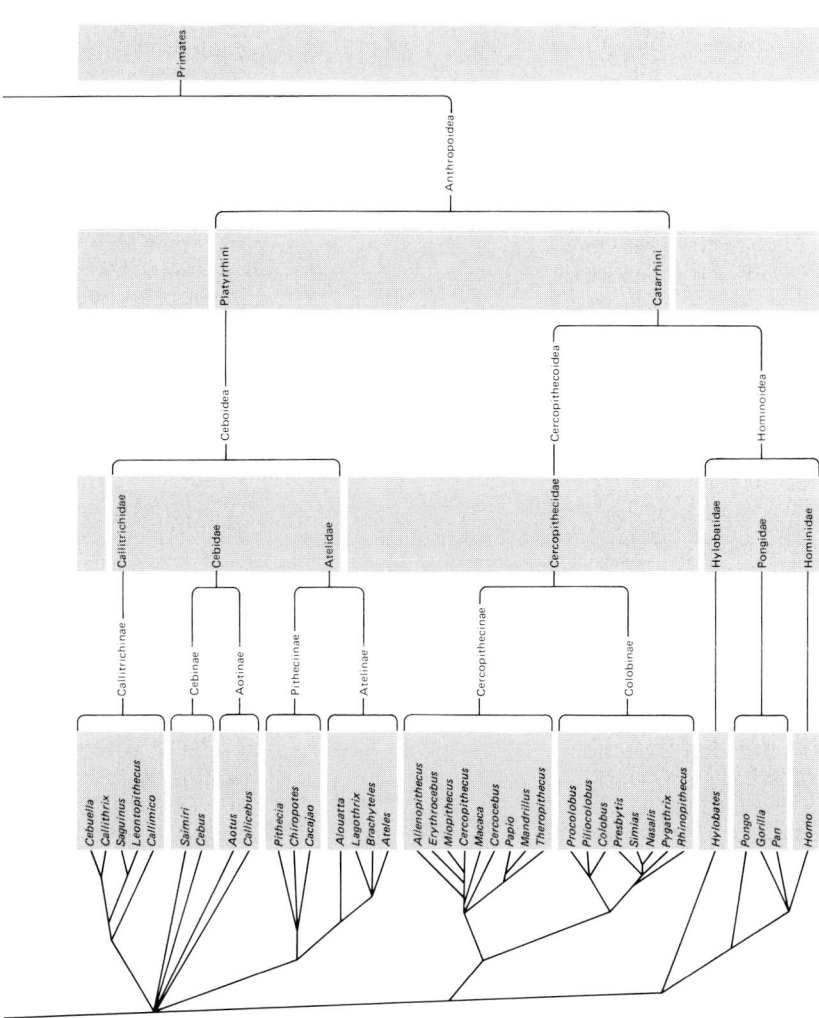

Fig. 1. An outline of one classification and hypothesis of phylogenetic relationships within the order Primates. (From Fleagle, 1988. With permission.)

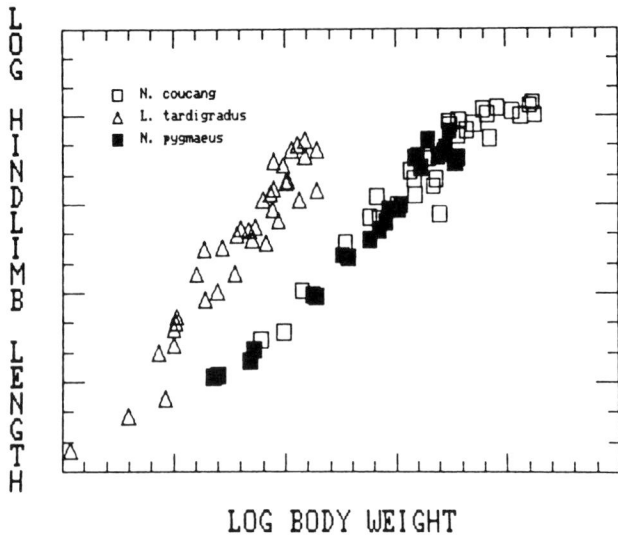

LOG BODY WEIGHT

Fig. 2. Patterns of ontogenetic allometry of hindlimb length in three lorisid species. Note that the proportion differences between *N. coucang* and *N. pygmaeus* result from ontogenetic scaling, while those between *L. tardigradus* and the two *Nycticebus* species clearly do not. (From Gomez, 1992. With permission.)

An alternative though somewhat less robust approach to the study of adaptation during growth is the comparative approach, where morphological differences are correlated with ecological variations or inferred functional differences. In such cases, the use of growth allometry provides the most effective and rigorous *criterion of subtraction* (Gould, 1966, 1975), since once again this approach contains more information than is available in static adult data sets. I have discussed the use of ontogenetic allometry as a criterion of subtraction, and provided selected examples from bone growth in primates, in Shea (1985a, 1988). Fig. 2 illustrates an example from Gomez (1989), nicely demonstrating that, while adult proportion differences between slow lorises (*Nycticebus coucang*) and pygmy slow lorises (*N. pygmaeus*) result from simple ontogenetic scaling, those adult proportion differences between the slow lorises and the slender loris (*Loris tardigradus*) represent nonsize-related shifts. The growth allometric approach thus highlights the latter proportion differences as potential special adaptations related to locomotor differences (Gomez, 1989).

An additional recent application of some of these approaches is seen in Ravosa's (1988, 1991a, b, c) work on circumorbital and brow ridge morphology in primates. This project was designed to test, via comparative allometric analyses, the many previous claims that variation in supraorbital morphology among primates is related to biomechanical variables thought

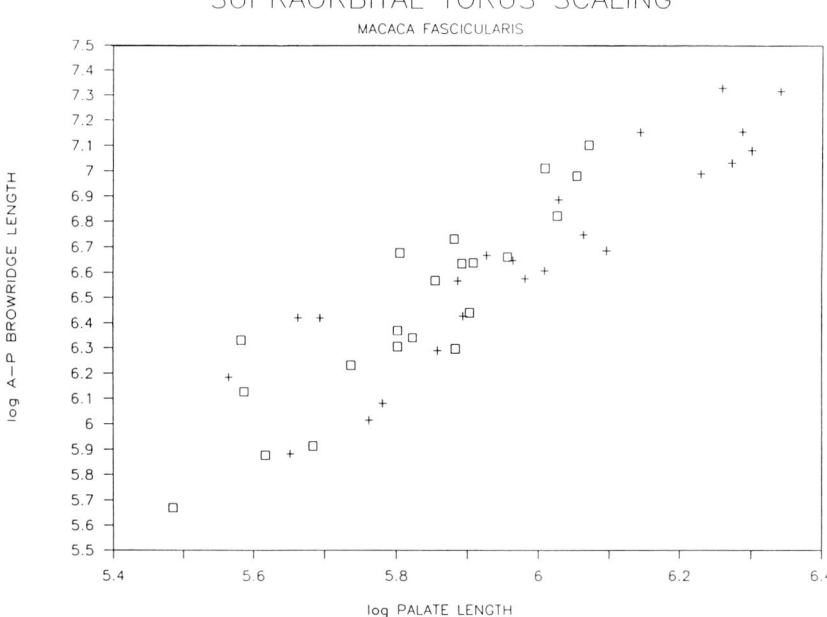

Fig. 3. Ontogenetic allometry of browridge length against overall skull size (palate length) in male and female *Macaca fascicularis*. (From Ravosa, 1991b. With permission.)

to reflect the stresses produced by anterior dental loading and other aspects of masticatory function. In particular, Oyen *et al.* (1979) have argued that the gross structure as well as the pattern and timing of bone deposition in the supraorbital region of growing baboons is directly responsive to changing stresses produced by shifts in load/lever relations of the gnathic region. Using size-corrected values of brow ridge form and variables reflecting potential biomechanical relations, Ravosa (1991a) concluded that simple allometric factors were the primary determinant of variation in brow ridge size among adult primates, with only one or two biomechanical variables exhibiting significant correlations. In an ontogenetic series of crab-eating macaques, *Macaca fascicularis*, Ravosa (1991b) found no correlation between regression-adjusted residuals of brow ridge size and residuals of composite biomechanical variables, again suggesting that overall body and skull size were the most important influences on brow ridge morphology. Fig. 3 illustrates the scaling of brow size against overall skull size in growth sequences of male and female macaques — the ontogenetic criterion of subtraction reveals that the relatively larger browridges of males result from their larger size, and not special intersexual differences (Ravosa, 1991b). Research integrating these growth allometric approaches with experimentally derived determinations of bite forces, muscle activity patterns, and bone strain levels would be a most valuable contribution.

Studies of growth allometry of the limb skeleton (measured either directly on dry bones or reflected in external anthropometrics between bony landmarks on living animals) have been used to make functional inferences about patterns of locomotion and support in primates. Jungers and Fleagle (1980) demonstrated contrasting patterns of postnatal growth allometry in two species of cebus monkeys, resulting in relatively shorter limbs in the stockier *Cebus apella* as compared to *C. albifrons*. They view these differences in growth trajectories and terminal proportions as adaptive modifications related to the more cursorial and mobile activities of *C. albifrons*, as contrasted with the powerful foraging and feeding behavior of *C. apella*. Other examples of primate limb growth studies from a functional perspective include Schultz (1930), Lumer (1939), Grand (1983), Shea (1981), Buschang (1982), Jantz and Owsley (1984), Jungers and Susman (1984), and Gomez (1989, 1992) (see also Allometry and Heterochrony).

Bone Growth and Phylogenetic Reconstruction

Investigations of bone growth can make important contributions to the study of phylogeny reconstruction in primates and other forms. Ontogenetic analyses are the primary means for distinguishing between similarity resulting from *homology* (shared features inherited from a common ancestor) and that due to *homoplasy* (shared features not inherited from a common ancestor and produced by parallelism, convergence, or reversals). Studies of growth allometry have also been used to control for size differences in assessing morphological features of systematic interest.

One of the most persistent and significant debates in primatology over the past several decades has involved the identification of bony synapomorphies defining the order, along with the important related classificatory issue of where (and why) to draw the ordinal boundary. Cartmill (1982) reviews these issues from a historical perspective. The formation of an auditory bulla as an outgrowth of the petrosal bone (see Fig. 4 for illustration of this and other structural configurations) has been given as an important defining characteristic of the order Primates (e.g., Szalay, 1972), though all workers agree that we know little about any potential functional significance regarding the different pathways seen in mammals for enclosing the middle ear region.

A recent contribution drawing on knowledge of bone formation and growth in the basicranium of primates and other mammals has advocated a rejection of the "petrosal bulla" as an acceptable defining characteristic of the primates (MacPhee *et al.*, 1983). The developmental justification for this de-

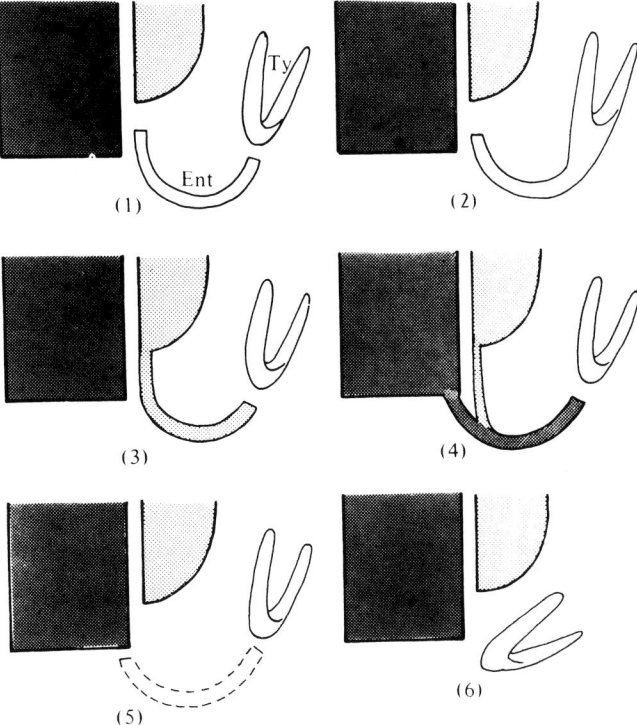

Fig. 4. A schematic diagram illustrating various structural configurations of the mammalian auditory bulla in coronal section. (1) Ossified entotympanic bulla; (2) tympanic bulla; (3) petrosal bulla; (4) basisphenoid or alisphenoid bulla; (5) cartilaginous bulla; (6) bulla absent (membranous bulla). Dark shading = basisphenoid or alisphenoid; light shading = periotic; broken outline = cartilage; Ent = entotympanic bone; Ty = tympanic bone. (After Novacek, 1977. With permission.)

cision essentially relates to the claim that we cannot determine the composition of the bulla from the adult bony morphology (which is all we have available in the fragmentary fossil forms of the Paleocene). Developmental studies of the basicranium have demonstrated that the bulla originates in the fetus as an outgrowth of the ossifying petrosal in all euprimates investigated (MacPhee, 1979, 1981). However, since some mammals develop a non-petrosal bulla that fuses seamlessly with the petrosal in later postnatal life, MacPhee *et al.* (1983) argue that we cannot reliably infer the bulla's origin from an absence of sutures in adults. On the basis of this and other evidence, they conclude that the fossil plesiadapiforms of the early Cenozoic of Europe and North America cannot be definitively linked with the "euprimates" (the first primates "of modern aspect" plus all extant primates), and they opt for an organization of primates into several major *grades*, a scheme compatible with Cartmill's (1972, 1974, 1982) earlier taxonomy where the plesiadapiforms are not included within the Order Primates. A detailed review of the relevant anatomy in primates and other taxa, as well as important discussion of related issues, is given in MacPhee and Cartmill (1986).

This example nicely illustrates how a knowledge of bone development and growth can provide a novel perspective on central issues in primate systematics. MacPhee's (1977) ontogenetic studies also clarify the transformational differences between the configurations characterizing the lemuriform (intrabullar tympanic) and lorisiform (extrabullar tympanic) primates. Basic differences in sutural tissue formation underlie the differences in adult configurations (fetal lemuriforms lack a tissue layer, thus making the suture between the petrosal plate and tympanic bone less "stable" and providing a simple mechanism for the transformation from intrabullar to extrabullar states). Of course, the detractors of MacPhee *et al.* (1983) will emphasize that their argument is essentially keyed to negative evidence, and one can always disrupt previously accepted phylogenetic linkages by simply hypothesizing (as opposed to demonstrating) that adult similarities might in fact not prove to be homologous once extensive developmental investigations are undertaken.

An additional example of the potential phylogenetic implications of divergent patterns of cranial bone growth is seen in discussions of paranasal sinuses in anthropoids. Bone growth in the face and skullbase is related to the development of paranasal and mastoid air sinuses, although many details of this relationship are unknown. Cave and Haines (1940) investigated the ontogenetic development of paranasal sinus formation in selected higher primates and produced evidence directly relevant to the important systematic issue of the relationships among the large-bodied hominoids. This debate has been rekindled through various inputs in recent years, including of course the biomolecular data (e.g., Sibley and Alquist, 1987), as well as specific suggestions which run counter to current orthodoxy, such as a linking of all the great apes to the exclusion of *Homo* (Kluge, 1983), or *Homo* plus *Pongo* to the exclusion of the other hominoids (Schwartz, 1985a, b). The usefulness of the developmental perspective of Cave and Haines (1940) emerges in a consideration of the frontal sinus as a synapomorphy linking African apes and humans to the exclusion of orangutans and the lesser apes (Fig. 5). African apes and humans appear to be the only groups which have an *ethmoidally derived* frontal sinus (even though some other forms, such as orangutans and *Proconsul africanus*, may exhibit considerable pneumatization of the frontal bone).

Schultz (1936) demonstrated that the timing of fusion of the developing wrist bones could be used to link chimpanzees, gorillas, and humans to the exclusion of the Asian hominoids (orangutans and gibbons). In the African

(a)   (b)

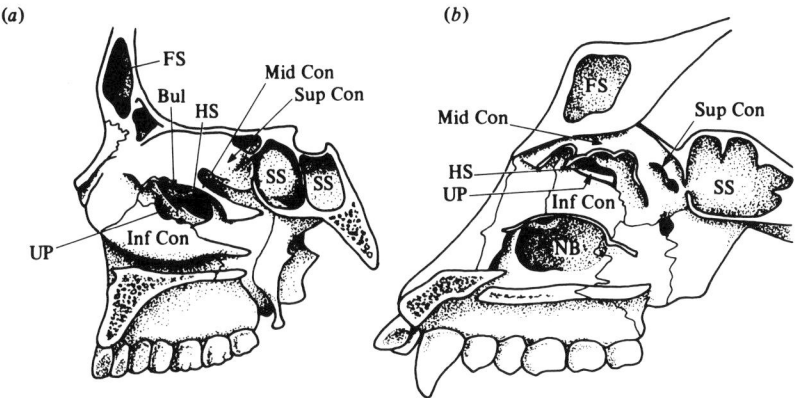

Fig. 5. Sagittal sections illustrating the right lateral wall of the nasal cavity in humans (a) and gorillas (b). The inferior, middle, and superior conchae have been resected. FS = frontal sinus; SS = sphenoid sinus; UP = uncinate process; HS = hiatus semilunaris; NB = nasolacrimal bulla; Bul = ethmoid bulla. (From Moore, 1981. With permission.)

group, the os centrale and navicular bones fuse early (usually prenatally), resulting in eight carpal bones; in orangutans and gibbons these bones fuse later in life, and in the monkeys not at all (Watts, 1986).

Bromage's (1985, 1990, 1992) use of scanning electron microscopy (SEM) to analyze facial remodeling during growth in fossil hominids and extant humans also illustrates the phylogenetic significance of ontogenetic studies. Although metric analyses of linear dimensions and proportions have indicated some similarity between skulls of the robust australopiths (*Australopithecus boisei*, *A. robustus*) and other early hominids thought to be more closely related to modern humans, Bromage's SEM analysis reveals fundamental differences in the ontogenetic patterns of facial resorption and deposition between members of our own lineage and our specialized robust relatives. These growth studies suggest that the proportional similarity is a result of homoplasy (parallelism) rather than homologous synapomorphy, and probably relates to the masticatory specializations of the robust australopiths.

A number of investigations have used basic patterns of growth allometry as input to systematic problems. Among the primates, we have no such striking examples of this utility as in the case of living and extinct reptiles, where growth allometry has been used to collapse multi-species and even multi-genera taxonomies into a potential single-species growth sequence (e.g., Dodson, 1975; Grine *et al.*, 1978; Tollman *et al.*, 1980). Nevertheless, in one of the earliest investigations of skeletal growth allometry in primates, Giles (1956) demonstrated that chimpanzees and gorillas shared common patterns of growth allometry to the exclusion of orangutans. Jungers and Hartman (1988) have also used skeletal growth data to assess phylogenetic relationships among extant large-bodied hominoids. They compared bivariate and multivariate patterns of growth allometry of the postcranial skeleton in orangutans, gorillas, chimpanzees, bonobos, and humans, and found natural "allometric clusters" which in fact did not coincide with the bulk of accumulated biomolecular and morphological data (in grouping the African apes with orangutans as opposed to humans, and chimpanzees with gorillas as opposed to bonobos). Rather, the clustering reflected functional associations and specializations, such as the positive allometry of hindlimb length in humans (Fig. 6). As the authors note, these findings suggest caution in drawing phylogenetic inferences from a limited set of data, and this warning is of course no more or less appropriate to growth allometric coefficients than to static adult proportions or characters.

My own studies of growth allometry in African apes were not set up as a test of phylogeny, and thus neither humans nor orangutans were included (Shea, 1981, 1982, 1983a, 1985a). Nevertheless, my results contrast with those of Jungers and Hartman (1988) in clearly linking bonobos with common chimpanzees to the exclusion of gorillas. This is true for both a comparison of postcranial skeletal growth allometric coefficients in bivariate comparisons (Shea, 1982) as well as bivariate and multivariate cranial comparisons (Figs. 7 and 8). These somewhat divergent results probably reflect the fact that Jungers and Hartman based their assessment of similarity of allometric patterns on bivariate and multivariate coefficients of growth allometry alone, as opposed to comparisons of both slope and position differences. It is differences in position ("y intercept") values which most clearly separate the growth allometries of *Gorilla* from the two species of *Pan*. A comparative growth allometric study of scapula dimensions also clearly links the two chimpanzees to the exclusion of gorillas (Shea, 1986a).

As a general rule, I would argue that the data derived from growth allometric comparisons are of superior value in studies of phylogeny construction, since they contain all the information present in the more traditional static adult data, but also include otherwise unavailable data reflecting dynamic growth processes. However, the diversity of structures and systems sampled, and the accurate recognition of homologies and polarities, will be the most significant determinants of the ultimate worth of the phylogenetic inference, just as in cases based solely on adult data. The ontogenetic data play a key role in this determination of homology and polarity.

Bone Growth and the Evolution of Growth Patterns

Investigation of the growth of the bony skeleton, as any other bodily system, may be undertaken for what it reveals about more general patterns of growth, development, and maturation. Much of Schultz's work on primate skeletal growth was integrated with life history data for this purpose. More

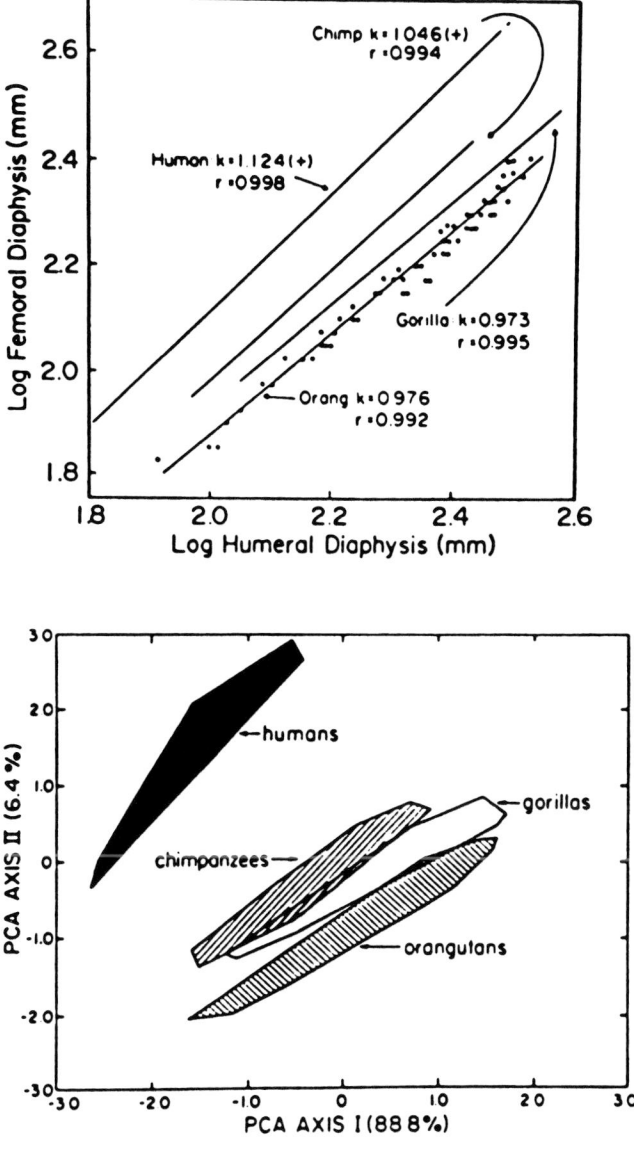

Fig. 6. Results from ontogenetic bivariate allometry (above) and multivariate principal components analyses (below), illustrating the distinctiveness of the human postcranium (and especially the lower limb) relative to the great apes. (From Jungers and Hartman, 1988. With permission.)

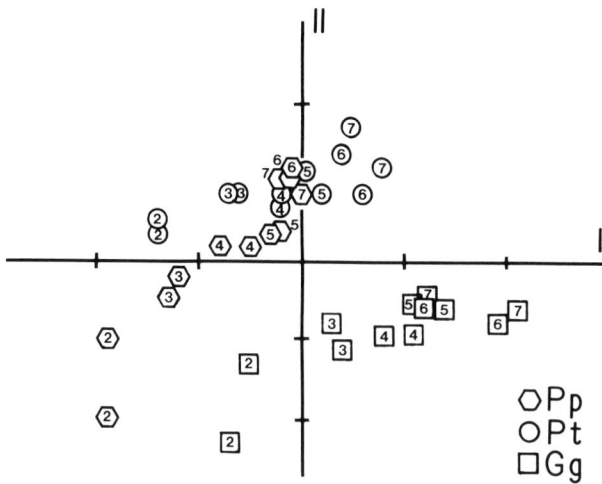

Fig. 7. Results of a principal components analysis of growth allometry in 55 cranial dimensions in *Pan paniscus* (Pp), *P. troglodytes* (Pt), and *Gorilla gorilla* (Gg). Note the clumping of the two chimpanzee species and the separation of the gorillas (see text and Shea, 1983a, for additional discussion). (From Shea, 1983a.)

recently, Watts (1986, 1988) has been a primary contributor to this research. Her excellent review paper on prenatal and postnatal skeletal development in primates (Watts, 1986) should be consulted for many further details and examples. The work of Schultz (1969), Watts, and many others has suggested that among catarrhine primates (Old World monkeys, apes, and humans) there exists a clear phylogenetic trend toward an overall delay in the timing of ossification, with relatively little divergence in the ossification sequences themselves. This pattern corresponds to other developmental and life history data (Schultz, 1969). However, a broader perspective suggests that this apparent trend may largely be a reflection of advanced skeletal ossification in cercopithecoid monkeys, since the degree of skeletal development in newborn humans, ceboid (New World) monkeys, tarsiers, and prosimians is quite comparable (Watts, 1986). Much additional empirical work is required, but such comparative studies highlight the evolutionary novelty of the cercopithecoid pattern and help establish a framework for further investigation in this group of monkeys.

Allometry and Heterochrony

One of the most promising areas for the application of studies of bone growth to problems in primate evolutionary biology lies in the investigation of heterochrony, or evolutionary changes resulting from shifts in the rate or

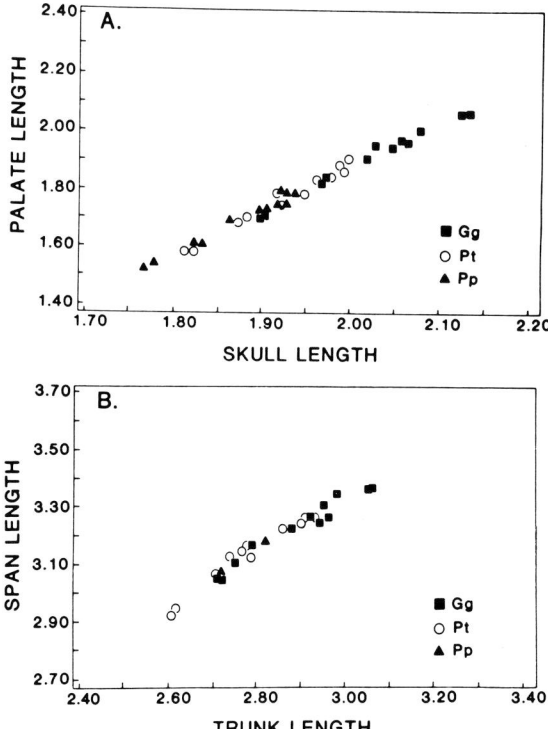

Fig. 8. Representative illustrations of ontogenetic scaling of cranial (A) and postcranial (B) proportions in pygmy chimpanzees (Pp), common chimpanzees (Pt), and gorillas (Gg). For B, span = maximum distance between the fingers of the outstretched arms in wild-shot animals and trunk = crown-rump length (see Shea, 1981).

timing of ancestral developmental patterns (DeBeer, 1930; Rensch, 1959; Gould, 1977; Alberch *et al.*, 1979). Although heterochronic approaches can make important contributions to various realms of evolutionary biology, including functional morphology and systematics, I see their primary application in the area of processes and patterns of both integration and change in morphologies and life histories. Heterochrony provides two particularly important insights for the morphologist — first, an understanding of when a series of integrated features change in concert as a result of selection on a particular developmental process (e.g., size change, rate of shape change) and, second, the realization that broad morphological transformations may result from selection for shifts in life history features (e.g., duration of growth, time to maturation). It is this focus on the dynamic processes underlying morphological integration, coordinated transformation, and diversification which is the strength of heterochronic approaches, though clearly we also need an understanding of the genetic and epigenetic mechanisms driving the processes of covariation and dissociation. For these reasons, I believe an approach based on allometry and heterochrony is preferable to the more descriptive framework utilized by Schultz and others in studies of bone growth, since such tends to treat bony dimensions or elements in isolation.

The work of Gould (1977) provided impetus for a resurgence of interest in the relationships between growth and patterns of adult morphological diversification among the primates, as with other groups of organisms. The bulk of my own research has focused on bone growth in the context of allometry and heterochrony. The empirical work for various body regions and taxa are presented in Shea (1981, 1983a to d, 1984, 1985a, b, 1986a, b), Shea et al. (1987), Shea and Gomez (1988), and several papers in preparation (Shea and Pagezy, 1988; Shea and Bailey, 1989). Other discussions which consider more of the broad evolutionary implications of this and related work are given in Shea (1985a, 1988, 1990b). Elsewhere (Shea, 1989) I have discussed in detail perhaps the best-known application of a heterochronic interpretation of primate evolutionary change, i.e., the long-debated case of human neoteny (see Gould, 1977 and Montagu, 1981, for historical reviews and proponents' views). I will not review my analysis here except to point out that it is really a better understanding of the processes and patterns of bony growth in humans and our close relatives that has produced much of the recent data which together suggests to me that pedomorphosis via neoteny has not played a central role in human evolution. Interestingly, these same recent results have actually strengthened heterochronic interpretations of other evolutionary transformations in primates (see Shea, 1988, and the present discussion).

This work has illustrated how a detailed knowledge of bone growth can elucidate interspecific and phylogenetic patterns of adult morphological diversification. Ontogenetic scaling, or the extension and truncation of common patterns of growth allometry (Gould, 1975), has been shown to play a prominent role in producing adult shape differences covariant with overall size changes. Fig. 8 illustrates two such cases, one of facial proportions in chimpanzees and gorillas, and one of postcranial proportions in chimpanzees and gorillas. Elsewhere, I have discussed these and additional cases in the African apes and other primates, and the reader is referred to Shea (1985a, 1988, 1990) for additional information.

A considerable body of work which analyzes patterns of growth allometry in interspecific primate series is now emerging, though much of it is in preparation or in the initial stages of publication. Some recent examples include studies of limb proportions in New World monkeys (Levitch, 1986; Leutenegger and Larson, 1985), bony proportions of the hominoid foot (Manley-Buser, 1986), cranial and postcranial proportions in cercopithecine monkeys of different sizes (Shea, 1988), and cranial proportions in lesser apes (Shea, 1988). Gomez (1992) has recently published results from an interesting study of growth allometry of the postcranial skeleton in three species of lorises (*Loris tardigradus*, the slender loris, *Nycticebus coucang*, the slow loris, and *N. pygmaeus*, the pygmy slow loris). Adults of these species differ significantly in various limb and body proportions, and these have previously been the basis for speculation concerning possible differences in locomotor adaptations among these lorisines. However, the comparative growth allometric approach revealed that the shape differences between adult slow lorises and pygmy slow lorises result from ontogenetic scaling, and thus directly result from the differences in terminal adult size. This study also nicely illustrates the value of growth allometric approaches in assessing non-size-related changes, since the shape differences between the adult slender lorises (*Loris*) and slow lorises (*Nycticebus*) were clearly not simple concomitants of ontogenetic scaling. Fig. 2 summarizes the results of Gomez's comparisons of these lorisines. This intriguing case study may also involve significant timing differences, since preliminary data suggest that adult *N. pygmaeus* mature earlier than *N. coucang* (Gomez, personal communication), thus providing a case of time hypomorphosis (Shea, 1983b), or progenesis (Gould, 1977). If further investigation corroborates these apparent differences, this will be the clearest example of this particular type of heterochronic and allometric transformation within the primates. The implications for our understanding of bone growth in primates are straightforward but fundamental — adult shape differences may be consequences of allometric growth patterns and shifts in terminal adult size, and this size change may itself be a secondary result of selection for earlier maturation and growth cessation.

A number of recent studies have also applied an allometric and heterochronic perspective to morphological differences in bony size and shape between the sexes, following the approach and rationale advocated by Shea (1983b, 1986b). Cochard (1985) examined male and female skull shape in *Macaca mulatta* using growth allometric approaches, and found that almost all the adult intersexual shape differences (save nuchal crest thickness and bizygomatic breadth) were the result of ontogenetic scaling, or the sharing of common patterns of growth allometry. In a subsequent study, Cheverud and Richtsmeier (1986) applied finite-element scaling methods to sexual dimorphism in skull growth in *M. mulatta*. As in Cochard's (1985) study, they found that females and males generally shared common patterns of size/shape change. Because males and females exhibited increases in bony dimensions for approximately the same length of time (with the males exhibiting a higher rate throughout), Cheverud and Richtsmeier (1986) characterized the size and shape differences in the facial region as resulting from rate hypermorphosis (Shea, 1983b).

Leigh and Cheverud (1989) report a comparable study of growth and sexual dimorphism in the baboon skull, which exhibits considerable shape differentiation between the sexes, particularly in the gnathic region. Results correspond to the macaque case in that males and females generally share comparable allometric trajectories, with males attaining larger terminal sizes. Timing of growth cessation (or at least marked slowing) exhibited clearer differences between the sexes than with the macaques. In heterochronic terminology, the allometric extrapolation and growth prolongation in the males would be an example of time hypermorphosis (Shea, 1983b), though of course there is also some contribution of rate differentiation (i.e., rate hypermorphosis) here. These findings support the claim, based on weight growth, that the increased sexual dimorphism in baboons as compared with the closely related macaques, involves a significant increase in sexual bimaturism (Shea, 1986b). It is worth pointing out in this context that the many studies of sexual dimorphism using (static adult) allometric approaches and explanations actually are implicitly underlain by assumptions about growth allometric patterns. Examples include Wood (1976) and Albrecht (1978). However, it is now well-appreciated that there are both theoretical and statistical problems associated with inferring growth allometries from static adult comparisons (see Shea, 1981, 1983c), and thus such studies would be more firmly based if they included full ontogenetic comparisons.

Work in progress by Ravosa (1991c) on the cercopithecine *M. fascicularis* and the colobine *Nasalis larvatus* demonstrates that within each species males and females typically follow identical ontogenetic trajectories. Here again, shape differences between adults of the two sexes result from hypermorphosis (reflecting predominantly or at least significantly time hypermorphosis). Recent work on cranial dimorphism in the orangutan by Leutenegger and Masterson (1989) also indicates a predominant component of size and shape differences resulting from ontogenetic scaling and an extension of duration of growth in males.

In the African apes, a heterochronic investigation of cross-sectional bone growth has suggested that the increased dimorphism in *Gorilla* as compared with *Pan* is primarily the result of an increase in sexual bimaturism (probably due both to prolonged male growth and truncated female growth, Shea, 1985b). In other cases, perhaps *Cercopithecus* monkeys and close relatives, increased dimorphism appears to be produced only by rate differentiation, with no increase in bimaturism. Leutenegger and Larson (1985) analyzed sexual dimorphism in the postcranial skeleton of cebus (*Cebus*) and squirrel (*Saimiri*) monkeys of the New World, and found that the primary intersexual differences of size and shape were the result of time hypermorphosis. Dwarf slow lorises, *Nycticebus pygmaeus*, exhibit marked dimorphism compared to their larger congeners, *N. coucang*, and this appears to result from increased bimaturism and time hypermorphosis, primarily reflecting early female maturation and growth truncation (Gomez, personal communication). This case bucks the common trend of increased dimorphism with greater body size, at least among close relatives (Rensch, 1959), and thus may prove to be a particularly interesting situation.

Elsewhere I have discussed some of the theoretical bases for analyzing sexual dimorphism from the perspective of growth and heterochrony (Shea, 1986b, 1988) and reviewed some other examples of primate dimorphism. The primary advantage of such an approach, whether focused on bone growth or growth of some other system, is that it elucidates the processes of differentiation which yield the terminal results of adult dimorphism. Because comparable terminal results may be underlain by quite different developmental processes, these reflecting divergent selective foci, life history strategies, and ecological contexts, it is imperative to maintain an ontogenetic perspective on differences between the sexes (Shea, 1986b). This will be an important area of future work in primatology, particularly if combined with longitudinal field studies of individual animals (Shea, 1990).

The order Primates is rife with possibilities for similar intraspecific and interspecific analyses of bone growth in allometric and heterochronic contexts. This is particularly true within the strepsirhine primates, since these have received much less attention than the haplorhines, which include tarsiers, monkeys, apes, and humans. Examples of interesting variation in size, shape, and timing parameters abound within various primate lineages, and there are also many as-yet unexamined cases of dwarfism and gigantism among closely related pairs. Analyses of bone growth in these instances will undoubtedly increase our understanding of both the patterns and processes of shape differentiation within our order, and also permit an elucidation of the fossil record (Shea, 1988, 1990).

The process of morphological diversification via ontogenetic scaling is intimately related to the various themes of developmental constraints (Maynard Smith et al., 1985), historical factors (Lauder, 1981), and structuralist approaches to morphological transformations (Wake and Larson, 1987). This is because underlying allometric relations may impart a directionality to evolutionary change, which helps explain why allometry was frequently involved in the classic cases of purported orthogenesis (see Simpson, 1953). More specifically, changes in overall size and/or duration of growth periods (due either to selection or random changes) will result in complex and novel shape configurations which are determined by the integrated covariation of growing parts inherited by descendants from their ancestors. Of course, it is important to stress that such patterns of size/shape covariation are probably not unrelated to changing function during ontogeny (see above and Shea, 1985a). Furthermore, such directional trends do not necessarily reflect especially strong or "deep" constraints, growth allometries themselves presumably being previously the product, and currently the potential target, of natural selection (Maynard Smith et al., 1985). The important themes of covariation and constraint point to the central issue of the genetic and epigenetic *controls* of bone growth, and how shifts in these controls produce integrated changes in bony morphology.

Control of Bone Growth — Evolutionary Implications

The investigation of both the intrinsic and extrinsic controls of bone growth is a fascinating area about which relatively little is known, but which will undoubtedly have important implications for our understanding of evolutionary processes and patterns. Studies of bone development and growth in primates have contributed relatively little to this area (Hall, 1982b), perhaps understandably, considering the size, expense, and duration of primate growth periods. However, it is certainly true that our general understanding of the controls of bone growth find important applications in the study of primate evolution, as with other taxonomic groupings.

Aspects of the control of bone growth have been reviewed by Moss (1972, 1973), Hall (1982a, b, c, 1983), Bryant and Simpson (1984), and Thomson (1988), among others. Hall (1982c) stresses two important points regarding an understanding of the differentiation, morphogenesis, and growth of bony structures: (1) these must be studied at all levels of biological organization, from molecules to whole organisms and (2) both intrinsic factors (such as intrinsic rate and polarization of cell division, initial number of stem cells in skeletal condensations, position-specific cell interactions, etc.) and extrinsic factors (such as division rates of chondroblasts, osteoblasts, and myoblasts mediated by hormones or epigenetic interaction with adjacent tissues, etc.) must be clearly explicated. Evolutionary changes in morphology can emerge from shifts in growth controls at any of these levels. Hall (1982b, c, 1984) utilizes the various known and potential developmental bases of changes in mandibular form in mammals and other animals as an example of the evolutionary implications of shifts in these developmental controls. It is probably generally true that changes in the controlling factors operative early in development will produce substantially greater morphological transformations than those occurring during later development. Thomson (1988) provides interesting general discussion of the evolutionary implications of changes at various points in morphogenesis.

The point I wish to stress here is that most of the allometric and heterochronic transformations discussed above probably result from shifts in extrinsic growth controls operating relatively late in development. Although Gould (1971) suggested that shifts in extrinsic control factors such as systemic growth hormones might underlie global dissociations of allometric patterns to produce generalized *isometric* transformations, accumulated evidence makes it more likely that shifts in growth hormone (GH) and insulin-like growth factor 1 (IGF-1) levels result in ontogenetic scaling, or global *allometric* transformations (Shea, 1988; Shea et al., 1987; Shea and Gomez, 1988). It remains to be investigated whether overall size differences within species, and among closely related species, can be linked directly to shifts in GH and IGF-1 levels, though existing data provide considerable evidence for such an association (Eigenmann et al., 1984a; Masoud et al., 1985;

Pidduck and Falconer, 1978; Althen and Gerrits, 1976; Sinha *et al.*, 1975; Merimee *et al.*, 1987; Palmiter *et al.*, 1983; Blair *et al.*, 1987). An understanding of the role that systemic growth control substances play in mediating complex and coordinated patterns of allometric growth during development elucidates the evolutionary patterns of ontogenetic scaling frequently seen in comparative series or the fossil record (Gould, 1966, 1977; Frazzetta, 1975; Shea, 1985a). As further advances are made in the study of the controls of bone growth at various levels of morphogenesis, we can expect to clarify many other aspects of changes in the size and shape of bones in evolutionary comparisons.

References

Alberch, P., Gould, S. J., Oster, G. F., and Wake, D. B. (1979). Size and shape in ontogeny and phylogeny. *Paleobiology*, **5**: 296–317.

Albrecht, G. H. (1978). The craniofacial morphology of the Sulawesi macaques. *Contr. Primatol.*, **13**: 1–111.

Althen, T. G. and Gerritts, R. J. (1976). Pituitary and serum growth hormone levels in Duroc and Yorkshire swine genetically selected for high and low backfat. *J. Anim. Sci.*, **42**: 1490–1497.

Arnold, S. (1983). Morphology, performance and fitness. *Am. Zool.*, **23**: 347–361.

Baird, D. M., Nalbandov, A. V., and Norton, H. W. (1952). Some physiological causes of genetically different rates of growth in swine. *J. Anim. Sci.*, **11**: 292–300.

Blair, H. T., McCutcheon, S. N., Mackenzie, D. D. S., Gluckman, P. D., and Ormsby, J. E. (1987). Variation in plasma concentration of insulin-like growth factor-1 and its covariation with liveweight in mice. *Aust. J. Biol. Sci.*, **40**: 287–293.

Bromage, T. G. (1990). Ontogeny and phylogeny of the human face. In: *Primate Life History and Evolution*. DeRousseau, J., Ed., Alan R. Liss, New York, 105–114.

Bromage, T. G. (1992). Ontogeny of *Pan troglodytes* craniofacial architectural relationships and their implications for early hominids. *J. Hum. Evol.*, **23**: 000–000.

Bryant, P. J. and Simpson, P. (1984). Intrinsic and extrinsic control of growth in developing organs. *Q. Rev. Biol.*, **59**: 387–415.

Buschang, P. H. (1982). The relative growth of the limb bones for *Homo sapiens* — as compared to anthropoid apes. *Primates*, **23**: 465–468.

Buss, L. W. (1987). *The Evolution of Individuality*. Princeton University Press, Princeton, New Jersey.

Carrier, D. R (1983). Postnatal ontogeny of the musculo-skeletal system in the black-tailed jack rabbit (*Lepus californicus*). *J. Zool.*, **201**: 27–55.

Cartmill, M. (1972). Arboreal adaptations and the origin of the order Primates. In: *The Functional and Evolutionary Biology of Primates*. Tuttle, R. H., Ed., Aldine, Chicago, 97–122.

Cartmill, M. (1974). Rethinking primate origins. *Science*, **184**: 436–443.

Cave, A. J. E. and Haines, R. W. (1940). The paranasal sinuses of the anthropoid apes. *J. Anat.*, **74**: 493–523.

Cheverud, J. M. and Richtsmeier, J. T. (1986). Finite-element scaling applied to sexual dimorphism in rhesus macaque (*Macaca mulatta*) facial growth. *Syst. Zool.*, **35**: 381–399.

Cochard, L. R. (1985). Ontogenetic allometry of the skull and dentition of the rhesus monkey (*Macaca mulatta*). In: *Size and Scaling in Primate Biology.* Jungers, W. L., Ed., Plenum Press, New York, 231–255.

DeBeer, G. R. (1930). *Embryology and Evolution.* Clarendon Press, Oxford.

Dodson, P. (1975). Taxonomic implications of relative growth in lambeosaurine hadrosaurs. *Syst. Zool.,* **24**: 37–54.

Eigenmann, J. E., Patterson, D. F., Zapf, J., and Froesch, E. R. (1984a). Insulin-like growth factor 1 in the dog: a study in different dog breeds and in dogs with growth hormone elevation. *Acta Endocrinol.,* **105**: 294–301.

Eigenmann, J. E., Zanesco, S., Arnold, U., and Froesch, E. R. (1984b). Growth hormone and insulin-like growth factor 1 in German Shepherd dwarf dogs. *Acta Endocrinol.,* **105**: 289–293.

Eigenmann, J. E., Patterson, D. F., and Froesch, E. R. (1984c). Body size parallels insulin-like growth factor 1 levels but not growth hormone secretory capacity. *Acta Endocrinol.,* **106**: 448–453.

Fleagle, J. G. (1988). *Primate Adaptation and Evolution.* Academic Press, New York.

Frazzetta, T. H. (1975). *Complex Adaptations in Evolving Populations.* Sinauer, Sunderland, MA.

Giles, E. (1956). Cranial allometry in the great apes. *Hum. Biol.,* **28**: 43–58.

Gomez, A. (1989). Allometric scaling of the limbs of three lorisid species. *Am. J. Phys. Anthropol.,* **78**: 229.

Gomez, A. M. (1989). Allometric scaling of the limbs of three lorisid species. *Am. J. Phys. Anthropol.,* **78**: 229.

Gomez, A. M. (1992). Primitive and derived patterns of relative growth among species of Lorisidae. *J. Hum. Evol.,* **23**: 000–000.

Gould, S. J. (1966). Allometry and size in ontogeny and phylogeny. *Biol. Rev.,* **41**: 587–640.

Gould, S. J. (1971). Geometric similarity in allometric growth: a contribution to the problem of scaling in the evolution of size. *Am. Nat.,* **105**: 113–136.

Gould, S. J. (1975). Allometry in primates, with emphasis on scaling and evolution of the brain. In: *Approaches to Primate Paleobiology.* Szalay, F. S., Ed., S. Karger, Basel, 244–292.

Gould, S. J. (1977). *Ontogeny and Phylogeny.* Harvard University Press, Cambridge.

Grand, T. I. (1983). The anatomy of growth and its relation to locomotor capacity in *Macaca.* In: *Advances in the Study of Mammalian Behavior.* Eisenberg, J. F. and Kleinman, D. G. Eds., American Society of Mammalogists, Special Publication No. 7, 5–23.

Grine, F. E., Hahn, B. D., and Gow, C. E. (1978). Aspects of relative growth and variability in *Diademodon* (Reptilia: Therapsida). *S. Afr. J. Sci.,* **74**: 50–58.

Hall, B. K. (1978). *Developmental and Cellular Skeletal Biology.* Academic Press, New York.

Hall, B. K. (1982a). The role of tissue interactions in the growth of bone. In: *Factors and Mechanisms Influencing Bone Growth.* Dixon, A. D. and Sarnat, B. G., Eds., Alan R. Liss, New York, 205–215.

Hall, B. K. (1982b). How is mandibular growth controlled during development and evolution? *J. Craniofac. Genet. Dev. Biol.,* **2**: 45–49.

Hall, B. K. (1982c). Mandibular morphogenesis and craniofacial malformations. *J. Craniofac. Genet. Dev. Biol.,* **2**: 309–322.

Hall, B. K. (1983). Epigenetic control in development and evolution. In: *Development and Evolution.* Goodwin, B. C., Holder, N., and Wylie, C. G., Eds., Cambridge University Press, Cambridge, 353–379.

Hall, B. K. (1984). Developmental processes underlying heterochrony as an evolutionary mechanism. *Can. J. Zool.,* **62**: 1–7.

Huxley, J. S. (1932). *Problems of Relative Growth.* MacVeagh, London.

Jantz, R. L. and Owsley, D. W. (1984). Temporal changes in limb proportionality among skeletal samples of Arikara Indians. *Ann. Hum. Biol.,* **11**: 157–163.

Jungers, W. L. and Fleagle, J. G. (1980). Postnatal growth allometry of the extremities in *Cebus albifrons* and *Cebus apella*: a longitudinal and comparative study. *Am. J. Phys. Anthropol.*, **53**: 471–478.

Jungers, W. L., and Hartman, S. E. (1988). Relative growth of the locomotor skeleton of orang-utans and other large-bodied hominoids. In: *Orangutan Biology*. Schwartz, J. H., Ed., Oxford University Press, Oxford, 347–360.

Jungers, W. L., and Susman, R. L. (1984). Body size and skeletal allometry in African apes. In: *The Pygmy Chimpanzee: Evolutionary Biology and Behavior*. Susman, R. L., Ed., Plenum Press, New York, 131–177.

Jungers, W. L., Cole, T. M., III, and Owsley, D. W. (1988). Multivariate analysis of relative growth in the limb bones of Arikara Indians.

Kluge, A. G. (1983). Cladistics and the classification of the great apes. In: *New Interpretations of Ape and Human Ancestry*. Ciochon, R. L. and Corruccini, R. S., Eds., Plenum Press, New York, 151–177.

Lauder, G. V. (1981). Form and function: structural analysis in evolutionary morphology. *Paleobiology*, **7**: 430–442.

Leigh, S. R. and Cheverud, J. M. (1989). A finite element scaling study of growth, allometry and sexual dimorphism in the baboon skull (*Papio* sp.). *Am. J. Phys. Anthropol.*, **78**: 259–260.

Leutenegger, W. and Larson, S. (1985). Sexual development of the postcranial skeleton of New World monkeys. *Folia Primatol.*, **44**: 82–95.

Levitch, L. C. (1986). Ontogenetic allometry of small-bodied platyrrhines. *Am. J. Phys. Anthropol.*, **69**: 230.

Lumer, H. (1939). Relative growth of the limb bones of anthropoid apes. *Hum. Biol.*, **11**: 379–392.

Lumer, H. and Schultz, A. H. (1941). Relative growth of the limb segments and tail in macaques. *Hum. Biol.*, **13**: 283–305.

Lumer, H. and Schultz, A. H. (1947). Relative growth of the limb segments and tail in *Ateles geoffroyi* and *Cebus capucinus*. *Hum. Biol.*, **19**: 53–67.

MacPhee, R. D. E. (1977). Ontogeny of the ectotympanic-petrosal plate relationship in strep-sirhine prosimians. *Folia Primatol.*, **27**: 245–283.

MacPhee, R. D. E. (1979). Entotympanics, ontogeny and primates. *Folia Primatol.*, **31**: 23–47.

MacPhee, R. D. E. (1981). Auditory regions of primates and eutherian insectivores: morphology, ontogeny and character analysis. *Contr. Primatol.*, **18**: 1–282.

MacPhee, R. D. E, and Cartmill, M. (1986). Basicranial structures and primate systematics. In: *Systematics, Evolution and Anatomy*. Comparative Primate Biology, Vol. 1, Swindler, D. R. and Erwin, J., Eds., Alan R. Liss, New York, 219–276.

MacPhee, R. D. E., Cartmill, M., and Gingerich, P. D. (1983). Palaeogene primate basicrania and definition of the order Primates. *Nature*, **301**: 509–511.

Manley-Buser, K. A. (1986). A heterochronic study of the human foot. *Am. J. Phys. Anthropol.*, **69**: 235.

Masoud, I. M., Moses, A. C., and Shapiro, F. D. (1985). Skeletal growth in the normal rabbit: a longitudinal study of serum somatomedin-C and skeletal development. In: *Normal and Abnormal Growth: Basic and Clinical Research*. Dixon, A. D. and Sarnat, B. G., Eds., Alan R. Liss, New York, 233–243.

Maynard Smith, J., Burian, R., Kauffmann, S., Alberch, P., Campbell, J., Goodwin, B., Lande, R., Raup, D., and Wolpert, L. (1985). Developmental constraints and evolution. *Q. Rev. Biol.*, **60**: 265–287.

Merimee, T. J., Zapf, J., and Froesch, E. R. (1987). Insulin-like growth factors in pygmies. The role of puberty in determining final stature. *N. Engl. J. Med.*, **316:** 906–911.

Montagu, A. (1981). *Growing Young*. McGraw-Hill, New York.

Moore, W. J. (1981). *The Mammalian Skull*. Cambridge University Press, Cambridge.

Moss, M. L. (1972). The regulation of skeletal growth. In: *Regulation of Organ and Tissue Growth*. Goss, R. J., Ed., Academic Press, New York, 127–142.

Moss, M. L. (1973). A functional cranial analysis of primate craniofacial growth. In: *Symp. 4th Int. Congr. Primat.*, Vol. 3, S. Karger, Basel, 191–208.

Novacek, M. J. (1977). Aspects of the problem of variation, origin, and evolution of the eutherian auditory bulla. *Mammal. Rev.*, **7**: 131–149.

Oyen, O. J., Walker, A. C., and Rice, R. W. (1979). Craniofacial growth in olive baboons (*Papio cynocephalus anubis*): browridge formation. *Growth*, **43**: 174–187.

Palmiter, R. D., Norstedt, G., Gelinas, R. E., Hammer, R. E., and Brinster, R. L. (1983). Metallothionein-human GH fusion genes stimulate growth of mice. *Science*, **222**: 809–814.

Pidduck, H. G. and Falconer, D. S. (1978). Growth hormone function in strains of mice selected for large and small size. *Genet. Res. Camb.*, **32**: 195–206.

Ravosa, M. J. (1988). Browridge development in Cercopithecidae: a test of two models. *Am. J. Phys. Anthropol.*, **76**: 535–555.

Ravosa, M. J (1991a). An interspecific perspective on mechanical and non-mechanical models of primate circumorbital morphology. *Am. J. Phys. Anthropol.*, submitted.

Ravosa, M. J. (1991b). Ontogenetic perspective on mechanical and non-mechanical models of primate circumorbital morphology. *Am. J. Phys. Anthropol.*, **85**: 95–112.

Ravosa, M. J. (1991c). The ontogeny of cranial sexual dimorphism in two Old World monkeys: *Macaca fascicularis* (Cercopithecinae), and *Nasalis larvatus* (Colobinae). *Int. J. Primatol.*, **121**: 403–426.

Rensch, B. (1959). *Evolution Above the Species Level*. Columbia University Press, New York.

Riedl, R. (1978). *Order in Living Organisms*. John Wiley & Sons, New York.

Schultz, A. H. (1936). Characters common to the higher primates and characters specific for man. *Q. Rev. Biol.*, **11**: 259–283.

Schultz, A. H. (1969). *The Life of Primates*. Universe Books, New York.

Schwartz, J. H. (1984a). The evolutionary relationships of man and orang-utans. *Nature*, **308**: 501–505.

Schwartz, J. H. (1984b). Hominoid evolution: a review and a reassessment. *Curr. Anthropol.*, **25**: 655–672.

Shea, B. T. (1981). Relative growth of the limbs and trunk in the African apes. *Am. J. Phys. Anthropol.*, **56**: 179–202.

Shea, B. T. (1982). Growth and Size Allometry in the African Pongidae: Cranial and Postcranial Analyses. Ph.D. thesis, Duke University, Durham, NC.

Shea, B. T. (1983a). Size and diet in the evolution of African ape craniodental form. *Folia Primatol.*, **40**: 32–68.

Shea, B. T. (1983b). Allometry and heterochrony in the African apes. *Am. J. Phys. Anthropol.*, **62**: 275–289.

Shea, B. T. (1983c). Phyletic size change and brain/body scaling: a consideration based on the African pongids and other primates. *Int. J. Primatol.*, **4**: 33–62.

Shea, B. T. (1983d). Paedomorphosis and neoteny in the pygmy chimpanzee, *Science*, **222**: 521–522.

Shea, B. T. (1984). An allometric perspective on the morphological and evolutionary relationships between pygmy (*Pan paniscus*) and common (*Pan troglodytes*) chimpanzees. In: *The Pygmy Chimpanzee: Evolutionary Biology and Behavior*. Susman, R. L., Ed., Plenum Press, New York, 89–130.

Shea, B. T. (1985a). Ontogenetic allometry and scaling: a discussion based on the growth and form of the skull in African apes. In: *Size and Scaling in Primate Biology*. Jungers, W. L., Ed., Plenum Press, New York, 175–206.

Shea, B. T. (1985b). The ontogeny of sexual dimorphism in the African apes. *Am. J. Primatol.*, **8**: 183–188.

Shea, B. T. (1986a). Scapula form and locomotion in chimpanzee evolution. *Am. J. Phys. Anthropol.*, **70**: 475–488.

Shea, B. T. (1986b). Ontogenetic approaches to sexual dimorphism in anthropoids. *Hum. Evol.*, **1**: 97–110.

Shea, B. T. (1988). Heterochrony in primates. In: *Heterochrony in Evolution: A Multidisciplinary Approach.* McKinney, M. L. Ed., Plenum Press, New York, 237–266.

Shea, B. T. (1989). Heterochrony and human evolution: the case for human neoteny reconsidered. *Yearb. Phys. Anthropol.*, **32**:69–101.

Shea, B. T. (1990). Dynamic morphology: growth, life history and ecology in primate evolution. In: *Primate Life History and Evolution.* DeRousseau, J., Ed., Alan R. Liss, New York, 325–352.

Shea, B. T. and Gomez, A. (1988). Tooth scaling and evolutionary dwarfism: an investigation of allometry in human pygmies. *Am. J. Phys. Anthropol.*, **75**: 117–132.

Shea, B. T. and Pagezy, H. (1988). Allometric analyses of body form in Central African pygmies. *Am. J. Phys. Anthropol.*, **75** (abstr.): 269–270.

Shea, B. T., Hammer, R. E., and Brinster, R. L. (1987). Growth allometry of the organs in giant transgenic mice. *Endocrinology*, **121**: 1924–1930.

Sibley, C. G. and Alquist, J. E. (1987). DNA hybridization evidence of hominoid phylogeny: results from an expanded data set. *J. Mol. Evol.*, **26**: 99–121.

Simpson, G. G. (1953). *The Major Features of Evolution.* Columbia University Press, New York.

Sinha, Y. N., Salocks, C. B., and Vanderlaan, W. P. (1975). Prolactin and growth hormone levels in different inbred strains of mice: patterns in association with estrous cycle, time of day, and perphenazine stimulation. *Endocrinology*, **95**: 1112–1122.

Szalay, F. S. (1972). Paleobiology of the earliest primates. In: *The Functional and Evolutionary Biology of Primates.* Tuttle, R. H., Ed., Aldine, Chicago, 3–35.

Thompson, D. W. (1917). *On Growth and Form.* Cambridge University Press, Cambridge.

Thomson, K. S. (1988). *Morphogenesis and Evolution.* Oxford University Press, Oxford.

Tollman, S. M., Grine, F. E., and Hahn, B. D. (1980). Ontogeny and sexual dimorphism in *Aulacephalodon* (Reptilia: Anomodontia). *Ann. S. Afr. Mus.*, **81**: 159–186.

Wake, D. B. and Larson, A. (1987). Multidimensional analysis of an evolving lineage. *Science*, **238**: 42–48.

Watts, E. S. (1986). Skeletal development. In: *Comparative Primate Biology*, Vol. 3. Dukelow, W. R., Ed., Alan R. Liss, New York, 1–25.

Watts, E. S. (1988). Evolutionary trends in primate growth and development. In: *Primate Life History and Evolution.* DeRousseau, C. J., Ed., Wiley-Liss, New York, 89–104.

Wood, B. A. (1976). The nature and basis of sexual dimorphism in the primate skeleton. *J. Zool.*, **180**: 15–34.

7

Bone Growth and Paleopathology

DONALD J. ORTNER

Department of Anthropology
National Museum of Natural History
Smithsonian Institution
Washington, D.C.

Introduction

The very substantial literature on human skeletal paleopathology reveals that virtually all the major categories of orthopedic disease known to the modern clinician have an antiquity that extends back for at least several centuries. Archeological cases of skeletal disease can reveal fine details of bone tissue pathology and the more general effects of disease on bone when the pathological process is multifocal. Dry-bone pathology also has much to demonstrate about normal bone tissue including factors that affect its growth and development.

At the cellular level, the abnormal bone tissue that results from pathological conditions is a response to well-known physiological processes including (1) active hyperemia that is associated with osteoclast activity and bone destruction and (2) passive hyperemia that is associated with osteoblast activity and bone formation. What remains much less well understood is what governs the specific local pathological expression of these basic and normal physiological processes.

Bone growth occurs in association with two types of precursor tissue. One of these is growth associated with a cartilage tissue model (endochondral ossification). Endochondral ossification is linked primarily with growth in the long axis of bones. (One exception is the growth of the vertebral body in which endochondral ossification is associated with the short axis.) The calcified cartilage that results from endochondral ossification normally is associated with growth of the individual. It is a very temporary tissue that is quickly replaced by bone formed within osteoid, the second of the two precursor tissues (intramembranous ossification). In addition, intramembranous ossification is responsible for growth in width (typically the short axis of bones) and much of the growth associated with the skull vault.

Skeletal paleopathology offers one avenue of research for achieving insight into growth processes associated with both types of ossification. The absence of soft-tissue histology and many elements of clinical history is an obvious limitation. There are, however, at least two very important advantages. The first is the ability to observe fine details of abnormal dry-bone tissue rarely seen in clinical X-ray films. The other is the potential to observe the distribution of abnormal skeletal manifestations of disease in virtually the entire skeleton, often in the context of a very substantial sample of cases from the same archeological site. Interpreting this information in the context of what is known about normal and pathological bone growth and development is an intriguing and potentially useful exercise.

Abnormal conditions affect bone directly as in fracture and primary tumors of bone. Abnormal dry-bone tissue can also result from the secondary effect of pathological processes in other organs and tissues. Both primary and secondary abnormal conditions can affect the growth of bone and both are well known in paleopathological materials.

In the following report I draw on the large biomedical human skeletal collection of the National Museum of Natural History (NMNH), Smithsonian Institution, to provide examples of skeletal pathology that either produce abnormal growth or that adversely affect the growth process. I focus on three general categories of disease: (1) infection, (2) anemia, and (3) congenital and metabolic disturbances of growth.

Infection

Most of the infectious agents that result in dry-bone changes are bacteria. Furthermore, most of the infectious diseases that affect bone are long-term, chronic conditions in which the host's immune response controls, but does not eliminate, the infectious agent. Often the organism is spread by hematogenous pathways; bone marrow is a common focus for infectious processes. Infectious disease of the bone marrow (osteomyelitis) may be the result of any one of several infectious agents. If osteomyelitis is present during the growth phase it may interfere with growth by disrupting endochondral ossification either at the growth plates or in epiphyseal ossification centers. This may result in deformed and shortened bones. Chronic infection may also create neurovascular conditions that stimulate excessive growth. In osteomyelitis, either or both endochondral and intramembranous ossification can be affected, resulting in bones that are longer and/or wider than normal.

An example of accelerated bone growth is apparent in a case of osteo-myelitis from an archeological site near La Oroya, Peru. (A more detailed report of this case can be found in Ortner and Putschar, 1981: 123–127.) The archeological date is uncertain but is likely to be pre-Columbian. The only bones recovered from this specimen were the right and left tibia (Figs. 1 and 2). The length of the normal right tibia suggests an age of about 9 years at the time of death. The pathological left tibia exhibits all the classic features of osteomyelitis including sequestra, cloacae, and involucrum. Most pertinent to this discussion, however, is the major increase in length of the pathological tibia (219 mm) in contrast to the normal left tibia (196 mm). Chronic inflammation associated with osteomyelitis has stimulated abnormal growth in the pathological tibia. Although growth in width has also occurred this is an indirect effect of the sequestration and death of the diaphysis and the formation of a new cortex to maintain mechanical function.

Three syndromes of treponematosis (venereal syphilis, yaws, and bejel) can affect the skeleton. Only one of these syndromes, syphilis, is known to result in congenital transmission. Congenital syphilis can result in bone changes and affect the development of teeth, including their overall size and shape and formation of enamel.

An intriguing question is why pregnant women with the other two syndromes, yaws and bejel, do not transmit the disease to the developing fetus. One possible reason for this is the age of onset of the three syndromes. Both yaws and bejel are typically acquired early in childhood and, if full recovery does not occur, have entered the chronic phase of the disease by the time childbearing occurs. Venereal syphilis normally is acquired later in adolescence or early adulthood, close to the time when childbearing begins. The disease is thus in an earlier stage of host/pathogen interaction when the immune response of the host may not be fully developed and thus less able to prevent transplacental infection of the fetus.

The effect of congenital syphilis on bone development is somewhat different from that seen in the case of osteomyelitis described above. Endochondral bone development is not normally affected. One typically sees activation of the periosteum and widening of the bones (intramembranous ossification) but this is not due to sequestration and formation of involucrum. Diaphyses remain alive and functioning throughout but vascular conditions stimulate appositional bone formation by the periosteum. There is generally no evidence of an abnormal change in bone length.

A possible archeological case of congenital syphilis is from the Fisher Site in Northern Virginia (NMNH 385786). (NMNH numbers refer to specimen numbers in the collection of the National Museum of Natural History). The

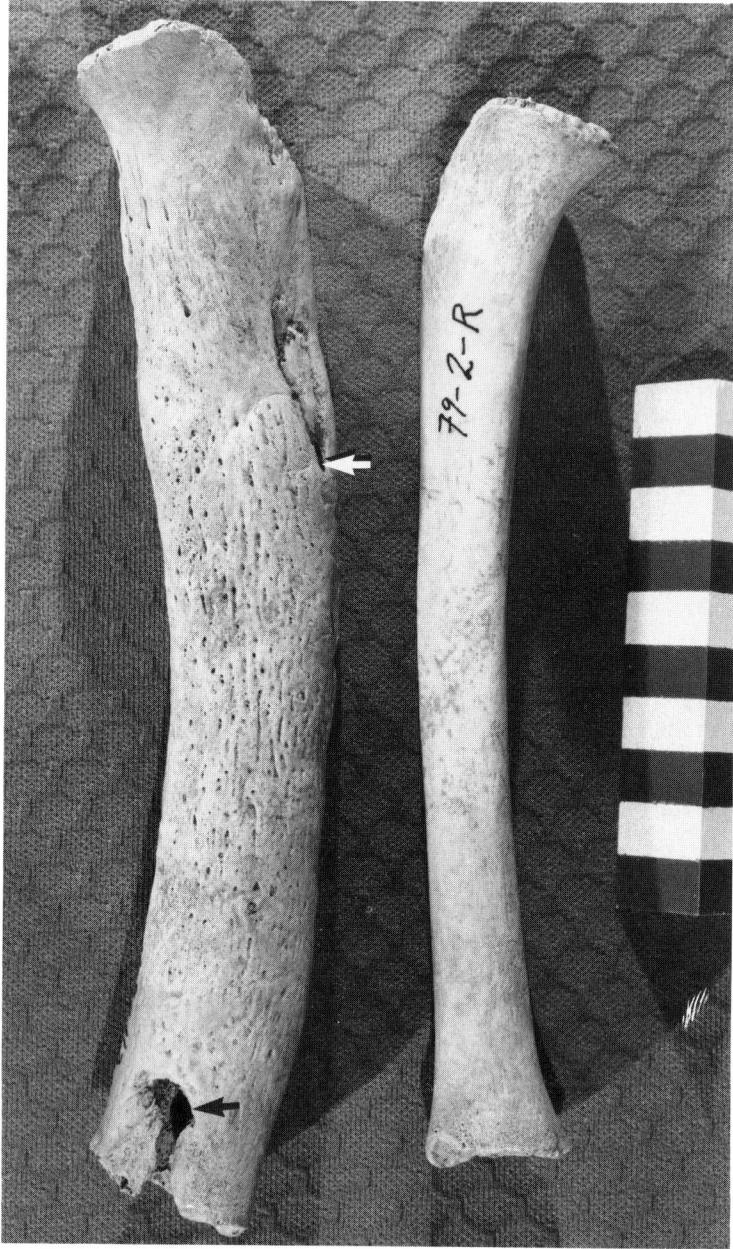

Fig. 1. Osteomyelitis of the left tibia compared with the normal right tibia. Specimen from a child about 9 years of age recovered from an archeological site near La Oroya, Peru. Medial view demonstrates the greater length of the pathological tibia. Also seen are cloacae (arrows) and a sequestrum in the proximal cloaca. Compare the width of the pathological left with the normal right tibia. The original cortex of the left tibia is necrotic and completely surrounded by involucrum formed by the periosteum to maintain biomechanical function of the lower limb. (NMNH 378243; scale in centimeters.)

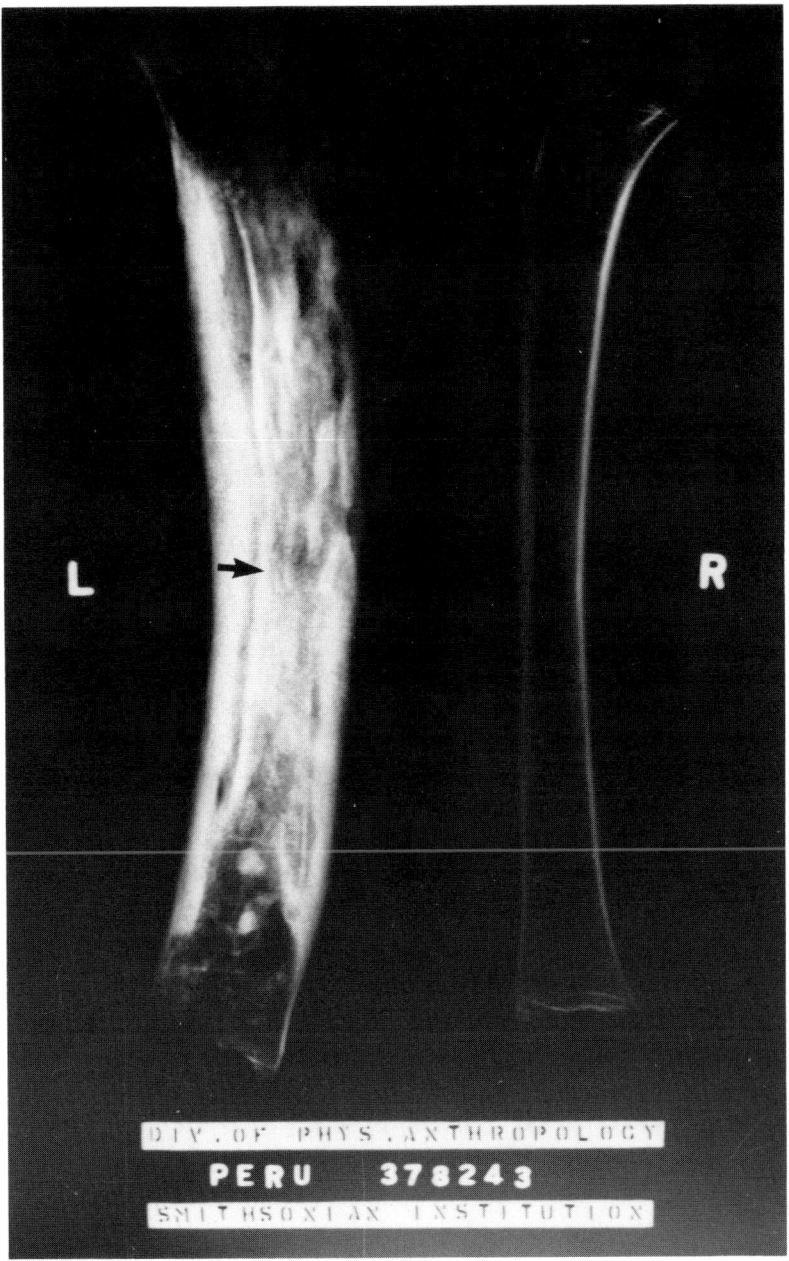

Fig. 2. Mediolateral X-ray film of pathological and normal tibiae seen in Fig. 1. The necrotic, sequestrated original cortex (arrow) is apparent within the involucrum.

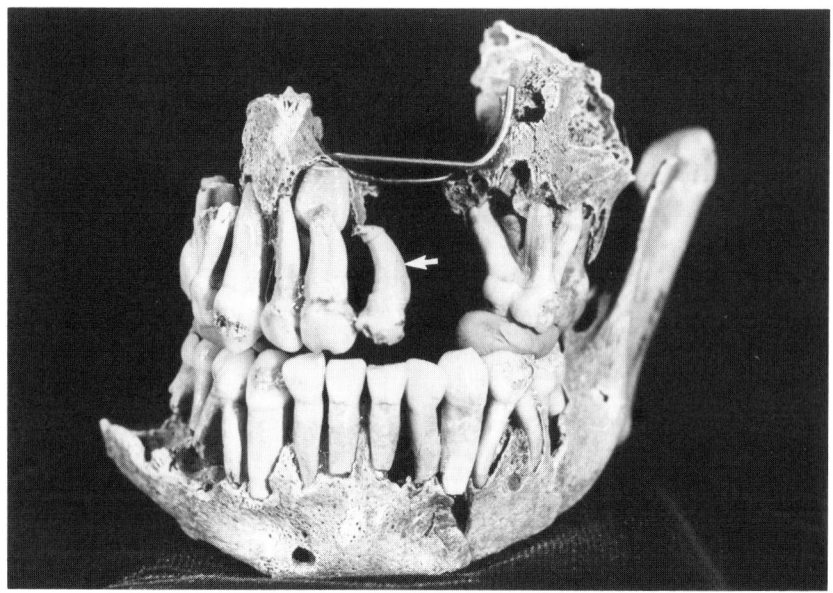

Fig. 3. Abnormal dental development of dental root (arrow) and hypoplastic enamel in a possible case of congenital syphilis. Specimen is a child about 2 to 3 years of age and from the Fisher Site in northern Virginia. Anterior view of dentition demonstrates the multifocal nature of the dental problems. (NMNH 385786.)

site has been dated by both the pottery typology and carbon-14 dating to between A.D. 1000 and 1400. An adult, male skeleton (NMNH 385788) from the same site exhibits the classic skeletal features of acquired treponematosis. It thus seems likely that treponematosis of some type was endemic when the community was active.

The specimen in question is that of a child between 3 and 4 years of age at the time of death. Bone preservation was poor but reconstruction of both dental arches was possible. Dental hypoplasia is apparent on most of the deciduous teeth (Figs. 3 and 4), although severity and location varies between the teeth. Dental involvement is sometimes, but not always, bilateral. If the condition is bilateral, the specific location and severity of the abnormality within the tooth tends to be variable. Bradlaw (1953) has made a similar observation on the sporadic distribution of dental lesions in modern cases of congenital syphilis.

The occurrence of dental hypoplasia on the deciduous incisors indicates the occurrence of pathology around the time of birth and possibly before. Both occlusal and smooth surfaces are affected and caries appears to have been a serious complicating factor in several teeth, particularly the lower

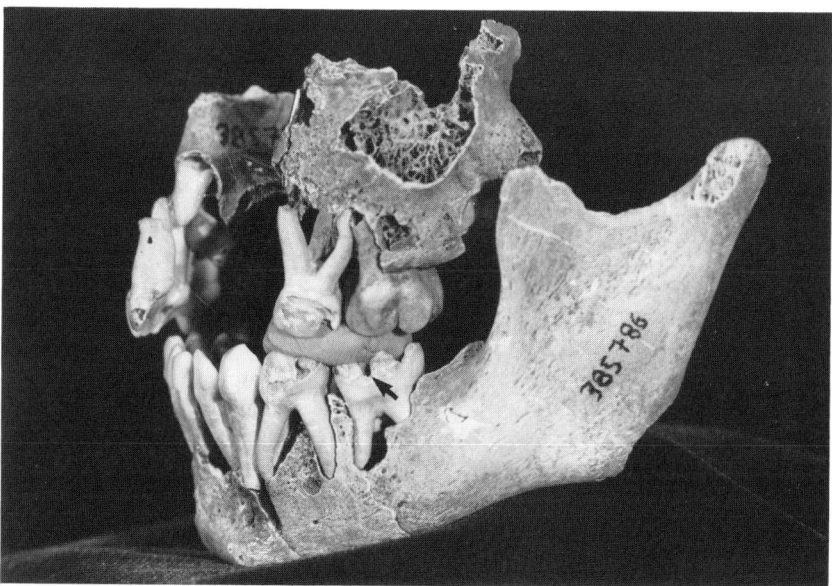

Fig. 4. Lateral view of specimen in Fig. 3. Note the severe defects in enamel formation and the effect of secondary caries particularly apparent in the lower second deciduous molar (arrow).

The postcranial skeleton is incomplete and fragmentary. There is, however, clear evidence of periosteal, reactive, appositional bone on several fragments. This is particularly apparent and extensive on the tibiae (Fig. 5). Both Caffey (1939) and Bauer (1944) report the presence of inflammatory periostitis on long bones in congenital syphilis. Caffey (1939), however, emphasizes that many infant and childhood diseases result in this bone pathology including anemia, osteomyelitis, rickets, and trauma.

The combination, in this case, of dental hypoplasia and evidence of a systemic inflammatory condition resulting in abnormal periosteal bone apposition is strongly suggestive of congenital syphilis. The clear presence of acquired treponematosis in another adult specimen from the same site makes this diagnosis even more plausible.

The stimulation of bone apposition by systemic inflammation is well demonstrated in this case. The tissue formed is fairly well-organized fiber bone that is porous in appearance. This is indicative of a moderate growth rate in the abnormal bone that is certainly faster than the rate of normal circumferential lamellar bone that underlies the abnormal tissue. The abnormal bone formation in this case appears to be exclusively intramembranous; there is no evidence of any effect on endochondral ossification.

second deciduous molars. The upper left central incisor exhibits a deformed and hypoplastic root along with the enamel defect.

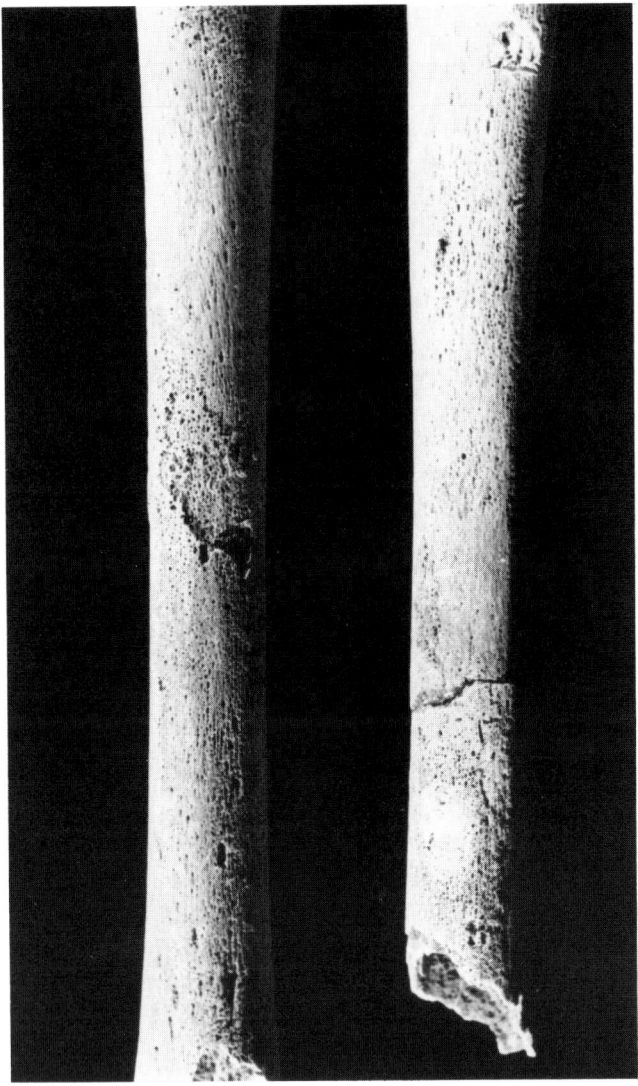

Fig. 5. Left and right tibias of specimen seen in Fig. 3. Note the porous reactive bone covering virtually the entire anterior diaphysis.

Anemia

Defective hemoglobin in red blood cells, a major factor in many anemias, may be the result of several factors. In sickle cell anemia, one of the genetically based hemolytic anemias, one amino acid (valine) is substituted for

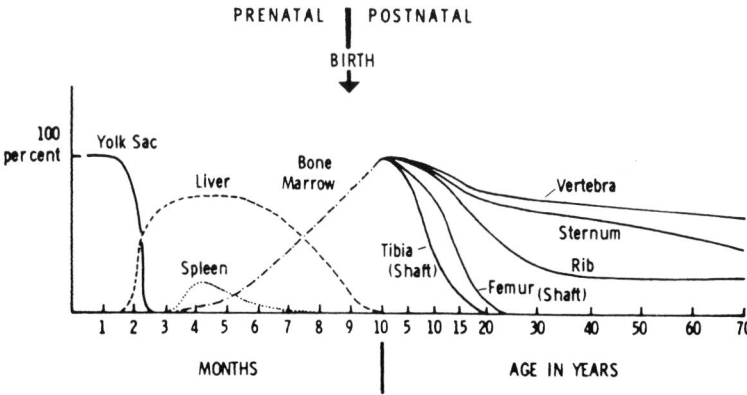

Fig. 6. Graph demonstrating the reduction of hematopoietic marrow in the tibia and femur during the growth phase. Vertebra continue to be site for red marrow throughout life. (Reproduced from Lewis (1981) and reprinted with the permission of the publisher, Appleton-Century-Crofts.)

the normal amino acid (glutamic acid) in the β-chain of the hemoglobin molecule (Resnick and Niwayama, 1988). In acquired anemia, such as iron deficiency anemia, inadequate availability of dietary iron results in abnormal hemoglobin. In either case the red blood cell is defective and has a shorter than normal life-span resulting in increased red cell turnover and greater demand for space for hematopoietic tissue. Most bone changes in anemia are a secondary effect of the need for increased hematopoietic tissue that greatly exceeds the normal volume of marrow at that particular age. In the adult the increased need for red marrow can be accommodated at the expense of space for fatty marrow.

If anemia occurs in infancy or early childhood, all marrow is already fully occupied with red hematopoietic tissue (Fig. 6) (Lewis, 1981). Normally, by adolescence the long bones contain minimal hematopoietic tissue which is now concentrated in the axial skeleton. In infancy and early childhood any increase in demand for hematopoietic tissue must occur in areas not normally associated with blood formation. In some cases of anemia this is done by increasing red marrow volume in bone. The factors that affect this are poorly understood. In long bones the increase is achieved at the expense of cortical bone and one sees increased marrow space and diminished cortical thickness. In the skull, the diplöe increases primarily at the expense of the outer table. The dry-bone appearance in the skull is characterized by a much thicker diplöe and an outer surface that is very porous. In the more recent literature on paleopathology the most common term used to describe porous enlargement of the skull is porotic hyperostosis (Angel, 1966). It is important to stress that other pathological conditions including cynotic congenital heart disease with secondary polycythemia (Ascenzi and Mari-nozzi, 1958), polycythemia vera (Dykstra and Halbertsma, 1940), infection, scurvy, and rickets (Ortner and Putschar, 1981) can produce an enlarged diplöe and a porous outer surface. However, if one sees clear evidence of generalized marrow enlargement, anemia is the most likely diagnostic option.

Angel (1966) links the archeological evidence for anemia in the Eastern Mediterranean to the presence of endemic malaria. He argues that the type of anemia is most likely thalassemia. The abnormal nature of the hemoglobin interferes with the life cycle of the malarial parasite and thus confers some immunity to the disease. Individuals having the homozygous form (thalassemia major), however, rarely live past early childhood (Ortner and Putschar, 1981). Individuals with the less-severe expressions of the disease have enough of the abnormal protein to inhibit the reproductive cycle of the malarial parasite. Such individuals are not, however, seriously anemic and have increased immunity to malaria. A similar mechanism exists for the sickle cell gene on the African continent.

Archeological evidence for anemia exists in geographical areas of the world where there is no evidence of malaria. One of these areas is the American Southwest. There, the most plausible explanation proposed thus far is iron-deficiency anemia. The heavy emphasis on maize in the diet appears to be a major factor. Phytates in maize flour combine with iron and reduce its dietary availability (El-Najjar et al., 1976; Mensforth et al., 1978). Iron is a critical element in hemoglobin. Dietary deficiency in iron results in abnormal hemoglobin and increased red cell turnover. The potential for skeletal tissue changes involves a similar mechanism to that seen in the genetic hemolytic anemias.

This condition is illustrated in a case from the pre-Columbian archeological site of Pueblo Bonito, NM (NMNH 327107). (A more complete description of this specimen and another like it is found in Ortner and Putschar 1981: 260–262.) The specimen consists of the partially complete skeleton of a child approximately 2 years of age at the time of death. Porous, enlarged bone tissue on the skull is largely limited to the parietals (Fig. 7). The inner table is much thinner than normal in the porous areas and the outer table is entirely replaced by an enlarged diploetic space (Fig. 8). The lesions avoid the sagittal suture and encroach only slightly on the occipital bone. The frontal bone is unaffected.

The long bones that are present in this case exhibit enlargement of the medullary cavity with the cortex being much thinner than normal. The cortex of the affected femur is less than 1 mm thick in contrast with unaffected femora from specimens from the same site and about the same age. These are 2 to 3 mm in cortical thickness (Fig. 9). Clearly red marrow space has increased greatly at the expense of cortical bone.

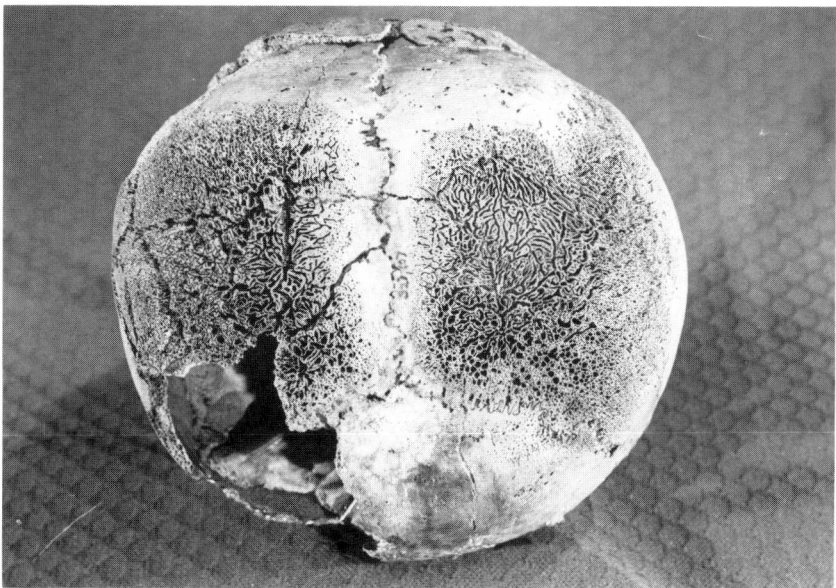

Fig. 7. Enlargement of hematopoietic marrow in the diplöe obliterating much of the outer table of the right and left parietal in a probable case of iron-deficiency anemia. Specimen is from the skeleton of a child about 2 years of age from the pre-Columbian site of Pueblo Bonito, NM. Note that the abnormal bone tends to avoid the tissue adjacent to the sagittal suture. There is only slight involvement of the occipital bone seen in the lower portion of the figure. (NMNH 327107.)

One of the intriguing questions in the context of the impact of pathology on bone growth and maturation is the relationship between biomechanical and physiological requirements and the potential conflict between them. On the skull the most serious expression of porotic hyperostosis avoids the major areas of muscle attachment, particularly that of the temporalis and trapezius muscles. This suggests that the physiological need for increased hemato-poietic space is met in areas of the skull in a way that minimizes biome-chanical problems.

Genetic and Metabolic Disturbances in Bone Growth

Both endochondral and intramembranous ossification are under relatively independent hormonal and genetic control. In normal bone growth, the balance between endochondral and intramembranous ossification is care-fully orchestrated by a complex interrelationship primarily involving the pituitary and thyroid glands. There are many abnormal metabolic and

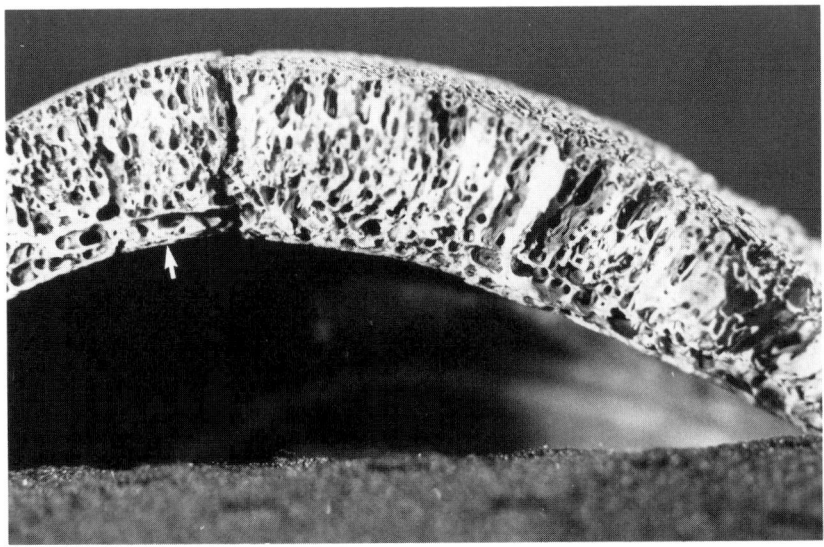

Fig. 8. Detail of a transverse, post-mortem break through the left parietal of the specimen seen in Fig. 7. The inner table (arrow) has only a very thin remnant left and the outer table has been entirely replaced by the abnormal growth of porous bone providing space for greatly increased hematopoietic marrow. The total thickness of the parietal is much greater than normal.

congenital conditions that can affect either or both of these mechanisms of bone growth.

In pituitary deficiency, for example, both endochondral and intramembranous ossification are diminished but the reduction in body and skeletal development is proportional. Long bones are both shorter and narrower but normal proportions between length and width are maintained. In contrast, the various genetically determined manifestations of osteogenesis imperfecta affect only intramembranous ossification. Both the quality and quantity of the osteoid is diminished but endochondral ossification and growth in the long axis is relatively normal. In severe cases of osteogenesis imperfecta the bone quality is so poor that fractures are common even in the protected environment of the uterus. Because of the combination of multiple fractures and complications in other organs, long-term survival of neonates with severe osteogenesis imperfecta is uncommon and particularly unlikely in an archeological context. However, some of the less-severe syndromes may be compatible with long-term survival.

At least one case of probable osteogenesis imperfecta has been recovered from an archeological site. This case (NMNH 384120) is from the Juhle site in Maryland and is dated to Late Prehistoric period between 1400 and 1500

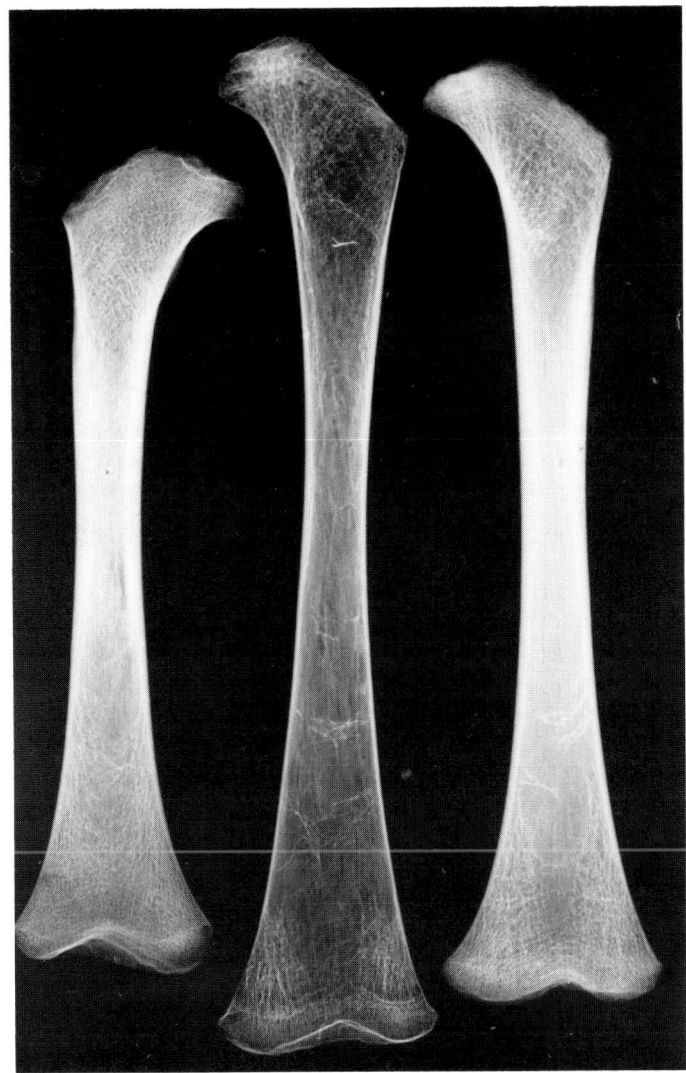

Fig. 9. X-ray film of right femur (center specimen in figure) from specimen seen in Fig. 7. Abnormal specimen is compared to two femora from other children's skeletons from the same site and approximately the same age. Note the much-thinner cortex and the wider marrow space in the abnormal femur.

A.D. The case includes most of the major long bones. The bone quality is poor, almost certainly a partial reflection of the ante-mortem, bone-tissue abnormality. The epiphyseal ends of the bones are particularly vulnerable to post-mortem breakage and loss in archeological skeletons. This is especially true in this case which, along with the abnormal shape, contributes to the difficulty in identifying the bones that are present.

The gross dry-bone morphology indicates relatively normal growth in length (Fig. 10) with the size indicative of late adolescence or adulthood. Long-bone width is markedly subnormal. The histology of compact bone reveals some evidence of osteon remodeling but far less than should be apparent in someone at or near adulthood (Fig. 11). One of the intriguing aspects of this case is that, despite the clear indication of deficient intramembranous ossification and poor bone quality, there is no evidence of healed fracture in any of the bones.

Defects in endochondral ossification can be the result of genetic abnormalities included in the broad disease category of bone dysplasias. Achondroplasia is probably the best-known example of the dysplasias. In this condition growth of endochondral bone is markedly deficient resulting in dwarfism. Bone thickness, however, is unaffected leading to the appearance of short but robust long bones. The extremities are relatively more affected than the axial skeleton. Different syndromes of the cartilage dysplasias affect different bones or groups of bones. (The known syndromes are described in Bergsma, 1979.)

Insufficient thyroid hormone can also result in deficient endochondral ossification and, in dry-bone specimens, may be difficult to differentiate from the cartilage dysplasias. Hypothyroidism occurs endemically because of an absence or inadequacy of dietary iodine, an essential element in thyroid hormone. In the earlier part of this century and before, it was well known in villages in the high Alps where both the soil and water lack iodine. (See Schinz *et al.*, 1951–1952 for an excellent review of skeletal manifestations in cases of endemic hypothyroidism from the Swiss Alps.)

Deficient thyroid hormone can also result from a congenital, partial-to-complete absence of the thyroid gland (sporadic hypothyroidism). Other conditions (e.g., tumors) that affect the normal production of thyroid hormone can also result in sporadic hypothyroidism. In an archeological context the complete absence of the thyroid gland would not be compatible with extended post-natal life.

An interesting case of possible hypothyroidism is seen in an adult female skeleton (NMNH 271813) from the archeological site of Kwastiyukwa, NM, in the southwestern region of the U.S. (described briefly in Ortner, 1986). The archeological dates for this site range from A.D. 1250 to 1700 and are thus well before any effective treatment would have been possible. The skeleton is well preserved and most of the bones are available for study. There has been some post-mortem loss of the smaller bones and some breakage of the epiphyseal ends of the long bones during excavation and subsequent handling.

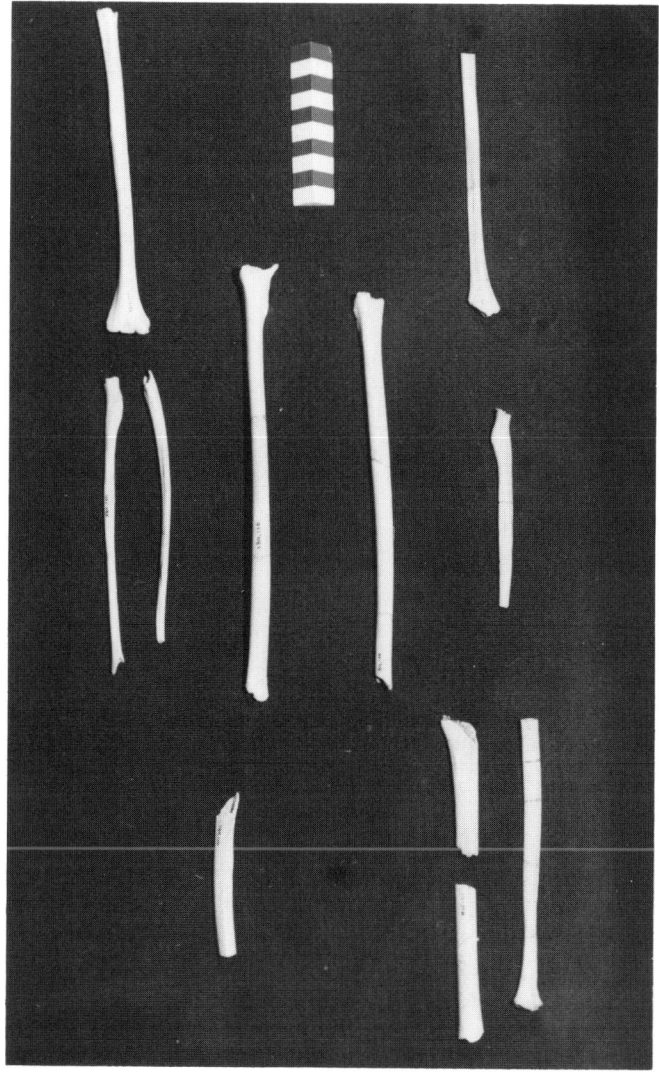

Fig. 10. Anterior view of the long bones available for study in a probable case of osteogenesis imperfecta. The bones are displayed in approximate anatomical position with the bones of the upper extremity arranged nearer the top of the figure and lateral to the two femora in the center of the figure. The length of the long bones is compatible with completed growth and an estimated age of at least 15 years. Intramembranous ossification (growth in diameter of the diaphysis) is markedly deficient. Surprisingly there is no evidence of ante-mortem, healed fracture. (NMNH 384120; scale in centimeters.)

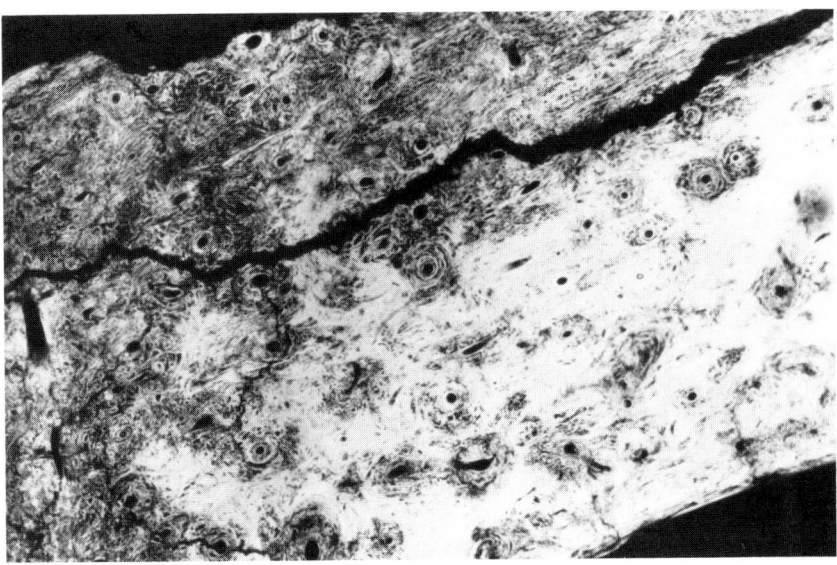

Fig. 11. Microradiograph of a compact bone section from the tibial diaphysis of the specimen seen in Fig. 10. Secondary osteons are present but much less frequent than would be seen in a section of normal compact bone in someone at least 15 years of age. The outer cortex is apparent in the lower right corner of the figure. The large crack apparent in the figure is an artifact of section preparation. The darker areas that obscure the histological detail, particularly seen in the left portion of the figure, are the result of post-mortem destruction of tissue, probably by fungi. (Approximately × 40.)

In general the abnormality in this case is due to deficient endochondral bone growth most obviously expressed as shortening of some long bones. There is also some shortening of the base of the skull resulting in a slightly depressed midfacial region but this is minimal. One of the important features of this case is that not all bones are affected. However, when a bone is affected the condition is bilateral. The inconsistent growth pattern is best demonstrated in the bones of the upper extremity (Fig. 12). The humeri are much shorter than normal and also have an abnormal shape, particularly at the distal end. There, the medial component is disproportionately shorter than the lateral, leading to an abnormal angulation of the elbow components. Both the ulnae and radii are normal in length with the ulna being virtually the same length as the humerus. The midshaft diameters of all long bones are normal indicating normal intramembranous ossification.

The clavicles, sternum, and first ribs exhibit subnormal growth. The reduced anteroposterior axis of the vertebral arch indicates that the disease process was present during early childhood before endochondral growth of the vertebral canal is completed (Roaf, 1960). Vertebral body height is

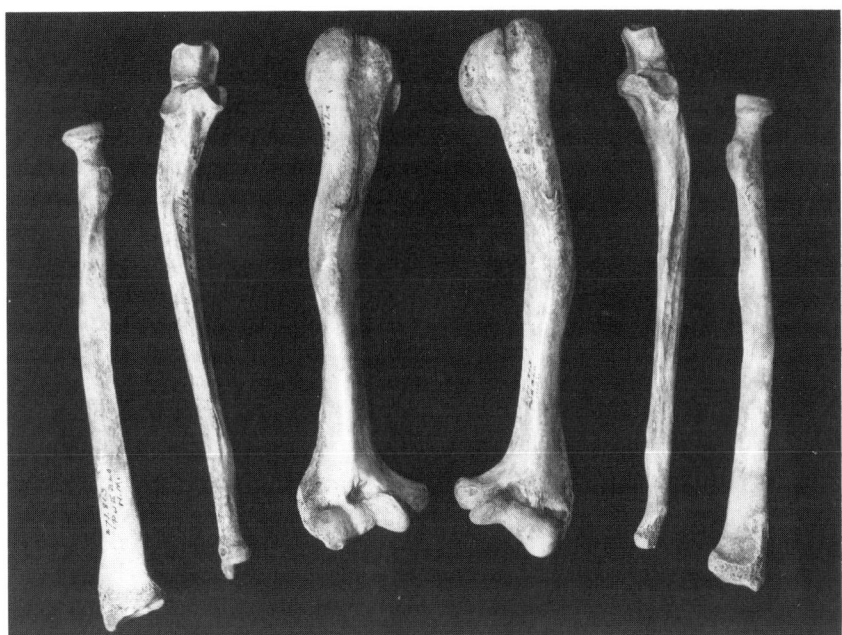

Fig. 12. Anterior view of the major long bones of the upper extremity in a possible case of sporadic hyperthyroidism. The specimen is from the skeleton of an adult female from the pre-Columbian archeological site of Kwastiyukwa, NM. The radii and ulnae are normal in length although the shape of the ulnae is somewhat abnormal. The humeri, in the center of the figure, are shorter than normal, particularly on the medial side. Note that the superior portion of the humeral head is below the plain of the greater tuberosity. Note also the abnormal angle of the distal articular surface relative to the long axis of the diaphysis. (NMNH 271813.)

somewhat subnormal but the great number of endochondral ossification centers and the typically slower rates of growth in the spine ensured a relatively normal overall height for the vertebral column. The pelvis, however, was markedly affected by the disease process, attaining only about two thirds the normal size. Also apparent in the innominate is an abnormally large and shallow acetabulum (Fig. 13) similar in appearance to hip dysplasia. Chronic dislocation of the hip was probably a problem throughout this individual's life.

The bones of the lower extremity are normal in length, although the femora are somewhat more bowed than normal. The femoral heads have had some post-mortem breakage but there is sufficient subchondral bone remaining to indicate that the articular surface was flattened superiorly and had a very irregular surface, as one would expect given the morphology of the acetabulum. The bones of the hands and feet that are present exhibit minimal abnormality.

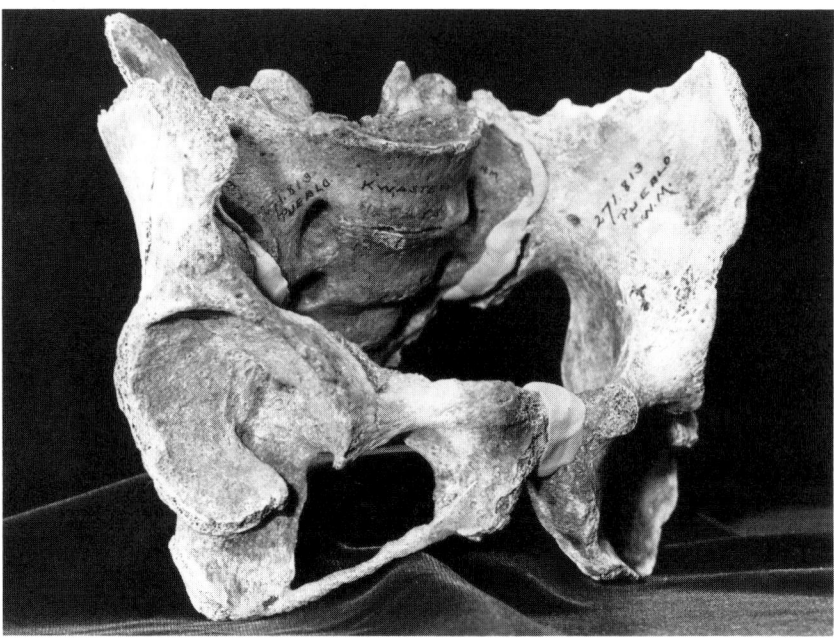

Fig. 13. Right, three-quarter view of the pelvis of specimen seen in Fig. 12. Note the diminished anterior-posterior diameter of the pelvic inlet and the greatly enlarged and shallow acetabulum.

In this case the clear evidence of abnormal endochondral ossification limits the probable diagnostic options to hypothyroidism or one of the rare chondrodysplasias. This skeleton exhibits an overall pattern of abnormal bone shape and size that fits fairly well with a diagnosis of hypothyroidism although there are some residual unresolved problems. Endemic hypothyroidism is not known to occur in this area of the American Southwest. If the case from New Mexico had hypothyroidism it would most likely be the result of a deficient thyroid gland (sporadic hypothyroidism). The disease process probably was present at birth but certainly would have begun by early childhood. Nevertheless, the fact that not all bones participated in the disease suggests that some thyroid hormone was produced. This probability is supported by the fact that there is no delay in epiphyseal union as would be the case if thyroid hormone deficiency was severe and continuous throughout life.

This case raises some intriguing questions. Since all the long bones are growing more or less proportionally, why are the humeri, clavicles, first ribs, sternum, and pelvis severely affected while most of the other long bones are not? In the humerus, why is the medial, distal component more deficient in length growth that the lateral? If the supply of thyroid hormone was deficient but constant throughout the growth and development of this case, different bones are differentially affected. Indeed one side of the distal humerus was more affected than the other.

Summary and Conclusions

I have reviewed three general paleopathological conditions in which the development of normal or abnormal bone tissue is affected directly by the pathological process. These conditions include (1) infection, (2) anemia, and (3) congenital and metabolic problems. Each of these conditions affects the development of bone tissue in different ways and involves different physiological and biomechanical mechanisms.

If infection of bone occurs during the growth phase it can inhibit or stimulate either abnormal endochondral or intramembranous ossification. This effect is primarily the secondary result of local inflammation resulting from the physiological response to infectious agents or their toxic by-products. Infection can directly inhibit bone growth in situations where the growth plate is partially or completely destroyed by the infective process.

In infants and young children, anemia can result in an abnormal increase in the need for space for hematopoietic tissue. This demand produces an increase of hematopoietic marrow at the expense of cortical bone. This can occur in the long bones but the process produces particularly dramatic effects in the skull where the diplöe enlarges and may completely replace the outer table of compact bone in some areas of the skull. The latter results in a very porous appearance in the skull of some dry-bone cases of anemia. An intriguing observation is that the increase of red marrow avoids, as long as possible, areas of muscle attachment and bone that has to withstand the greatest biomechanical stress.

The abnormal pattern of bone growth seen in the possible subacute case of sporadic hyperthyroidism suggests that thyroid hormone affects the growth process of some bones and some areas within bones more than others. This argues for the presence of a threshold effect that may vary in different, bilateral, bone groups and within some bones such as we have seen in the humerus. For the bones that were affected in this case, the amount of thyroid hormone was inadequate for normal growth. However, for most of the bones in the specimen, the available thyroid hormone met the necessary minimum threshold amount needed for relatively normal endochondral bone growth.

The paleopathological specimens described in this report demonstrate the well known principle that pathology teaches us much about the normal. In paleopathological cases, we often have access to all or most of the bones of a specimen. Such dry-bone, biomedical research materials provide insight regarding patterns of bone involvement in disease and also the fine details of bone reaction to pathological conditions.

Acknowledgments

I should like to acknowledge, with deep appreciation, the editorial assistance of Mrs. Agnes Stix, Department of Anthropology, National Museum of Natural History, Smithsonian Institution, who also contributed significantly to the quality of the illustrations. Dr. James Krakker, of the same department, provided critical information on the archeological context of the specimens. I am also grateful to Appleton-Century-Crofts for permission to reproduce the graph demonstrating the age-associated changes in the normal distribution of hematopoietic tissue. Research for this report was supported in part by a grant from the National Institutes of Health (Grant No. HHS-1RO1 AM34250).

References

Ascenzi, A. and Marinozzi, V. (1958). Sur le Crane en Bosse au Cours des polyglobulie secondaires a l'hypoxemie chronique. *Acta Haematol.*, **19**: 253–262.

Angel, J. L. (1966). Porotic hyperostosis, anemias, malarias and marshes in the prehistoric Eastern Mediterranean. *Science*, **153**: 760–763.

Bauer, W. H. (1944). Tooth buds and jaws in patients with congenital syphilis. *Am. J. Pathol.*, **20**: 297–319.

Bergsma, D., Ed. (1979). *Birth Defects Compendium*, 2nd ed., Alan R. Liss, New York.

Bradlaw, R. V. (1953). The dental stigmata of prenatal syphilis. *Oral Surg.*, **6**: 147–158.

Caffey, J. (1939). Syphilis of the skeleton in early infancy. *Am. J. Roentgenol. Radium Ther.*, **42**: 637–655.

Dykstra, O. H. and Halbertsma, J. (1940). Polycythemia vera in childhood: report of a case with changes in the skull. *Am. J. Dis. Child.*, **60**: 907–916.

El-Najjar, M. Y., Ryan, D. J., Turner, C. G., and Lozoff, B. (1976). The etiology of porotic hyperostosis among the prehistoric and historic Anasazi Indians of the Southwestern United States. *Am. J. Phys. Anthropol.*, **44**: 477–488.

Lewis, S. M. (1981). Erythropoiesis. In: *Postgraduate Haematology*, 2nd ed., Hoffbrand, A. V., Lewis, S. M., Eds., Appleton-Century-Crofts, New York, 1–34.

Mensforth, R. P., Lovejoy, C. O., Lallo, J. W., and Armelagos, G. J. (1978). The role of constitutional factors, diet, and infectious disease in the etiology of porotic hyperostosis and periosteal reactions in prehistoric infants and children. *Med. Anthropol.*, **2**: 1–59.

Ortner, D. J. (1986). Metabolic and endocrine disorders in human skeletal paleopathology. In: *6th Eur. Meet. Paleopathology Association, Proceedings*. Bellard, F. G. and Sanchez, J. A., Eds., Universidad Compultense de Madrid, Madrid, 17–24.

Ortner, D. J. and Putschar, W. G. J. (1981). *Identification of Pathological Conditions in Human Skeletal Remains*. Smithsonian Contributions to Anthropology No. 28. Smithsonian Institution Press, Washington, D.C.

Resnick, D. and Niwayama, G. (1988). *Diagnosis of Bone and Joint Disorders.* 2nd ed., W. B. Saunders, Philadelphia.

Roaf, P. (1960). Vertebral growth and its mechanical control. *J. Bone Jt. Surg.*, **42B**: 40–59.

Schinz, H. R., Baensch, W. E., Friedl, E., and Uehlinger, E. (1951–1952). *Roentgen Diagnostics: Skeleton.* Vol. 1 and 2, English translation by J. T. Case. Grune and Stratton, New York.

8

Drugs and Bone Growth

MARTHA E. SUCHESTON

Department of Cell Biology, Neurobiology and Anatomy
The Ohio State University
Columbus, Ohio

Introduction
Analgesics
Anesthetics
Anticonvulsants
Anti-infective
    Antibiotic agents
    Antiviral agents
    Antiparasitic agents
Chemotherapeutic
    Alkalating agents
    Antimetabolites
    Antibiotics
    Miscellaneous
Diuretics
Psychotropics
    Tranquilizers
    Antidepressants
    Sedatives
Vitamins
Summary
References

Introduction

In 1941 Gregg identified German measles (rubella virus) as the cause of congenital malformations in children whose mothers had been exposed to the virus during pregnancy. Twenty years later, the sedative thalidomide was a perfect example of a causal relationship between a specific environmental teratogen and human malformations (Lenz, 1961; McBride, 1961). In 1971 Herbst *et al.* noted the relationship between young women with vaginal adenocarcinoma and the drug diethylstilbestrol (DES), which had been prescribed to their mothers during the pregnancy. This drew interest to the possible carcinogenic action of drugs on the developing fetus. More recently, study has been directed toward the effect on the developing fetus of maternal alcohol consumption during pregnancy. These incidents, coupled with the fact that individuals have become increasingly dependent on drugs, have focused the attention of the medical community on the potential hazards of drugs to the developing fetus.

The purpose of this chapter is to review the *in utero* effect drugs have on fetal growth and the developing skeletal system. The selected list of drugs is limited to those that are classified as therapeutic agents and have been proved or are suspected to constitute a potential or actual teratogenic risk to the growth and the development of the skeletal system in the human and/or laboratory animal. Whereas many drugs have a variety of actions, the drugs in this chapter have been classified on the basis of their primary pharmacological activity. The list of references, by no means complete, is considered by the author to be the most relevant in characterizing and identifying the teratogenic potential of a given drug or group of drugs as related to bone growth and/or development.

Analgesics

The analgesics, in particular the salicylates, are the most frequently ingested drugs in the general human population (Schardein, 1976). This, coupled with animal studies in which fetal malformations have been produced as a result of maternal ingestion of analgesics, has led clinicians to try and determine if a correlation exists between analgesic, salicylate, or narcotic ingestion during pregnancy and an increased incidence of malformations.

Nelson and Forfar (1971), in a survey of 458 mothers of children with defects, found that significantly more of them took aspirin during the first trimester. A later study by Saxen (1975) of 599 children observed that 14.9% of mothers with malformed children took salicylates during pregnancy compared to 5.6% of mothers with normal children who did not take salicylates. Sayli and co-workers (1966) described a patient who had taken aspirin before and during two of her pregnancies; both children were born with phocomelia; however, the authors were hesitant to attribute the limb defects to aspirin ingestion rather than to consanguinity. McNiel (1973) studied several patients who had taken salicylates singularly or in combination with other drugs (e.g., antihistamines, tetracyclines) during pregnancy. An increased incidence of limb deformities (e.g., polydactyly, syndactyly, shortened limbs) was noted in their offspring; however, these defects were not statistically significant.

Eriksson *et al.* (1973), in a comparative study of strong narcotics as opposed to mild analgesics that were taken by pregnant women, found very few adverse effects in offspring of either group. The most consistent finding was low birth weight, especially in the narcotic group. A significant decrease in birth weight, with an increase in perinatal mortality and no significant increase in congenital anomalies, was observed by Turner and Collins (1975) in their clinical studies on regular salicylate ingestion in pregnant women. Collins (1981), in a study on the effects in the mother and fetus of nonnarcotic analgesics, acetaminophen, and salicylates, noted an increase in fetal resorptions and reduced fetal growth. At this time, there is limited evidence of a direct causal relationship to birth defects or teratogenic potential in the human of either the salicylates or narcotic analgesics.

Salicylates and other analgesics, however, have been recognized as teratogens in laboratory animals since Warkany and Takacs (1959) reported on the effects of methyl and sodium salicylate in pregnant rats given a subcutaneous injection on day 9, 10, or 11 of gestation. Increased resorptions and skeletal abnormalities of the ribs, cranium, vertebral column, and limbs were noted in the treated fetuses. Other rat studies on salicylate teratogenicity (McColl *et al.*, 1965; Kimmel *et al.*, 1971; Klein *et al.*, 1981; Mitala *et al.*, 1984) recorded (1) an increase in fetal mortality, fetal resorption, skeletal variations, and abnormalities and (2) a decrease in fetal weight depending upon the day of treatment and/or dosage. Studies by Gabrielsson and Larsson (1987) stressed the need for physiological and pharmacokinetic models in the assessment of the teratogenic potential of drugs such as salicylic acid.

The results of another study of the teratogenic and postnatal development of rats receiving the narcotic analgesic, morphine, indicated that — in the absence of respiratory depression — high doses of this drug are not teratogenic (Fujinaga and Mazze, 1988). Previous investigators, for the most part, gave bolus doses of morphine and found that it caused deleterious effects on growth and neurobehavioral development of offspring (Smith and Joffe, 1975; Sobrian, 1977). Some, however, have reported that the drug is teratogenic (Zagon and McLaughlin, 1977; Ciociola and Gautieri, 1983). There is very little information available concerning the narcotic analgesics in laboratory or clinical studies and what there is is contradictory.

Strain differences to salicylate ingestion have been observed in mouse studies. Larsson and Bostrom (1965) noted a 52.2% increase in rib defects and a 33.3% increase in vertebral defects in the A/Jax mouse treated with the sodium salt of salicylic acid compared to 16 and 4%, respectively, in the CBA strain. Trasler (1965), on the other hand, observed microcephaly, polydactyly, syndactyly, spina bifida, and rib fusions in both C57BL/6 and A/Jax mouse exposed to sodium or methyl salicylate on day 6 of gestation to term. Chronic toxicity studies of analgesic and antipyretic drugs and congeners, however, showed no significant increase in fetal defects through several generations of ABC-A mice (Wright, 1967).

Comparative teratogenic studies in mouse and rabbit (Szabo and Kang, 1969), rat and monkey (Wilson, 1971; Tanimura, 1972; Wilson et al., 1977), and monkey and guinea pig (Kromka and Hoar, 1973) showed that the mouse and rat were more susceptible to salicylate insult than other species. This was reflected in their low birth weight and multiple skeletal problems.

Very few studies have reported the effects that analgesics have in combination with other agents. Aspirin and food restriction have been shown to produce a 25.8% incidence of malformations in rat fetuses whose mothers were treated on days 7 to 10 of gestation (Beall and Klein, 1977). Another study (Knight and Roe, 1978), on the effect of salicylamide and protein restriction in the rat, identified the salicylamide as the teratogenic agent and showed that protein restriction had no significant effect on the developing centers of ossification. The incidence of skeletal malformations was independent of the diet. In addition, the percentage of skeletal malformations was inversely related to the number of centers of ossification present. The gestational day of treatment was also found to be important.

Ungvary et al. (1983) studied the combined embryotoxic action of toluene and acetylsalicylic acid in CFY rats. Acetylsalicylic acid-treated fetuses were weight and skeletal retarded. With increasing dosages of acetylsalicylic acid, the rate of skeletal anomalies also increased. Toluene was found to potentiate the toxic effect of the acid. Another study by Guy and Sucheston (1986) demonstrated an additive effect of ethanol and aspirin in the CD-1 mouse. They found a significant increase in anomalies plus delayed ossification in the groups treated with the aspirin/ethanol combination.

Some species of laboratory animals (e.g., hamster, dog, cat) are not regularly used for teratogenic screening, although they have shown sensitivity to some teratogens. LaPointe and Harvey (1964), in studies on the effect of salicylamide-induced anomalies in hamster embryos, noted subdermal hemorrhages and increased resorptions. These subdermal hemorrhages and thin-walled, blood-filled capsules were also observed in fetal A/Jax mice exposed to salicylates in utero (Larsson et al., 1963). The authors felt that these hemorrhaged areas in the mouse represented the precursor to tissue breakdown that would eventually produce a malformation.

Increased abortion rate, retarded ossification, and several types of limb anomalies were observed in cat fetuses whose mothers were treated with methotrexate, aminopterin, or acetylsalicylic acid (Khera, 1975). In the cat there appeared to be no significant decrease in fetal weight, and no single anomaly predominated. Robertson et al. (1979) studied beagle dog fetuses that had been exposed in utero to aspirin. They gave either 100 or 400 mg/kg/d of aspirin to the bitches on days 15 to 22 or 23 to 30 of gestation. The investigators noted that resorption and malformation rates were time and dose related. No obvious effect on fetal weight, however, was noted in either dosage group. Skeletal abnormalities included missing or fused vertebrae, accessory ribs, and sternebral variations. As with most drug testing in animals, it is difficult to relate the effects of analgesics in animals to humans. In light of these animal studies, however, the possibility of risk for women of childbearing age taking large therapeutic doses of analgesics, e.g., aspirin, during pregnancy should not be discounted.

Anesthetics

Epidemiologic surveys (Smith, 1968; Corbett, 1972; Cohen *et al.*, 1974; Vessey and Nunn, 1980) have suggested that anesthetic agents may lead to increased incidences of abortion, premature onset of labor, perinatal mortality, and congenital defects in the offspring of operating room personnel and in women who have surgery during pregnancy. It has been suggested that several factors may be responsible for the fetal toxicity sometimes associated with anesthetic agents: (1) hypoxia as a result of the anesthetic; (2) hypercapnia, which may allow a higher concentration of the anesthetic to reach the fetal cellular level; and (3) alteration of maternal physiology and/or direct drug action (Smith, 1968).

Corbett (1972) and co-workers (1974) reported a spontaneous abortion rate of 30 to 38% among pregnant women working in an operating room environment compared to only a 10% incidence in regular duty hospital personnel. One study found a 2% increase in musculoskeletal problems in offspring of operating room personnel (Smith, 1974). These problems included congenital dislocated hip and pectus excavatum. Cohen and co-workers (1971) and Cohen (1974) also noted an increased risk of congenital defects in offspring of unexposed wives of male operating room personnel, leading some investigators (Rosenberg and Kirves, 1973; Spence *et al.*, 1974) to feel that stress may play a more important role than the anesthetic in fetal toxicity. In addition to environmentally exposed hospital personnel, it has been estimated that approximately 50,000 pregnant women per year are exposed to a regional or general anesthetic sometime during pregnancy (Mazze *et al.*, 1985). A direct association, however, between anesthetics and growth retardation, delayed ossification, and variations or defects of the skeletal system has not been observed in either exposed group to date.

Laboratory animal studies of anesthetic agents have demonstrated both positive and negative teratogenic results. Fink *et al.* (1967) and Basford and Fink (1968) studied the effect of the gases halothane and nitrous oxide in the rat. A decrease in fetal weight indicative of growth retardation was not observed, but there was an increased incidence of extra ribs and delayed fusion of vertebral ossification centers. A recent study by Fujinaga *et al.* (1989), on the susceptible period of nitrous oxide teratogenicity in rats, found that skeletal abnormalities of the ribs and vertebrae were increased following exposure on day 9 of gestation. Cervical ribs, though, were observed only after exposure on day 8 of gestation. Yet Mazze *et al.* (1986), in their study of nitrous oxide and halothane plus isoflurane and enflurane in Sprague-Dawley rats, found no significant teratogenic effect.

In a series of articles (Mazze *et al.*, 1982, 1985; Wharton *et al.*, 1979, 1980, 1981) on the effect of various inhalation anesthetics on mouse development, the authors ranked the agents studied in the following decreasing order of toxicity: isoflurane > enflurane > halothane > methoxyflurane > nitrous oxide. The authors noted, though, that these studies were from only one mouse strain, and extrapolation to the pregnant patient was not appropriate. The most often-cited effects to bone and bone growth were extra ribs, bifid sternum, malpositioned limbs, and decreased ossification of the skull. In addition, Mazze *et al.* (1982, 1984) found that none of the agents was toxic at the trace concentrations usually found in operating rooms.

In a very extensive study Smith (1968, 1974) examined several different anesthetic agents as well as premedicants and supplemental drugs used before and after surgery. He compared the effect of these drugs in several species: mouse, rat, rabbit, and chick. The most common finding was an increased resorption rate in all species; there was no statistical evidence for anomalies in any specific system. Defects of the skeletal system, when they occurred, were associated with extra, fused, or wavy ribs and delayed fusion of vertebral ossification centers. The chick was the only species that showed stunted growth. Thompson *et al.* (1974), in a comparative study of the effects of orally administered chloroform on rats and rabbits, noted that general retardation of ossification did not occur. Skeletal variations in the form of extra ribs, split sternebrae, absent bones, and unossified or malaligned skulls were found. The administration of thiopental sodium to pregnant mice on day 11 of gestation resulted in decreased fetal weight, but no significant increase in skeletal defects (Tanimura *et al.*, 1967). Fused ribs, increased number of ribs, and delayed ossification of the phalanges, however, were recorded. Fujinaga *et al.* (1967), employing osmotic minipumps in their study of fentanyl, noted no major or minor reproductive abnormalities or teratogenic findings in any treated group of rats.

Most researchers agree that there is no evidence that links any hazard of anesthetics to the developing fetus. Because of the wide variety of anesthetic agents in use today, the contradictory findings in laboratory animal studies, and the inability to extrapolate these findings to the pregnant patient, it seems advisable to limit the exposure to anesthetics during pregnancy.

Anticonvulsants

Clinical evidence has shown that children of epileptic mothers have a higher incidence of malformations than children of nonepileptic mothers (Meadow, 1968; Speidel and Meadow, 1974; Committee on Drugs, 1979; Janz, 1982; Robert and Guibaud, 1982; Bjerkedal *et al.*, 1982; DiLiberti *et al.*, 1984; Lindhout and Meinardi, 1984; Jeavons, 1984; Tein and Mac-Gregor, 1985; Rating *et al.*, 1987). Controversy continues as to whether the increased risk of malformation is due to the seizure (accompanied by hypoxia) or to the anticonvulsant therapy used in the treatment of epilepsy (Persaud *et al.*, 1985). It is now recognized, however, that anticonvulsants are potential human teratogens (Center for Disease Control, 1982). Anticonvulsant syndromes have been described in newborns whose mothers were treated with the drugs trimethadione (German *et al.*, 1970; Zackai *et al.*, 1975), diphenylhydantoin (Hanson and Smith, 1975), phenobarbitol (Bethenod and Frederich, 1975; Seip, 1976), and more recently sodium valproate (Koch *et al.*, 1983; Robert and Rosa, 1983; DiLiberti *et al.*, 1984; Hanson *et al.*, 1984; Lindhout and Meinardi, 1984). These syndromes share several features, including intrauterine growth retardation, minor dysmorphology primarily of the facies, central nervous system dysfunction, and multiple minor skeletal abnormalities.

A possible primidone embryopathy has been described by Rudd and Freedom (1979) in an infant with features similar to the fetal hydantoin syndrome. Carbamazepine (CBZ), in contrast to the numerous references to other anticonvulsants as teratogens, has not been studied as extensively nor are the reported results in complete agreement. It has been stated that combinations of anticonvulsants, including CBZ, result in a 6.8% malformation rate. Other reports, though, have indicated that CBZ produces a protective effect (Lowe, 1973; Schardein, 1976; Hiilesmaa *et al.*, 1981; Batz, 1983). Starreveld-Zimmerman *et al.* (1973) found no evidence of malformations in 50 children born to epileptic mothers receiving CBZ.

Hill *et al.* (1974), in a study of 1653 infants whose mothers received anticonvulsants during pregnancy, noted a 1.9% incidence of skeletal defects. The skeletal defects were second in order of occurrence behind cleft lip and/or palate; intrauterine growth retardation was last with an incidence of 0.2%. Some of the more common skeletal problems observed in the offspring of epileptic mothers were delayed ossification, vertebral fusion (usually in the lumbar region), scoliosis, club foot, spina bifida, congenital dislocated hip, and minimal camptodactyly.

A number of theories have been proposed to account for the teratogenic activity of anticonvulsants: genetic factors, folic acid deficiency, reduced uterine circulation with fetal hypoxia, maternally produced metabolites, and/or direct toxic action of the drug. Very little is known, however, concerning the mechanism or the site of action of anticonvulsant agents in the fetus. One of the major concerns in determining the teratogenic risk of a particular anticonvulsant therapy during pregnancy is the common method of treating epileptics with two or more anticonvulsant agents. This method of treatment makes it more difficult for a causal association to be made between a particular malformation and a specific agent.

Experimental studies with laboratory animals have confirmed the association between anticonvulsants and congenital malformations. Exposure to anticonvulsants early in animal development usually results in low birth weight and skeletal defects, representing a delay or retardation in growth. Of the compounds used in the effective treatment of epilepsy, phenobarbital has been in continuous use the longest. Experimental work with rodents (Fahim et al., 1970; Sullivan and McElhatton, 1975, 1977; Fritz et al., 1976; Finnell et al., 1987a, b) suggested that phenobarbital was a weak teratogen with little or no effect on growth or skeletal development. Finnell et al. (1987b), though, in a study comparing the effects of phenobarbital in three strains of mice, noted marked strain differences in malformations. They observed a decrease in fetal weight in the C57BL/6J strain; the weight of the SWV and LM/Bc fetal mice was not affected at any treatment level. Ossification delays in facial bones, occipital bones, sternebrae, vertebrae, and distal phalanges were observed in 47.1% of the C57BL/6J fetuses exposed to the highest concentration of phenobarbital. All strains showed a significant increase in skeletal defects. These findings are consistent with the pattern of anomalies referred to as the phenobarbital syndrome in the human.

Animal studies on trimethadione (Poswillo, 1972; Rifkind, 1974; Buttar et al., 1976, 1978) and its metabolites have shown a dose-related decrease in fetal weight and an increased incidence of nonspecific skeletal defects such as retarded ossification of the calvaria, extra or wavy ribs, sternal variations, and bowing of the long bones in the limbs. The trimethadione syndrome identified in the human has not to date been reproduced in an animal model.

Malformations associated with the human fetal hydantoin syndrome have been reported in animal studies (Massey, 1966; Gibson and Becker, 1968; Harbison and Becker, 1969, 1972; Mercier-Parot and Tuchmann-Duplessis, 1974; Sulik et al., 1979). Yet it was not until 1981 that Finnell produced an animal model of the fetal hydantoin syndrome that closely paralleled the human disorder. Treating the SWV, C_3H, and C57BL/6J inbred strains of mice with diphenylhydantoin (DPH), he observed a growth deficiency evidenced by low fetal weights and incomplete ossification plus skeletal defects in the offspring of the treated animals. Using this animal model, Finnell postulated that the drug phenytoin, not the presence of a maternal seizure disorder, was responsible for the defects.

Rat studies by Elmazar and Sullivan (1981) and Lorente *et al.* (1981) also noted growth retardation in fetuses whose mothers were treated with phenytoin. In a study by Zengel *et al.* (1989), pregnant rats were treated with phenytoin on days 9, 11, and 13 of gestation and allowed to deliver. An equal number of male and female offspring were observed until postnatal day 135. The authors suggested that *in utero* exposure to phenytoin may interfere with normal dimorphism based on gender. They also confirmed the toxic effect of this drug on postnatal growth, adult body proportion, and craniofacial geometry. Phenytoin studies (McClain and Langhoff, 1980) in rabbits have produced a pattern of malformations that are similar to those observed in mice and rats. The malformations included shortened or curved long bones, shortened ribs, club foot, syndactyly, adactyly, and delayed ossification of the skull and phalanges. The average fetal body weights and crown-rump lengths in treated groups of rabbits, however, were not significantly different from those of the control group.

Administration of DPH to cultured mouse embryos during organogenesis produced growth and developmentally retarded embryos as indicated by the decrease in protein and DNA content and the reduction in somite number, crown-rump length, and yolk sac diameter (Bruckner *et al.*, 1983). Chick embryos (Singh and Shah, 1989) that had received a single dose of phenytoin were found to have limb, craniofacial, abdominal, and occular defects in addition to deficiencies in growth. The skeletal defects included hypoplasia of digital phalanges and nails and shortened wings.

In contrast to the numerous references to the hydantoins as animal teratogens, CBZ has not been studied as extensively (Brown *et al.*, 1979) nor are the reported results in complete agreement. Administration of a low dose of CBZ to mice did not produce a teratogenic effect (Fritz *et al.*, 1976). Yet in a comparative study of six anticonvulsants, the teratogenic effects of CBZ were second only to DPH (Sullivan and McEllhatton, 1977). In a pilot study by Eluma *et al.* (1981), a low incidence of craniofacial malformations in the CD-1 mouse fetus was observed. Similar results have been reported for studies in the A/J mouse (Wray *et al.*, 1982).

Teratogenic effects have been reported in mice, rats, and rabbits that were given valproic acid (VA) or its salt during pregnancy (Whittle, 1976; Sucheston *et al.*, 1979, 1986; Brown *et al.*, 1980; Nau *et al.*, 1981, 1984; Bruckner *et al.*, 1983; Chatot *et al.*, 1984; Paulson *et al.*, 1985, 1988, 1989; Coakley and Brown, 1986; Petrere *et al.*, 1986; Nau and Scott, 1987; Ritter *et al.*, 1987; Vorhees, 1987; Naruse *et al.*, 1988; Turner *et al.*, 1989). Studies by Kao *et al.* (1981) of the CD-1 mouse treated on days 8 to 10 of gestation with VA have shown a dose-related decrease in fetal weight along with rib and vertebral anomalies. *In vitro* studies by the same investigators, using CD-1 mouse fetuses grown in serum containing VA, indicated a notable reduction in growth and irregular segmentation of somites. Paulson *et al.*

(1985), also studying the CD-1 mouse fetus that had been exposed to VA *in utero*, observed fore- and hindlimb defects in the form of syndactyly and partial hemimelia in addition to a significant dose-dependent decrease in fetal weight. Further studies by Paulson *et al.* (1988, 1989) used osmotic minipumps, which controlled the maternal VA plasma levels and varying oxygen levels. The investigators noted decreased fetal weight and delayed skeletal ossification in some of the cranial bones in fetuses under hypoxic conditions.

Collins *et al.* (1990) exposed A/J mice to dimethadione, sodium valproate, or sodium diphenylhydantoin on day 9.5 of gestation and found that all three anticonvulsants produced postaxial forelimb ectrodactyly, located predominately on the right side. Rats (Vorhees, 1987), which were treated on gestational days 7 to 18 with 400 mg/kg of VA, produced fetuses with a 68% incidence of skeletal malformations while fetal weight was reduced by 43%. A low dose of 200 mg/kg of VA produced no reduction in fetal weight and few skeletal defects. The embryotoxic and teratogenic potential of VA also has been investigated in the rhesus monkey (Mast *et al.*, 1986, 1987; Hendrickx *et al.*, 1988). These authors noted intrauterine growth retardation in addition to the reduction of fetal dimensions: crown-rump, crown-hip, foot length, head width, and circumference. There were also widespread malformations of the craniofacial, axial, and appendicular skeleton. Esaki *et al.* (1975) also recorded fetal growth retardation, but reported no malformations in their study of rhesus monkeys treated with VA. The lack of reported defects in this study may be due to the termination of the pregnancies prior to complete skeletal ossification. In all experimental animal models, malformations of the skeletal system are the most consistent finding of VA exposure and are an appropriate teratogenic endpoint for species comparisons.

Both *in vivo* and *in vitro* comparative studies of various anticonvulsant agents (Bruckner *et al.*, 1983; Vorhees, 1983; Chatot *et al.*, 1984; Eluma *et al.*, 1984; Lindhout *et al.*, 1984; Sucheston *et al.*, 1986) have led several investigators to rank those most commonly used agents. The following agents are listed in order of the severity, greatest to least, of their teratogenic response on growth and skeletal development: valproic acid > diphenylhydantoin > carbamazepine > trimethadione > phenobarbitol.

Anti-Infective

It has been well established that maternal infection in the human can prove harmful to the developing embryo and fetus. Such infections may result in congenital malformations, intrauterine growth retardation, abortion, or disease in the newborn (Alford and Pass, 1981; Williams *et al.*, 1981; Yanoff *et al.*, 1982; U.S. Department of Health and Human Services, 1983;

Rathbun, 1983; Remington and Klein, 1983; Amstey, 1984; Plotkin, 1984). It is therefore of interest to determine if anti-infective agents used in treating maternal infections constitute an additional risk to the fetus.

Antibiotic Agents

Tetracycline antibiotics are among this large group of anti-infective agents that have shown teratogenic activity associated with bone growth (Ravid and Toaff, 1972). The wide range of antibacterial activity of these drugs, although their therapeutic and toxic properties are similar, has led to their identification as "broad-spectrum" antibiotics.

Andre (1956) and Milch *et al.* (1957) established that deposits of tetracyclines can be found in the skeleton. Later studies showed that the drugs were fixed to mineralizing tissues, producing a yellowish fluorescence, in addition to their association with enamel and dentine (Bevelander *et al.*, 1961), ossification (Bevelander, 1964), and calcification (Hansson, 1967). Wilson (1962) noticed webbing and absent digits in children exposed *in utero* to a broad-spectrum antibiotic. Carter and Wilson (1963), in a study of 327 infants whose mothers had received antibiotics during pregnancy, observed that 47% of the infants were malformed while only 3% of the controls showed any defects. In addition, Bevelander and Cohlan (1962) noted a decrease in fetal weight and fetal size in newborns exposed to tetracyclines between 10 and 12 weeks of gestation. Cohlan *et al.* (1963) studied 19 premature infants of whom 7 had received tetracycline therapy postnatally for a period of 9 to 12 days. Six of the 19 infants received the drug for 3 additional time periods of 9 to 12 days, and 6 infants served as controls. Upon measuring the fibular growth, the authors noted a 40% growth retardation in the treated infants. Growth rates returned to normal after the drug was discontinued.

Mennie (1962), however, found no medical evidence for tetracycline teratogenicity in the human. In another study (Walford, 1963) of over 700 newborns, no statistically significant increase in malformations was noted in infants whose mothers had been prescribed antibiotics during the first 12 weeks of pregnancy.

Several reports in the literature concern the discoloration of infants teeth caused by the maternal use of tetracyclines during the 4th to 9th months of pregnancy (Wallman and Hilton, 1962; Rendle-Short, 1962; Kline *et al.*, 1964; Toaff and Ravid, 1966; Demers *et al.*, 1968). The drugs stained the dental enamel of primary teeth and the crowns of permanent teeth (Persaud *et al.*, 1985). In addition, the drugs were also observed to affect the teeth when given to children up to 8 years of age.

Although congenital bone malformations have not been cited as an effect of tetracycline exposure in the human, studies have not been conclusive. Skeletal malformations have been noted in chick, rat, mouse, and monkey fetuses exposed to tetracyclines during development. Rolle and Bevelander (1966) injected tetracycline into the yolk sac of chick embryos. They examined the femurs and mandibles at regular intervals between 10 and 17 days of embryonic age. The drug appeared to affect intramembranous bone formation in the mandible and femur primarily by retarding or temporarily inhibiting the rate of mineralization. The investigators concluded that the effects produced by the drug were dependent upon the concentration of the drug and not upon the time of administration. Another study (Carter and Wilson, 1962) involving the chick noted that tetracyclines produced limb defects similar to those observed with thalidomide.

Further studies by Carter and Wilson (1963), on the effect of tetracyclines, penicillin, and streptomycin in the fetal rat at human therapeutic doses, noted no teratogenic effect of any of the drugs tested. Postnatal rat studies (Engesaeter and Skar, 1978) showed that human therapeutic doses of oxytetracycline produced a significant decrease in weight, length of bones, and bending strength of both tibia and fibula. One to three weeks following treatment, however, no differences were observed between treated and control groups of rats. In a study testing the teratogenic effects of methacycline on rabbits (Hansson et al., 1968), it was noted that the drug was deposited in the mineralizing tissues in the same way as the other tetracyclines. In addition, this drug was shown to interfere with the normal calcification process. Monkey studies (Yen and Shaw, 1972) of tetracyclines, in particular chlortetracycline, oxytetracycline, and demethylchlortetracycline, were observed to arrest bone growth in very young animals. The growth appeared to recover its normal pattern after drug administration was stopped. This pattern of arrested development, with a normal recovery after drug therapy ceases, is very similar to what has been observed in human infants.

In vitro studies (Bennett et al., 1967; Norton et al., 1968) of long bone growth in rats established that tetracyclines in the medium depress long bone growth. This inhibitory effect proved to be independent of calcification. Saxén (1965) also noted an inhibitory effect on the mineralization of mouse embryonic bones but did not feel that this finding was applicable at the clinical level.

The inhibitory effects of tetracyclines on bone growth have been assessed in experiments with animals and in humans mainly through studies of general body growth, density and linear measurements of long bones, and size of embryo, fetus, and/or newborn. This retarding effect on growth (although there appears to be a recovery period), in addition to the permanent damage to the enamel of an infant's teeth, suggests that this class of drugs is teratogenic. Chemotherapeutic antibiotics are discussed later in this chapter.

Antiviral Agents

Another group of drugs, the antiviral agents, has not been shown to be teratogenic in the human. Several of them, however, have been identified as potent animal teratogens. In addition to their antiviral activity, a few of these drugs are used as antitumor agents. The skeletal system is particularly susceptible to these antiproliferative agents.

The antiviral agents iodo- (IDU) and fluoro- (FDU) deoxyuridine have both been shown to affect limb development in the ICR mouse. Skalko and Packard (1973) found that treatment with IDU on days 7, 9, and 10 of gestation produced polydactyly, syndactyly, and ectrodactyly, respectively. Knudsen and Kochhar (1981), after injecting a single dose of FDU on days 10 to 13 of gestation, noted that the hindlimbs were more sensitive to the drug than the forelimbs and showed dose-dependent long bone reductions. Treatment on day 11 produced specific long bone reductions accompanied by preaxial polydactyly, while treatment on day 12 produced ectrodactyly, but no long bone reductions. In addition to the major limb defects observed, defects also occurred in the ribs and vertebral column. The authors did not observe a significant reduction in fetal weight. Dagg and Kallio (1962), in their studies on mice injected with FDU at dose levels of 10, 20, or 30 mg/kg on day 10 of gestation, noted that 14, 39, and 72% of the fetuses, respectively, had malformed hindfeet. Other studies have shown that IDU is also teratogenic in the rabbit as exhibited by clubbed forepaws (Itoi, 1975), but not in the rat (Murphy, 1965; Itoi, 1975).

Using varying routes of drug administration over several periods of gestation, Schardein et al. (1977) studied the effects of vidarabine (VIRA-A®, adenine arabinoside, and ara-A) on the offspring of rats, rabbits, and monkeys. The authors found that the drug produced malformations of the skeletal system in the rat and rabbit when treated intramuscularly and in the rabbit when treated topically. The most frequent skeletal malformations that occurred were ectrodactyly, polydactyly, and clubfoot and malformed ribs, skull, sternebrae, and vertebrae. Intravaginal administration of the drug in rats produced no defects in the offspring. There was no demonstrable teratogenic effect observed in the monkey. Cytosine arabinoside was studied by Chaube and Murphy (1965) in the pregnant rat. A single dose of 2.5 to 500 mg/kg was given on days 9 to 12 of gestation. They found that the lowest dose producing an effect was 20 mg/kg. At 100 mg/kg, 33 to 49% of the survivors were abnormal on days 10 and 12 and 80% on day 11. Skeletal abnormalities included general stunting, clubbed feet, ectrodactyly, and polydactylous paws.

The drug ribavirin (1-β-D-ribofuranosyl-1,2,4-triazole-3-carboxamide; Virazole®) is used for both human and animal viral infections. Ferm et al. (1978) studied this synthetic nucleoside in hamster and rat embryos. The hamsters were treated on day 7, 8, or 9 of gestation by a single intraperitoneal (i.p.) injection or on day 8 with either a single intravenous (i.v.) injection or an oral dose of the drug. Rats were treated i.p. on day 9 of gestation with three different dose levels of ribavirin or a single oral dose of two drug levels. Abnormalities of the limbs were one of the most common defects found in the hamster. The i.v. route of drug administration produced 100% malformed upper and lower limbs. The i.p. route of oral drug administration produced time-dependent upper limb defects and spina bifida on day 8 with lower limbs affected on day 9. A higher dose was required to induce defects in the rat compared to the hamster. Defects in the rat were primarily in the head region. Oral drug administration appeared to produce a greater teratogenic effect.

Marks and Poppe (1988) conducted two rat experiments on the effect of oral administration of bropirimine on days 7 to 15 of gestation. Their first experiment using 100, 200, and 400 mg/kg of the drug found a significant increase in delayed fetal ossification and skeletal variations. This was also true of the second experiment where animals received 25, 50, or 100 mg/kg of the drug. Bropirimine is being studied for potential use against cancer and serious viral infections. Other antiviral agents that have been studied, in particular tilorone and trifluorothymidine, have only been studied in the rabbit and as yet have not shown any teratogenic activity (Rohovsky et al., 1971; Itoi et al., 1975).

Inasmuch as reports of teratogenic activity of antiviral agents in the human are lacking, caution should be used in extrapolating the animal results discussed in this section to the human situation.

Antiparasitic Agents

Another large group of anti-infective agents are those drugs used in the treatment of parasitic infections in both human and veterinary practice. Included in this group are the antimalarials, anthelmintics (for the treatment of worms), and antifungal agents.

Antimalarial

The antimalarial agents of these three categories are the only drugs that have shown teratogenic activity in the human (Taylor, 1937; Forbes, 1940; Reed et al., 1955; Maier, 1964; McKinna, 1966; Zolcinski et al., 1966; Tanimura and Lee, 1972). In epidemiological surveys, though, the majority of the malformations noted were in those fetuses whose mothers had taken antimalarial drugs, in particular quinine, as an abortifacient. Few fetal defects have been reported when these drugs have been used at therapeutic levels. In addition to quinine, three other drugs in this category showing questionable teratogenic activity in the human are quinacrine (Verera and

Zatloukal, 1964), pyrimethamine (Pap and Tarakhovsky, 1967; Sfetsos, 1970; Hengst, 1972), and chloroquin (Hart and Naunton, 1964). The most frequently observed defect was deafness related to eighth nerve damage. Defects of limbs were also recorded.

Results of animal experiments so far reported are also inconclusive. Tanimura (1972) and Tanimura and Lee (1972) in studies on monkeys noted that quinine produced no fetal growth retardation or malformations. In studies on pregnant ICR-JCL mice that had received high doses of quinine via gastric tube, the authors found a significant increase in embryolethality and/or growth retardation with no malformations. Thiersch *et al.* (1954), in studying the Long-Evans rats whose mothers received quinine during pregnancy, noted stunting and cranial bone defects in the offspring. Rat studies by Bovet-Nitti and Bovet (1959) showed that a high dose of quinine increased the maternal mortality rate and that low doses produced fetal damage.

Anthelmintic

A number of antiparasitic agents have shown teratogenic properties in animals. An international study on the effects of the anthelmintic drug parabendazole demonstrated variable results dependent upon dose and species of animal. Lemon and Hancock (1974), Middleton *et al.* (1974), Saunders *et al.* (1974), and Szabo *et al.* (1974) studied the effect of this drug at varying doses and on different treatment days in lambs. The South African, U.S., and Australian study found that multiple defects of the skeletal system occurred at two times (60 mg/kg) the normal therapeutic dose. The most common malformations were of the joints and digits. In addition, abnormalities of the vertebral column, long bones, and pelvis were noted. The U.K. study, though, found no teratogenic effect on lambs at the therapeutic drug level. A study by Miller *et al.* (1974) on the pregnant cow found no fetal teratogenic effect at both the 30 and 60 mg/kg drug levels. The studies on the sow (Hancock and Poulter, 1974) and rabbit (Duncan *et al.*, 1974), included in this international survey, showed no fetal effect in those animals whose mothers had received the drug during critical teratogenic periods of development. The study of two strains of rats (Duncan and Lemon, 1974), treated with 10 mg/kg or above of the drug on days 6 to 15 of gestation, showed fetuses with low birth weight, while 50 mg/kg and above of the drug produced fetuses with malformations.

Another common anthelmintic drug, sodium arsenate, has been shown to produce exencephaly, micrognathia, rib defects, increased fetal resorptions, and decreased fetal weight in Swiss-Webster mouse fetuses treated on day 9 of gestation with 35 and 50 mg/kg of the drug (Hood and Pike, 1972). In another study (Hood and Bishop, 1972) using the same mouse species and injecting with 45 mg/kg of sodium arsenate on days 7 and 9 of gestation, the authors noted a decrease in fetal weight, ectrodactyly, micromelia, twisted limbs, fused vertebrae, and fused and forked ribs. They concluded that the widespread and varied effects indicated that arsenate was probably a general, rather than a specific, teratogen. Beaudoin (1974) injected pregnant Wistar rats with various doses of sodium arsenate on one of days 7 to 12 of gestation. The dose of 30 mg/kg at day 8, 9, or 10 produced optimal effects. The ribs and vertebrae were the most susceptible skeletal elements to treatment. The atlas was rudimentary or missing in 63% of the experimental fetuses examined for skeletal defects. Ferm (1972) found that arsenate produced no teratogenic effect in the fetal cat, rabbit, or hamster.

The anthelmintic cadmium has been shown to be a potent teratogen in hamsters (Ferm and Carpenter, 1968), in rats (Barr, 1973; White et al., 1986; Holt and Webb, 1987), and in mice (Keino and Yamamura, 1974). Depending upon the time of administration during gestation, this drug can produce defects of the central nervous system, face, and limbs and intrauterine growth retardation. The most common limb defects observed in the C57BL/6J mouse are forelimb postaxial reduction and hindlimb preaxial reduction hypertrophy, syndactyly, and polydactyly (Messerle and Webster, 1982). Layton and Ferm (1980) have shown that administration of cadmium in the same strain of pregnant mice prior to the sensitive period can protect against a subsequent teratogenic dose administered during the sensitive period. This effect may be important in the evaluation of teratogenic risks to human populations chronically exposed to metals. Autoradiographic studies (Christley and Webster, 1983), on the C57BL/6J mouse given a single i.p. dose at three dose levels, showed that the teratogenic dose of cadmium (2400 mg/kg) was localized in cells of the neural tube, limb buds, and gut. Fenston and Scott (1985) proposed that cadmium induces forelimb ectrodactyly in the mouse by creating an acidotic embryonic environment and that the yolk sac might be the primary site of cadmium's teratogenic activity.

Exencephaly and axial skeletal dysmorphogenesis were also observed in the MF1 mouse exposed to cadmium in utero (Padmanabhan and Hameed, 1986). These authors felt that the abnormalities they observed clearly (1) established the association between neural tube and axial mesoderm abnormalities and (2) emphasized the relationship of the neuroectoderm to the mesoderm in normal morphogenesis. Naruse and Hayashi (1989) noted that maternal pretreatment with bismuth nitrate prior to a single i.p. injection of cadmium sulfate ameliorated the teratogenicity of cadimum, including exencephaly and abnormalities of the axial skeleton. Barr (1973) investigated two different rat stocks that received cadmium chloride during pregnancy. He noted that subcutaneous (s.c.) dosages were not teratogenic while i.p. injections were highly teratogenic in both stocks. Cadmium on day 10 produced reduction deformities of forelimb similar to that reported for the acetazolamide syndrome. Ferm (1972), though, noted no teratogenic effect of cadmium in the hamster.

A study was made of the schistosomicidal agent, hycanthone, which has been used by the human population both in Africa and Brazil (Rosi *et al.*, 1965; World Health Organization, 1972). In animal studies results indicated that hycanthone was both embryolethal and teratogenic, particularly to the axial skeleton, in the mouse and rabbit (Sieber *et al.*, 1974).

Antifungal

There have been few reports of antifungal agents administered to pregnant women, and none has suggested a relationship to fetal defects (Harris, 1966; Vartiainen and Tervila, 1970; Patel, 1973; Culbertson, 1974). In addition, few of these agents have been shown to be teratogenic in animals. Robens (1969), in a study on the effect of thiram on pregnant hamsters, rabbits, and guinea pigs, found no major growth or skeletal problems. Roll's (1971) research on NMRI and SW mice noted that treatment between gestational days 6 and 17 produced increased resorptions, early decreased fetal development, and a syndrome of skeletal malformations — cleft palate, wavy ribs, curved long bones, and micrognathia. Days 12 and 13 were the most susceptible to teratogenic insult. Another antifungal antibiotic, griseofulvin (Slonitskaya, 1969; Gillick and Bulmer, 1972), has been shown to be teratogenic in the cat and rat at doses below those used therapeutically in the human. At present, there does not appear to be any conclusive evidence of teratogenic activity of the antiparasitical drugs in the human. These drugs, not unlike the other anti-infective agents discussed in this unit, can be used in the pregnant woman, with the possible exception of the tetracyclines and quinine, if the potential benefit warrants a potential risk to the fetus.

Chemotherapeutic

Chemotherapeutic drugs interfere with the growth of actively dividing normal and neoplastic cells. These drugs work primarily by affecting nucleic acid and protein synthesis, by destroying enzyme functions, and by modifying cellular metabolism. Since these drugs are normally given at the maximum tolerated dosage, the risk of congenital defects is great. These drugs are classified in this chapter into alkylating agents, antimetabolites, antibiotics, and a miscellaneous category. Four comprehensive review articles have been published on the effects of this large group of drugs in the human and in animal models (Murphy, 1962; Chaube and Murphy, 1968; Mirkes, 1985; Schardein, 1985).

Alkylating Agents

Some of the more commonly used drugs in this group are nitrogen mustard, chlorambucil, cyclophosphamide, and busulfan. The first known mustard was used as a poisonous gas in World War I. Its nitrogen-containing analogue, nitrogen mustard (HN2), has been widely used for treatment of cancer in the human. Garrett (1974) studied a male infant whose mother had received a combination of chemotherapeutic drugs, including HN2. The infant had digital defects such as four toes on each foot and webbing of the third and fourth toe on the right foot. Mennuti et al. (1975), however, noted no growth or skeletal defects in an infant exposed to a similar drug regimen. Other reports of human studies have been negative (Barry et al., 1962; Boland, 1951). This drug, though, has been shown to be a potent skeletal teratogen in all animal species studied. Mice (Danforth et al., 1954) treated by i.p. doses of HN2 on days 10 to 12 of gestation produced offspring with foot deficiencies and limb reductions. The authors noted that the defects were more prevalent on the left side of the body than the right. In studies on the mouse and chick, Jurand (1961) noted that the HN2 derivatives, acetyl and fluorine, were toxic to the mesodermal cells in both species. In the mouse these derivatives appeared to cause shortening of the limbs. Haskin (1948) observed bowing of the long bones, adactyly, missing toes, and digital deformities in albino rats whose mothers were treated by s.c. injections of HN2 on day 12, 13, 14, or 15 of gestation. Gottschewski (1964) treated pregnant rabbits for 9 days every 12 h beginning 19 h after mating with either HN2 or cyclophosphamide. He found that treatment on days 7 to 9 produced abnormal somites and limbs in the offspring.

Chlorambucil has not been shown to be teratogenic to the growth and development of the skeletal system in the human. It has been shown, however, to affect the skeletal development in laboratory animals. Sadler and Kochhor (1975) gave a single oral dose of this drug to ICR/DUB mice on day 10, 11, 12, or 13 of gestation. The offspring, whose mothers were treated on day 11 or 12, had a variety of limb defects (e.g., long bone reduction, absence of one or more bony components, absence of ossification centers, and ectro-, brachy-, syn-, and/or polydactyly). They also noted retarded development and cartilaginous defects in limb buds from 12-day-old embryos cultured in this drug.

Brummett and Johnson (1979a, b) in a series of studies examined the biochemical factors related to initial mineralization and its alteration in limbs of rats receiving chlorambucil during the period of cartilage-model calcification. They noted that the level of alkaline phosphatase increased in association with normal cartilage formation while the increase was only half as great in abnormal limbs. In addition, the pyrophosphatan and acid phosphatase in both normal and abnormal limbs did not change. The defects they observed were irregular mineralization of the humerus, bowing of the radius and ulna, angulated ribs, and fibular hemimelia while the controls were normal. Kernis (1972) treated pregnant rats with an i.p. dose of chlorambucil on day 12, 14, or 15 of gestation. The author observed an increase in fetal mortality in those fetuses whose mothers were treated on day 12 of gestation. Other defects cited were syndactyly and hemimelia of both fore- and hindpaws with phocomelia present only in the forelimb and polydactyly and clubfoot present only in the hindlimb. Murphy *et al.* (1958) injected chlorambucil into the yolk sac of a 4-d-old chick embryo. The most significant effect noted was a decrease in fetal weight. In studies on mice and rabbits, Didcock *et al.* (1956) noted that this drug produced increased abortions in both species.

There have been few reports in the literature on human teratogenesis of one of the most widely used antitumor agents, cyclophosphamide (CP). One such report (Greenburg and Tanka, 1964) was of a mother who was being treated for Hodgkin's disease and whose infant was born with bilateral absence of the big toe, cleft palate, and a hypoplastic middle phalynx of the fifth finger. In other cases involving treatment of Hodgkin's patients, Jacobs *et al.* (1981) noted only one infant (whose mother was being treated with CP) bore defects of the hands, feet, palate, and uvula. In another instance an infant was born with a single left coronary artery and the absence of all toes (Toledo *et al.*, 1971). Pizzuto *et al.* (1980) discovered, though, that in nine patients treated for acute leukemia with CP no defects in the offspring were observed. From the small number of cases so far reported, the conclusion that CP is a human teratogen is not warranted. In addition, in two of the reported cases the mothers were also exposed to X-ray treatment. However, in all animal species tested except sheep (Dolnick *et al.*, 1970) the drug has been shown to be teratogenic.

A CP syndrome was identified by von Kreylig (1965) in rat fetuses whose mothers had received the drug during pregnancy. This syndrome included limb, facial, and CNS defects and disturbances in ossification. Chaube *et al.* (1967) found CP to be teratogenic only when given on gestation days 11 and 12 in the rat. In addition to retarded development, the primary defects they observed were associated with the limbs (e.g., clubbed foot, ectro-, syn-, or polydactyly). Singh (1971) and Singh and Sanyal (1974) studied the effect of time of treatment with CP on the development and ossification of the limbs in the Wistar rat. They found that day 12 was the most sensitive to malformations of the digits and day 15 or 16 to limb and skeletal deformities. Ashby *et al.* (1976), in studying the same strain of rat treated with CP, found no defects prior to day 6.5 or after day 14.5 of gestation.

Decreased growth and characteristic morphologic lesions that had been observed in *in vivo* studies using CP also occurred in the *in vitro* studies of rat embryos (Schmid et. al., 1981). Sanyal *et al.* (1981), however, found no effect on day 11 CD rat fetuses treated *in vitro* for 2 days with CP. Kitchin *et al.* (1981) found that CP did not inhibit embryonic growth until they added a microsomal activating/embryo culture system. The researchers then noted decreased yolk sac size, embryonic protein, DNA content, and somite number. These findings were supported by the study of Mirkes *et al.* (1981) of rat embryos cultured from days 10 to 11 of gestation with CP. When Satish *et al.* (1985) cultured 11-day-old rat embryos in a CP metabolite, phosphoramide mustard, the embryos showed retarded embryonic growth and CNS anomalies. The forelimb, though, was unaffected by local injection of the agent into somitic tissue adjacent to the presumptive limb-bud region. From the *in vitro* studies in the rat and other species (Wiger *et al.*, 1989), it was observed that the parent compound, CP, must be metabolically activated to produce malformations in limbs developed in culture. This activation of the compound is by the hepatic P-450 system.

Shogi and Ohzu (1965) were among the first to report on the teratogenicity of CP in the mouse. They found that mice treated on days 11 to 14 of gestation had offspring with cleft palate, syndactyly, and kinky tail. Gibson and Becker (1968b) noted that fetal mice were most sensitive to this agent on days 10 to 12 of gestation. The skeletal defects they noted were of the digits, including adactyly, syndactyly, and polydactyly. Gebhardt (1970) confirmed their studies using the Swiss strain of mouse. Reiners *et al.* (1987) compared drug injection with drug infusion of CP in NMRI mice and found that not only the rates but also the pattern of malformations differed between the two regimens. A single injection of 20 mg/kg induced a malformation rate of 100%, while the same dose by constant rate infusion resulted in only 16% malformation rate. Defects observed were vertebral, rib, phalanges, and fibula. *In vitro* mouse studies (Manson and Smith, 1977; Hales and Jain, 1986) using hepatic P-450 generated metabolite(s) of CP in the culture noted preaxial ectrodactyly and hemimelia in the treated embryos.

Several studies of CP in the rabbit (Gerlinger, 1964; Fritz and Hess, 1971; Claussen *et al.*, 1980) have shown that the induction of the various skeletal defects observed was dependent upon the time of drug administration during the pregnancy. Days 11 to 13 were found to be most sensitive to teratogenic insult to the limbs. McClure *et al.* (1979), in studies on the *Macaca mullata* species of monkey, noted that the offspring of mothers treated with intramuscular doses of CP on days 25 to 43 of gestation were born with cleft lip/palate, craniofacial dysmorphia, ectrosyndactyly, and other skeletal variations. The combination of defects that they noted in the monkey is similar to that described as the CP syndrome by von Kreyhig (1965) in the rat fetus.

There have been conflicting reports with regard to the teratogenic potential of busulfan in the human treated prior to conception or during the first trimester of pregancy (Diamond *et al.*, 1960; Dennis and Stein, 1965; Nicholson, 1968; Johnson, 1972; Abramovici *et al.*, 1978). Results from experiments with laboratory animals have shown that busulfan is teratogenic in the mouse (Machado, 1968), rat (Murphy *et al.*, 1958; Weingarten *et al.*, 1971), and chick (Swartz, 1980). Swartz felt that the alteration of the vascular system, which affects the differentiation of the mesenchymal cells in the limb, may account for the abnormalities that were observed.

One other alkalating agent that has been studied for its teratogenicity in the mouse is N-Methyl-N'-nitro-N-nitroso-guanidine (MNNG) (Inouye and Murakami, 1978). Pregnant mice were treated on one of gestational days 7 to 12 with an i.p. dose of MNNG. When the fetuses were examined on day 18 of gestation, vertebral, long-bone, and fore- and hindlimb defects were noted. Ectrodactyly and microdactyly appeared with greater frequency on the left side of the body, while polydactyly appeared more frequently as a bilateral defect. Central nervous system and cleft palate defects were also present. In a study by Faustman *et al.* (1989), five direct-acting alkylating agents were studied in rat cultures of postimplantation embryos. The authors noted that in all five agents there was a significant dose-related decrease in protein, DNA, crown-rump length, and somites; minimal changes occurred in limb size.

Antimetabolites

The antimetabolites are structural analogues of substances required for normal physiological function. These antimetabolites interfere with or replace an essential metabolite by causing its deficiency or substituting for it *in vivo* . Other terms that have been applied to these substances are metabolic antagonists, enzyme antagonists, and competitive antagonists.

Folic Acid

The folic acid antagonists, aminopterin and methotrexate (MTX), have been identified as human teratogens and used to induce abortions during the first trimester. Thiersch (1952) described 12 cases of therapeutic abortion in which aminopterin was used, in two of which the attempted abortion did not succeed, and the infants were delivered at term. In each case the infant had gross multiple anomalies. The offspring of women who have received a folic acid antagonist during pregnancy have certain characteristic features in common, including pre- and postnatal growth deficiency, lack of ossification of various cranial bones, shortened forearms, hand anomalies, congenital dislocated hip, clubfoot, lambdoidal and coronal suture synostosis, and an upswept frontal hair pattern (Melzer, 1956; Thiersch, 1956; Warkany *et al.*, 1959; Emerson, 1962; Milunsky *et al.*, 1968; Powell and Ekert, 1971; Shaw, 1972; Warkany, 1981). This consistent pattern of malformations led Gellis and coworkers (1979) to identify an aminopterin embryopathy syndrome.

Laboratory studies have indicated that aminopterin is not a particularly potent teratogen. It has been shown to produce skeletal defects in the chick (Karnofsky *et al.*, 1949), rat (Thiersch and Philips, 1950), and sheep (James and Keeler, 1968). MTX, however, has proved to have a greater effect on pregnant animals, inducing malformations in fetal rats, rabbits, cats, and (to a much lesser degree) fetal mice and monkeys. In a comparative study, Wilson (1971) noted that in the rat MTX produced a resorption rate of 64% while 30% of the live fetuses were malformed. In the pregnant monkey, though, the only effect noted from MTX treatment was an increase in spontaneous abortions. Thiersch and Philips (1950), in studying two strains of rats, theorized that the mesenchyme was the site of action of this drug. In this same study CFW mouse fetuses showed no effects from the drug except an increase in the number of fetal deaths. These findings were confirmed by a later study using ICR mice (Skalko and Gold, 1974). In other studies carried out on the rat, Thiersch (1954) and Berry (1971) showed that the teratogenic effects of MTX can be prevented by treatment with folinic acid.

Woo *et al.* (1978) studied the augmentation of MTX-induced embryotoxicity by aspirin in rats. They found that the frequency of fetal malformations was not affected and fetal weight loss was not additive in the combined treatment. Pretreatment with aspirin, however, enhanced the embryolethality of the drug given on day 12 of gestation. The findings of a low incidence of teratogenic effects of MTX in this study are in accord with the view that the drug is highly fetotoxic and only moderately teratogenic in rats (Wilson, 1971; Jordan *et al.*, 1977). Intravenous injection of MTX into pregnant New Zealand white rabbits caused 50% of the fetuses to die, while 25% of the offspring that survived were malformed (Jordan *et al.*, 1970). The dosage used in this was 45 times that used in rats to produce an 80% resorption rate. The investigators proposed that the discrepancy in dosages between species may be the result of the lack of MTX inactivation in the rat, thus allowing for a build up of the drug to teratogenic levels.

In the rabbit the drug is rapidly inactivated before teratogenic levels are reached. In a later study by Jordan *et al.* (1977) using the same two species, the authors noted that rabbit embryos were more resistant to small doses of MTX than rats. When MTX was given intravenously on days 10 to 15 of gestation, the rabbit offspring exhibited a constant spectrum of malformations that included skull defects and severe fore- and hindlimb dysplasias. Khera (1975) treated pregnant cats with an oral dose of MTX on days 11 to 14, 14 to 17, or 17 to 20 of gestation. Test fetuses exposed on days 11 to 14 or 14 to 17 had the highest incidence of malformations, including retarded ossification of the calvarium.

Brewton and MacCabe (1990) using an avian model showed that MTX, when administered *in vivo* at stages 18 to 22 and examined on day 11 incubation, produced malformed wings in a stage-dependent manner while the chick legs were affected similarly at each stage studied. *In vitro* studies of the tissues did not show any measurable toxicity, suggesting that MTX may be metabolized differently *in vitro*. They suggested that limb malformations may be caused by a transient inhibition of cell division rather than an increase in cell death.

Another folic acid antagonist, 9-methyl pteroylglutamic acid (9MePGA), has been shown to be teratogenic in rats. Chepenik *et al.* (1970) showed that this agent significantly decreased the ATP levels and total adenine levels in the tissues of the developing rat. The authors felt that the failure of chondrogenesis may be the direct result of decreased ATP. *In vitro* rat studies by Schmidt *et al.* (1977) indicated that administration of 9MePGA on days 11 to 14 of gestation resulted in a variety of skeletal malformations, particularly of the long bones of the limbs. In a later *in vitro* study by Schmidt *et al.* (1982), a significant increase in the accumulation of labeled glycosaminoglycan was observed in the treated fetal forelimbs, but not in the hindlimbs. According to the authors, however, the significance of this increase is unknown.

While the remaining antimetabolites discussed in this section have not been shown to be teratogenic in the human, several have been suspect because of the increased incidence of offspring who are small-for-date in mothers who received one or more of these agents during pregnancy (Diamond *et al.*, 1960; Gilliland and Weinstein, 1983). The majority of these drugs, though, have been shown to be teratogenic in several laboratory species.

Purines

Four out of the eight purine analogues tested by Kury *et al.* (1968) in the rat on day 11 of gestation were found to be teratogenic. The gross external malformations observed were cleft lip/palate and deformed appendages and tail in fetuses treated with mercaptopurine, mercaptopurine riboside, mercaptopurine-3-*N*-oxide, or 6-hydroxyl-aminopurine. The malformations of the appendages were clubbing, adactyly, ectrodactyly, syndactyly, or brachydactyly. Of these four, mercaptopurine (used in the treatment of leukemia) has also been shown to produce developmental anomalies in the frog (Bieber *et al.*, 1952), chick (Karnofsky, 1960), and rat (Murphy and Chaube, 1962; Amemiya *et al.*, 1989). In the human, however, mercaptopurine has not had an adverse effect on fetal development (Huch *et al.*, 1984).

Electron microscopic studies on the cytotoxic effects of mercaptopurine on the limb-bud blastemal cell of rat embryos showed extensive damage to the limb blastemal cells on day $12 + 3$ h, the critical period when cartilage is beginning to develop (Merker *et al.*, 1975). It should be noted that the mechanism leading to this necrosis was not identified. Scott *et al.* (1980)

injected the pregnant rat with mercaptopurine riboside on day 11 of gestation. A high percentage of preaxial polydactyly of the hindlimb was observed. Their study provides further evidence that delayed ectodermal cell death is a cause of polydactyly; see Scott *et al.* (1977) for a review of the mechanism involved in the production of polydactyly. Amemiya *et al.* (1986, 1989) felt that mercaptopurine-induced alterations in mineral metabolism, in particular zinc, copper, iron, calcium, and magnesium, may affect reproduction and embryogenesis in the rat. The most common defects that they observed in rat fetuses treated with this drug were fewer ossification sites in the digits and vertebrae, polydactyly, syndactyly, phocomelia, and club foot. The purine agents that tested negative for the production of defects in the rat in Kury's study were methylmercaptopurine riboside, hydroxyl-amino-purine riboside, xanthine-3-*N*-oxide, and guanine-3-*N*-oxide.

In addition to the agents studied by Kury *et al.* (1968), the skeletal system of the chick has been shown to be sensitive to the purines azaserine and deoxyguanosine (dGUR) (Karnofsky and Lacon, 1964). Day 4 azaserine-treated chick embryos were found at hatching to have facial and palatal clefting and appendicular defects of both wings and the legs, including micromelia, hypophalangy, ectrodactyly, and hemimelia. This same myriad of defects has been observed in chicks treated with mercaptopurine (Grubb and Montigel, 1975). Adenine has been shown to prevent the action of azaserine on the skeleton of the chick embryo. Joint anomalies are the primary defect in treatment with dGUR on day 4, 5, or 6, but by the 7th day of development the drug is no longer a potent teratogen to the skeletal system. Injection of deoxycytidine into the chick embryo was shown to prevent the teratogenic effects of dGUR.

Pyrimidines

Several pyrimidine analogs also have teratogenic capability. Ritter *et al.* (1973) studied the pattern of cell death in relation to malformations in the rat limb. Rat embryos were exposed on day 12 of gestation to one of three cytotoxic drugs — hydroxyurea, cytosine arabinoside, and cytosine arabinoside palmitate. The last two drugs are pyrimidine analogs, while hydroxyurea is discussed under the miscellaneous group of chemotherapeutic agents. All three drugs produced varying patterns of ectrodactyly and adactyly. The authors felt that the particular digital malformations were a function of when cytotoxic damage occurred rather than the time of drug administration.

Kochhar *et al.* (1978) also found that a single dose of cytosine arabinoside injected i.p. into pregnant ICR mice produced a pattern of reduction defects of the limbs specific for each developmental stage at which treatment was given. Deoxycytidine injected simultaneously at doses eight times larger than cytosine arabinoside afforded virtually complete protection against the teratogenic effect of ectrodactyly. An increase in polydactyly, however, was found in protected fetuses leading the authors to theorize that there may be a common cellular basis underlying these two types of digital defects. Naruse and Kameyama (1986) found that cytosine arabinoside at a subteratogenic dose prevented the genetic expression of polydactyly in almost all $Pdn/^+$ and in some cases of Pdn/Pdn mice.

It is well-known that 5-bromodeoxyuridine (BudR), when injected into pregnant animals, may cause exencephaly, cleft palate, and limb anomalies (Bannigan and Langman, 1979). It produces preaxial polydactyly in most rodent species: mice (DiPaolo, 1964; Skalko et al., 1971; Roetz and Michels, 1977), hamsters (Ruffolo and Ferm, 1965), and rats (Scott et al., 1978, 1981). The halogenated pyrimidine BudR has also been shown to significantly inhibit chondrogenesis in the forelimb of mouse embryos treated in vitro (Agnish and Kochhar, 1976). If embryos are at a very early stage of limb development when exposed to BudR, limb differentiation is permanently and irreversibly damaged.

Treatment of C57BL/10 mice by various dosages of 5-fluoro-2'-deoxycytidine (FUDR), a fluoropyrimidine, on day 9 or 11 produces varying patterns of limb aplasias, synostoses, synchondroses, and inhibition of calcification (Kleinebrecht et al., 1972). This is in addition to supernumerary distal limb elements (Kleinebrecht et al., 1974). Bro-Rasmussen et al. (1971) administered FUDR on day 11 of gestation in mice and found extravasation of blood in the extremities on day 12. These areas of extravasation were later observed to become hematomas. This necrosis of blood vessels may account for the lack of normal limb development.

Chick studies using FUDR and fluorouracil (FU) have shown that these agents do not produce many defects in embryos surviving to 18 days, except for duplication of the first toe (Karnofsky and Lacon, 1964). Hall (1987), in a study of the mandibular skeleton of the chick exposed to FUDR, found that growth of the entire mandibular process was delayed. This differs from that of the rat in which FUDR inhibits the differentiation of Meckel's cartilage (Ferguson, 1978); catch-up growth, though, restored growth of the mandible to normal. Ferguson (1985) also administered FUDR to alligator embryos in vitro and found that the drug inhibited mandibular growth, but Meckel's cartilage differentiated normally. He attributed this to FUDR's action in migratory neural crest-derived cells. It is well known that a high percentage of digital malformations, including preaxial polydactyly, can be induced by 5-FU (Dagg, 1960; Kameyama et al., 1974; Scott, 1979). Mouse studies using FU on day 10, 11, 12, or 13 of gestation showed a variety of limb defects in two inbred strains. The tail region was the most sensitive, while the most common defects of the limbs were macrodactyly, polydactyly, limb reduction, phocomelia, and oligodactyly (Dagg, 1960). Forsthaefel (1972) reported that 5-FU increases the expression of the limb-skeletal effects of Strong's luxoid gene when injected intraperitoneally on days 8 to 11 of gestation.

The antimetabolite 6-amino-nicotinamide (6-AN) has been widely used as an experimental teratogen in combination with the protective agent nicotinomide (NAM). Landauer (1957) conducted studies with chicks, Murphy et al. (1957) with chicks and rats, and Pinsky and Fraser (1959) with mice. Chamberlain (1970) found that in vivo treatment with 6-AN resulted in decreased growth and congenital anomalies in rats. Since ATP is required for the synthesis of active sulfate (necessary for chondrogenesis and for synthesis of cyclic AMP), the observation by Ritter et al. (1975) on the inhibition or reduction of ATP synthesis in rat fetuses associated with 6-AN treatment in pregnant rats may help explain the production of limb defects in addition to other malformations.

Antibiotics

Ametantrone acetate is an antineoplastic antibiotic with antitumor activity against a variety of murine neoplasias (Johnson et al., 1979). Studies by Petrere et al. (1986), using rats and rabbits, noted that this drug was not teratogenic in the rat, while rabbit fetuses showed an increase in malformed litters. Fetal body weights, however, were not affected, and few skeletal defects occurred in the malformed litters. These findings are in contrast to studies on other antineoplastic antibiotics in which the rat is more sensitive. Thompson et al. (1978) studied adriamycin and daunomycin in rats and rabbits. Both drugs were teratogenic in the rat, causing a significant decrease in fetal weight and digital defects, but not in the rabbit. Daunomycin caused rib fusions, but less frequent digital defects in the rat. A high incidence of abortion occurred in rabbits treated with adriomycin; the primary defects were of the soft tissue type. Oguro et al. (1973) noted that adriomycin was not teratogenic in rats and mice.

Other antiobiotic agents that have been shown to be teratogenic are antinomycin C in the rat (Wilson, 1964), mitomycin in the mouse (Tanimura, 1961), and L-alanosine which induced scoliosis, forelimb, and other skeletal defects in the rat. Actinobolin, actidione, mithramycin, and nogalomycin have not been shown to produce defects in the rat (Murphy, 1962; Chaube and Murphy, 1968).

There have been no reports to date of birth defects in children whose mothers were treated with chemotherapeutic antibiotic drugs during pregnancy.

Miscellaneous

Thiadiazole

Murphy et al. (1957) were the first to report on the teratogenic action of this agent. They injected rats on day 9, 11, or 12 of gestation with

2-ethylamino-1,3,4-thiadiazole. Only day 11 treatment produced fetal defects of the axial skeleton. Beaudoin (1972), in studying 2-amino-1,3,4-thiadiazole in Wistar rats, showed that there were two periods of susceptibility to this drug. The first, day 5, showed a significant increase in the resorption rate while the second, days 9 to 13, produced major malformations, including ectrodactyly and syndactyly. Simultaneous treatment with nicotinamide produced a dramatic reduction as seen in both resorptions (37 to 6%) and in malformations (94 to 0%). Beaudoin (1973) extended his first study to include treatment of the pregnant rats with 2-amino-1,3,4-thiadiazole hydrochloride from days 1 to 16 of gestation. He supplemented the treatment with nicotinamide on days 5, 11, 12, and 13. This regimen markedly diminished the teratogenic and lethal effects of thiadiazole. Treatment on day 11 completely abolished the teratogenic effect. Scott et al. (1972) confirmed that simultaneous injection of nicotinamide with its antagonist aminothiadiazole protected the rat embryo and helped prevent reduction deformities of the digits. Wotring and Beaudoin (1980) studied the cartilaginous fusions, DNA synthesis, and protein synthesis, in embryonic rat limbs after injection of aminothiadiazole. They found abnormal cartilaginous continuities between various cartilage elements in 99% of the treated limbs. Cotreatment with nicotinamide, though, prevented fusion and depression of DNA synthesis.

Hadacidin

Because of the general metabolic effect that this drug exerts on the body, it is not suprising that halacidin causes a wide range of embryonic abnormalities, including growth deficiencies and skeletal defects. Hadacidin produces abnormalities of skeletal differentiation by disrupting morphogenetic rather than the initiative phases of development of particular elements in the rat, mouse, hamster, and chick (Murphy, 1962; Lejour-Jeanty, 1966; Roux and Horvath, 1971; Kollar, 1976; Shah, 1977; Jaskoll et al., 1978). The most frequent defects are abnormal extremities, thickened or distorted ribs, fused vertebrae, and abnormal long bones.

Hydroxyurea

This agent induces a high percentage of multiple defects in the craniofacial and trunk regions as well as the axial and appendicular skeleton in the rat, mouse, pig, dog, chick, hamster, and monkey (Murphy and Chaube, 1962, 1964; Ferm, 1965, 1966; Chaube and Murphy, 1966, 1973; Szabo and Kang, 1969; Wilson, 1971; Earl et al., 1973; Theisen et al., 1973; DeSesso and Jordan, 1977). Millicovsky and DeSesso (1980) noted apparent collapse of the vasculature of the forelimb bud and facial region in the fetal rabbit after a teratogenic dose of hydroxyurea. An intact vasculature is thought to be necessary for normal skeletal development. DeSesso (1981a, b), in a comparative ultrastructural study of rabbit limb buds treated with hydroxyurea or methotrexate, found that the primary morphologic site of action of these two drugs was different. He noted that with hydroxyurea treatment there was an increase in cell death and intercellular spaces. Methotrexate, however, caused a breakdown of intercellular junctions; an increase in cell death was not apparent.

Sugrue and DeSesso (1982) studied the alterations in glycosaminoglycan composition of embryonic rat forelimbs that had been exposed to hydroxyurea. They noted that beginning at 12 h posttreatment, an elevated hyaluronic acid/chondroitin sulfate ratio allowed for increased proliferation and reorganization of mesenchymal cells, thus indicating a recovery phase to the pathogenesis of hydroxyurea treatment.

Urethane

Defects of the CNS and limbs have been demonstrated in fetal rats (Hall, 1953; Murphy and Chaube, 1964), mice (Sinclair, 1950; Yasuda, 1977), and hamsters (Ferm, 1966) treated *in utero* with urethane. Yasuda (1977) noted that digital anomalies produced *in vivo* by treatment of pregnant ICR/JCL mice with urethane can also be produced in embryonic limbs cultured on days 11, 12, and 13 of gestation.

Vincristine

Some plant-derived antitumor agents, such as vincristine, colchicine, maytansine, VP-16-213, and VM-26, have been shown to be teratogenic in mice (Sieber *et al.*, 1978). These researchers observed that, at teratogenic doses, all compounds induced various cranial abnormalities as well as major skeletal defects.

Because virtually all anticancer agents are teratogenic in at least one laboratory animal species, the risk involved in treatment with these agents in the human during the first trimester of pregnancy must be weighed against the expected benefit to the mother.

Diuretics

At present, a relationship between the use of diuretics during pregnancy and congenital malformations in the human has not been shown. Diuretic agents carry, however, the warning that they should not be used in pregnancy, especially during the first trimester, unless the benefits outweigh the potential adverse effects that have been demonstrated in animal studies.

The routine use of diuretics during pregnancy is inappropriate as they do not prevent development of toxemia of pregnancy. Diuretics should be used only to treat pathologic causes of edema, not edema arising from the physiological or mechanical problems caused by pregnancy.

Animal studies involving the following diuretics — amiloride, dichlorphenamide, furosemide, hydrachlorothiazide, spironolactone, theophylline, and triamterene — have not shown a significant increase in bone defects in fetuses who have been exposed to these drugs *in utero*. Acetazolamide (ACE) used in humans since 1953, however, is the one diuretic that consistently produces skeletal defects in several of the animal models studied. The majority of animal studies have used ACE because of the unique teratological picture that this drug produces, first reported in 1965 by Layton and Hallesy. These investigators fed the drug to rats and mice throughout the pregnancy. The defect produced by the drug was postaxial ectrodactyly of the right forelimb. Even when the defect was found to occur bilaterally, it was more severe on the right side. These authors (Hallesy and Layton, 1967) also studied Sherman rats treated throughout the gestation period with dichlorphenamide, another carbonic anhydrase inhibitor. They found that this diuretic produced the same defects as found in ACE-treated animals. Wilson *et al.* (1968) further characterized ACE and ethoxzolamide teratogenesis in Wistar rats, determining that the susceptible period for producing a reduction deformity of the forelimbs was between days 10 and 11 of gestation. The technique used by Scott (1970) of intrauterine administration of ACE in rats eliminated maternal metabolism as a causative factor in the drug's teratogenesis. Scott *et al.* (1972) also noted in rats that a significant number of late fetal and term live births, affected by distal postaxial deficiency of the right forelimb, were female. Holmes *et al.* (1988), working with C57BL/ 6J mice, noted that males were significantly more likely to be malformed than females at all dose levels. They also found that the occurrence of limb defects did not correlate with maternal weight loss, fetal birth weight, or fetal position *in utero*.

Kimmel and Wilson (1973) examined several skeletal variations (e.g., ribs, vertebral centra, sternebrae) that occur spontaneously in rats. They wanted to determine if these variations could be increased by either manipulations associated with sham treatment of controls or by various doses of known teratogenic agents, one of which was ACE. Their data did not show that these variations could serve as a signal of teratogenic potential. Muther *et al.* (1977) felt that the injection vehicle combined with ACE would potentiate the drug's teratogenicity in the rat. The frequency of hemimelia, micromelia, and bilateral limb defects was greater in litters exposed to high pH ACE or to the epinephrine-acetazolamide combination. The researchers postulated that the reduction of uterine blood flow may be responsible for the potentiation of teratogenicity. Ugen and Scott (1985) also stated that a decrease in uterine blood flow may be a mechanism for production of these defects. In working with Wistar rats, they found that the vasoactive agents serotonin, ergotamine, nicotine, and phenylephrine potentiate ACE-induced forelimb ectrodactyly. Pretreatment with phenoxybenzamine and prazosin, α-adrenergic antagonists, prevented the phenylephrine-induced increase in limb defects. In addition, physical clamping of uterine horns plus ACE increased the frequency of forelimb ectrodactyly. In another study on potentiated response of ACE plus other agents, Ritter et al. (1982) administered ACE and inhibitors of DNA synthesis, RNA synthesis, and protein synthesis to pregnant rats together with caffeine at doses where each agent alone caused minimal embryotoxicity. Caffeine coadministered with any of the other agents caused a potentiated response. It was not known if much lower doses of caffeine, as normally found in humans, would potentiate the toxicity of other drugs.

Schreiner et al. (1981) studied the distribution of carbonic anhydrase and its inhibition by ACE in the rat, CBA/J mouse, and SWV mouse embryos. The authors noted that the forelimb buds of resistant and sensitive embryos had carbonic anhydrase activity in the area between the ectoderm and mesenchyma. There was no localization of enzyme activity corresponding to the malformation seen in ACE teratogenesis. They suggested that carbonic anhydrase in the forelimb was not the primary site of action for ACE. Castro-Correia et al. (1974) gave CR mice s.c. doses of sodium ACE on days 8 to 12 of gestation. They found that the drug had low maternal toxicity and embryolethality. In the fetuses, right forelimb postaxial polydactyly was more frequent than postaxial ectrodactyly. The fetuses were more sensitive on day 8 of gestation and not sensitive after gestational day 10. Other defects noted were exencephaly and macroglassia. Holmes and Trelstad (1979) examined histologic sections of mouse limbs exposed in utero to ACE. The authors were first able to identify the postaxial deformity on day 10.9 of gestation. There was a postaxial deficiency of mesenchyme without cell necrosis. Since the deformity was present prior to the aggregation of the mesenchymal cell stage of chondrogensis and the cell orientation was normal, they postulated that the primary effect was not on the formation of precartilage aggregates.

Tellone et al. (1980), working with CD-1 mice, noted rib, vertebral, ectrodactyly, and tail defects in fetuses treated with the drug. In addition, there was a reduction in fetal weight and crown-rump length and an increase in resorption rate in treated litters. Beck (1983), also using the CD-1 mouse, devised an assay system that was able to give a postnatal assessment of prenatal exposure to ACE in adult skeletons, even in the absence of gross abnormalities. In later work (Beck, 1989), using several toxic agents, including ACE noted that prenatal ossification of cervical centra was an excellent indicator of prenatal exposure to noxious substances.

Several studies of ACE teratogenicity have compared the effect of this drug on different strains of mice. One such study by Green et al. (1973) found that i.p. administration of ACE on day 9 or 10 of gestation in several inbred strains of mice produced postaxial abnormalities of the forelimb. A high frequency of defects was found in the CBA/J and C57BL/6J strains. An intermediate frequency in the A/J and DBA/2J was most susceptible on day 10 of gestation, the A/J on days 9 and 10, and the C57BL/6J and C3H/HeJ on day 9 of gestation. They also noted no reduction of amniotic fluid. Biddle (1975), in studies on the teratogenesis of ACE in the CBA/J and SWV strains of mice, found that SWV mice were totally resistant to the teratogenic and embryolethal actions of the drug. Hackman and Hurley (1983) discussed the interaction of dietary zinc, genetic strain, and ACE in CBA (sensitive) and SWV (resistant) mice. They found that the magnitude of the response was strongly influenced by the strain. Kuczuk and Scott (1984), also working with the SWV strain and the C57BL/6J mouse strain, treated both groups with cadium sulfate, ACE, and a combination of the two. Both drugs are carbonic anhydrase inhibitors. In the C57BL/6J fetuses treatment with both drugs independently plus in combination produced forelimb defects. $CdSO_4$, however, produced more left-sided and bilateral defects of the forelimb in addition to hindlimb defects. Kinky tail and rib defects were also noted. The SWV strain showed no limb defects, but kinky tail and rib abnormalities were present.

Milaire (1985), also working with the C57BL mouse and a combination of $CdSO_4$ and ACE, identified nine different morphological types of postaxial defects. Milaire's colony, though, was particularly resistant to ACE. Biddle (1988) studied 11 inbred strains of mice to determine the genetic differences in the frequency of ACE-induced ectrodactyly. ACE treatment produced limb defects in all strains. He also noted that ACE induced a spectrum of malformations in the mouse, including cleft palate, microphthalmia, exencephaly, and other skeletal abnormalities.

An SEM and TEM study by Datu et al. (1985), using Jcl:ICR mice treated with ACE, noted that the apical ectodermal ridge (AER) did not extend as far postaxially as in the control animals. The mesenchymal cell processes beneath the malformed ridge were denser than the controls. The authors felt that the disturbance of the AER-mesenchymal interactions may be the mechanism involved in the production of the limb defects associated with ACE. Brown et al. (1989) studied asymmetric developmental limb defects induced by treatment either in utero with ACE or in culture with misonidazole. The researchers noted that in situs inversus in mice the right limb defects were induced in situs solitus embryos, and left-sided defects were produced in situs inversus.

Layton (1971), working with the golden hamster, found that fetuses exposed to ACE on day 9 of gestation exhibited postaxial limb defects. These defects were, however, different from those seen in mice and rats. Both forelimbs were affected equally, and the left hindlimb showed preaxial deformity. The first external signs of the deformity were seen as a flattening of postaxial margins of the limb bud 24 h after the drug was administered. Landauer and Wakasugi (1967) injected either ACE or *N*-ethylnicotinamide into the yolk sac of the chick at 24 and 96 h of incubation. These diuretics in the chick produced nonspecific beak and skeletal defects.

Studies of the regenerating urodele limb are often considered to be an analog of limb development. It has been postulated that the urodele limb should be susceptible to teratogens, which selectively disrupt the developing limb. Dinsmore and Maren (1986), however, showed that ACE was toxic to the redbacked salamander. They noted that it did not have the same teratogenic effect on limb regeneration as seen in mammalian limb development.

DeSesso and Jordan (1977) found a high percentage of hypoplasia and lack of ossification of the first metacarpal in the rabbit, which accompanied generalized growth retardation. The authors indicated that ACE inhibition of carbonic anhydrase was the most likely mechanism of induced defects. Yet studies by Layton and Hallesy (1965) and Scott *et al.* (1981) noted that rabbits were resistant to ACE teratogenicity. Scott and co-workers also noted that rhesus monkeys showed no ACE-related defects.

Some studies are beginning to appear on the effect of "loop" diuretics in pregnant animals. Robertson *et al.* (1981) indicated that the loss of potassium could be a causative factor for skeletal malformations in rats treated with the loop diuretic, indacrinone. CRCD rats were treated with three doses of indacrinone on days 6 to 17 of gestation. There was a dose-related increase in wavy ribs and scapular and humerus defects in all drug-treated groups. One percent of KCl during the drug-dosing period reduced the incidence of wavy ribs and eliminated scapular and limb defects. These authors also noted that another diuretic, furosemide, produced the same defects. In a study of the loop diuretic, furosemide, in Sprague-Dawley rats [Crj:CD(SD)], Nakatsuka (1988) observed an increased incidence of wavy ribs, but no limb defects. He proposed that the wavy ribs could be caused by intrinsic factors, fetal musculature, or extrinsic factors, such as uterine musculature coupled with a decrease in amniotic fluid. Toxicity testing in rats, rabbits, dogs, hamsters, and baboons of bumetanide (McClain and Dammers, 1981), a potent diuretic agent, indicated that it was well tolerated in these various species. The toxicity that was observed is similar to that produced by other loop diuretics.

Dichlorphenamide, another carbonic anhydrase inhibitor, when used as treatment in Sherman rats throughout the gestation period, produced the same defects as found in ACE-treated animals (Hallesy and Layton, 1967).

Psychotropics

A review of the literature on therapeutic drug treatment for psychosis during pregnancy reveals a limited number of studies of the effect on the fetus. The drugs of this group have antiemetic and sedative properties as well as psychotropic properties. These therapeutic drugs include tranquilizers (antianxiety and antipsychotic agents), antidepressants, and sedatives. Also in this group are the anticonvulsants that have already been discussed. There have been several review articles (Linden and Rich, 1983; Martin, 1984; Spielvogel and Wile, 1986; Robinson *et al.*, 1986; Halbreich and Carson, 1989; Nurnberg, 1989; Cohen, 1989; Cohen *et al.*, 1989; Mortola, 1989) that describe the use and management of psychotrophic drugs in the pregnant patient, but few articles have alluded to the teratogenicity of this class of drug (Chan, 1984; Gal and Sharpless, 1984; Kellogg, 1985; Elia *et al.*, 1987; Warkany, 1988).

Tranquilizers

Antianxiety Agents

As a group, these minor tranquilizers rank as one of the most frequently prescribed drugs in use today. Daube and Chou (1966) attributed the brain defects observed in a child to the drug meprobamate, which the mother had taken during the first 3 months of pregnancy. Milkovich and van den Berg (1974), in a prospective study of 19,044 live births from 1959 to 1966, noted that the tranquilizers meprobamate and chlordiazepoxide (Librium®) accounted for almost 75% of the nonbarbiturates used by the mothers of these infants. The investigators noted that there was an increase in defects 12.1/100 and 11.4/100, respectively, compared with 2.6/100 children with no-drug cohorts. They also observed that if these two drugs were taken after the 6th week of pregnancy, there was no statistically significant increase in the rate of anomalies. The only bone or skeletal defects found were deformed joints and microcephaly.

Crombie *et al.* (1975), in a study of the drugs chlordiazepoxide, diazepam (Valium®), meprobamate, and other carbamates, noted an association between meprobamate and teratogenicity. They did not, however, describe what the teratogenic outcome was. In contrast Belafsky *et al.* (1969), in a retrospective study of 800 pregnant women who received meprobamate during one or more trimesters of pregnancy, did not observe any defects attributable to this drug. Hartz *et al.* (1975), though, found no evidence that either meprobamate or chlordiazepoxide taken at any time during pregnancy was teratogenic.

Patel and Patel (1980), in a case report of an infant exposed *in utero* to clorazepate (SCH 12041), observed that the infant was born with multiple anomalies. These anomalies included shortening of the right femur, bifid left foot, abnormal big toes, shortened digits, absent right fibula, and deformed sacrum. Unilateral duplication of the femur plus myelomeningocele was present in an infant whose mother had ingested the drug hydroxyzine during pregnancy (Balog and Skinner, 1984).

Although not skeletal in origin, the most consistent defect found in human and animal studies of tranquilizers was the presence of cleft lip and/or palate and/or dysmorphic features in newborns whose mothers had been exposed to diazepam during pregnancy (Aarskog, 1975; Safra and Oakley, 1975; Saxén and Saxén, 1975; Czeizel, 1976; Laegreid *et al.*, 1987). The one feature in these newborns that may show an impact on skeletal system development is growth retardation associated with maternal drug use. In a letter to the editor, Istvan (1970) noted that he had delivered a female infant with complete absence of thumbs, including the metacarpal bone, and with congenital dislocation of the head of the radius. He felt that these defects could be due to the diazepam and/or hydroxprogesterone that the mother had received during pregnancy. Ringrose (1972) presented the case of an infant with congenital absence of the left forearm and the radial two digits, syndactyly of the ulnar three digits, left femur hypoplasia, and syndactyly of the left fourth and fifth toes whose mother had taken diazepam and propoxyphene HCL (Darvon®) during the first 2 months of pregnancy. A second infant also had multiple defects including sternal cleft and dysplastic hips. This mother had received propoxyphene HCL and meprobamate during the second week of pregnancy.

Laegreid *et al.* (1987), in a prospective study of 37 women who regularly took oxazepam or diazepam throughout pregnancy, noted that 7 of the 37 children born had growth retardation, dysmorphic features, and multiple malformations. Jick *et al.* (1981), however, found no significant difference between newborns who had been exposed *in utero* to diazepam and flurazepam, and those not exposed to the drugs. In addition, DeLaney (1983) noted no malformations among offspring exposed to i.v. doses of diazepam in combination with an anesthetic. Rosenberg *et al.* (1983), in comparing infants exposed to diazepam to those not exposed, discovered that the drug did not affect the risk of facial clefts. Bergman (1990), however, in a study of diazepam, oxazepam, and nitrazepam did not conclude that these drugs were teratogenic.

As in most drug studies where a combination of drugs is being used by the patient, it is difficult to ascribe a cause/effect relationship to the production of congenital defects to one specific drug of the combination.

In animal studies on the drug chlordiazepoxide, Zbinden (1961) observed no effect on the offspring of rats fed this drug during gestation. Other research (Buttar *et al.*, 1979), though, showed a decrease in fetal weight and an increase in rib defects. Buttar (1980), in examining the drug used in combination with alcohol and alone, observed a decrease in fetal weight, retarded calvaria ossification, and sternal and rib defects. He also noted that the combination of alcohol and chlordiazepoxide had no more effect than chlordiazepoxide alone. Buttar and Moffatt (1983) studied the pre- and postnatal development of Wistar rats treated with propoxyphene (anesthetic) and chlordiazepoxide. The anesthetic alone produced no defects. The combination of drugs produced increased absorptions, decreased fetal weight, retarded ossification of skull bones, and sternal defects. Gill *et al.* (1981) injected hamsters with either chlordiazepoxide or diazepam on day 8 of gestation. The main defects observed were exencephaly and craniorachichisis. The researchers, however, did not observe a dose-related increase in frequency of malformed fetuses in either treatment group. Beyer *et al.* (1984) studied the potentiation of fetal anomalies resulting from treating the golden hamster with chlordiazepoxide and the antidepressant amitriptyline alone and in combination. The authors gave a single i.p. injection and sacrificed the animals on day 15 of gestation. The drugs given in combination produced several different cranial defects — anencephaly, exencephaly, and encephalocele — as well as missing digits and bent tail. When given alone, amitriptyline produced the greatest number of defects.

In a study by Owen *et al.* (1970), male and female rats were treated with oxazepam before and throughout two mating cycles on days 8 to 16 of gestation. Female mice were treated 7 days prior to mating and throughout gestation, and pregnant rabbits were treated on days 8 to 16. No significant differences were observed in the offspring as compared to the controls in any one of the three species.

A large number of the animal studies have involved the effect of diazepam, or a combination of diazepam with other drug(s), on the developing embryo. Miller and Becker (1971) compared the effects of diphenylhydantoin, a known teratogen, and diazepam in the Swiss-Webster mouse. A significant increase in skeletal abnormalities was not observed; however, cleft palate was common to both drugs. In later studies by the same authors (1973, 1975) on diazepam and its metabolites, a decrease in fetal weight, an increase of fetal absorptions, and cleft palate were found. Beall (1972) treated pregnant rats with diazepam and a related compound clorazepate (SCH 12041) (anticonvulsant) on days 6 to 15 of gestation. Neither drug was shown to be teratogenic. A study by the same author using albino rabbits found clorazepate to be nonteratogenic in this species also. Corwin and DeMeyer (1980) injected Long Evans rats with clorazepate on days 8, 9, and 10. No statistical differences were found between the treated and controls in external, visceral, or skeletal malformations. Stenchever and Parks (1975) fed diazepam to two groups of pregnant mice on days 1 to 9 and 5 to 12. No gross fetal anomalies were observed.

Katz (1988) investigated the effect of diazepam on palate formation in the Sprague-Dawley rat. The pregnant dams received 1 of 5 different dose levels of diazepam. Dams in each dosage group were sacrificed between 16.9 and 17.9 days of gestation. The results demonstrated that with an increased dose there was an increased delay in palatal shelf elevation and a decrease in crown rump length. This strain, however, showed a rapid prenatal recovery of the defects. Nagele *et al.* (1981) grew chick embryos in progressively larger doses of diazepam. There was a dose-related inhibition of neural tube closure, blastodermal expansion, and somite formation. Lee *et al.* (1984) studied the effect of diazepam on stage eight explanted chick embryos. They noted that the primary effect was on neuralation. Ramamurthy and Chaudhry (1979) injected pregnant hamsters with i.p. doses of diazepam on days 11, 12, and 13. No cleft lip and/or palate was observed, but the treated fetuses were smaller in size and weight.

Several of the studies on tranquilizers have involved a comparison of different species with several different drugs. One such study by Walker and Patterson (1974) used A/J, C3H, and CD-1 mouse strains to study the effects of the antianxiety agents chlordiazepoxide and hydroxyzine, the antipsychotic agent chlorpromazine, and the barbiturate sedatives pentobarbital, barbital, and phenobarbital on the pregnant dams. The most susceptible strains to the drugs were the A/J and CD-1, while the most teratogenic drugs were phenobarbital and hydroxyzine. The major defect observed was cleft palate, with no reporting of skeletal malformations.

Another comparative study was by Brunand (1975), who observed no teratogenic effects in newborn rats, mice, or rabbits whose mothers had received tetrazepam, clorazepate, or nitrazepam during pregnancy. Other studies by Guerriero and Fox (1977) fed pregnant mice one of six different benzodiazepines in their food from 21 days before mating until birth of the litters. The investigators observed no gross defects. Tuchman-Duplessis (1984) investigated several benzodiazepines (bromazepam, flurazepam, triazolam) in rats, mice, and rabbits and found no teratogenic effects. Saito *et al.* (1984) studied the fetal toxicity of the benzodiazepine derivatives, nitrazepam, oxazepam, nimetazepam, clonazepam, diazepam, and chlordiazepoxide, in Sprague-Dawley rats. They noted that (1) nimetazepam was highly toxic; (2) nitrazepam was less toxic, but showed an increase in fetal malformations; and (3) diazepam showed weak toxicity. Oxazepam and chlordiazepoxide showed no change from controls. The skeletal defects noted were ectrodactyly and club foot.

Antipsychotic Agents

This large group of drugs consists of the widely used phenothiazines as well as drugs with varying chemical structure, all of which are used as major tranquilizers. Because the drugs of this group have psychotropic properties as well as antiemetic and sedative properties, they are often prescribed during pregnancy and have been implicated in the production of birth defects.

In a survey by the Canadian Food and Drug Directorate (1962), eight cases of congenital malformations were associated with mothers who had taken trifluoperazine (Stelazine) during pregnancy. The malformations included polydactyly and clubbed feet. Corner (1962) in the same year reported skeletal abnormalities in twins whose mother had taken the drug during the first 6 months of pregnancy. In addition, Hall (1963) presented a case of phocomelia of the upper limb in a child who had been exposed *in utero* to this drug. A retrospective study by Moriarty and Nance (1963), however, of 472 women who had taken trifluoperazine during pregnancy, found no evidence of increased malformations when compared to a control population.

Several investigators have shown a negative correlation between the intake during pregnancy of the drug chlorpromazine (Thorazine®) and the production of malformations (Sobel, 1961; Kris, 1965; Favre-Tissot, 1967; Reider et al., 1975; Milkovich and van den Berg, 1976; Slone *et al.*, 1977; Nurnberg and Prudic, 1984). However, O'Leary and O'Leary (1964), in examining a newborn, associated the amelia of the lower limb with chlorpromazine that was taken by the mother during pregnancy. In addition, a large prospective survey (Rumeau-Rouquette *et al.*, 1977) of 12,764 women who had used phenothiazines during pregnancy was carried out by the French National Institute of Health and Medical Research. The result of this survey showed a significant increase in malformed infants, especially those exposed to chlorpromazine during the first trimester. The skeletal defects included clubfoot, reduction deformities, polydactyly, syndactyly, and spina bifida.

An increase has also been reported in severe limb anomalies in infants who had been exposed *in utero* to prochlorperazine (Hall, 1963; Freeman, 1972; Ho *et al.*, 1975; Edlund and Craig, 1984; Rafla, 1987).

Haloperidol has been indicated as a possible human teratogen in two cases (Dienlangard and Coignet, 1966; Kopelman *et al.*, 1975). In both of these cases limb development was affected. A retrospective study by van Waes and van de Velde (1969) of 91 cases of women who had received haloperidol during pregnancy did not substantiate (with respect to the induction of congenital defects) the claim that this drug was a potential teratogen.

The widespread use of lithium carbonate in treating manic-depressive patients has led to its scrutiny as a possible teratogen. Several human studies (Goldfield and Weinstein, 1973; Nora *et al.*, 1974; Pitts, 1983; Linden and Rich, 1983; Kallen and Tandberg, 1983; Gelenberg, 1988; Chapman, 1989) have shown that this drug is teratogenic. The primary target, however, is the cardiovascular rather than the skeletal system.

Animal studies involving the antipsychotic agents discussed in the human studies have shown no teratogenic activity in rabbits, hamsters, or chick embryos (Moriarity, 1963; Khan and Azam, 1969; Sherry, 1977; Szabo and Brent, 1974). Variable results have been reported in mice and rats (Roizin *et al.*, 1966; Szabo, 1970; Beall, 1972; Druga *et al.*, 1980; Gill *et al.*, 1982; Rodriquez and Friman, 1985; Sharma and Rawat, 1986; Jurand, 1988, Yu *et al.*, 1988; Hansen *et al.*, 1990; Jurand and Martin, 1990). The skeletal malformations that have been reported for the rat are micromelia and digital defects. In the mouse craniorachischisis, rachischisis, decreased fetal weight, deformed limbs, and syndactyly have been noted. One study (Sing and Padmanabhan, 1979) in particular addressed the effect chlorpromazine has on skeletogenesis in the rat. The investigators noted delayed ossification by 1 to 3 days in the long bones of the extremities, by 1 day in the scapulae, and by 2 to 3 days in the ilium. The ribs also showed a significant delay in maturity. Ossification of the skull bones was also delayed as evidenced by the wide sutures in the treated animals. The number and range of ossified vertebral bodies and arches in the treated group were always less than those in the control group. The greatest effect of the drug was on the sternebrae.

Antidepressants

There has been considerable controversy as to whether antidepressant drugs, particularly the tricyclic compounds, are teratogenic. This controversy was heightened by McBride's report (1972) of amelia associated with maternal use of imipramine during pregnancy. Two additional cases were subsequently reported associating this drug with limb defects (Barson, 1972; Freeman, 1972). In addition, several single case reports (Freeman, 1972; Goldman and Perman, 1980; Abramovici *et al.*, 1981) of absent fibula, hypoplastic tibia, and foot defects have been associated with maternal use of tricyclics during pregnancy.

Other reports (Banister *et al.*, 1972; Crombie *et al.*, 1972; Rachelefsky *et al.*, 1972; Wilson, 1972; Australian Drug Evaluation Committee, 1973; Bracken and Holford, 1981) did not confirm a correlation between teratogenicity, primarily limb reduction, and antidepressants. Other studies by Idänpään-Heikkilä and Saxén (1973) found it difficult to assess the effect of imipramine and chloropramine in pregnant women because of multiple drug use by the patient.

Many women are prescribed antidepressants before and during pregnancy, causing many infants to have been exposed to these drugs during critical periods of development. The apparent lack of an increase in reported major defects attests to the relative safety of this class of drugs.

Teratogenic properties of antidepressants have been shown in some animal models. Robson and Sullivan (1963), Harper *et al.* (1965), Alppli (1969), and Tucker (1983), in studying rabbit fetuses, found a significant increase in skeletal defects in those treated with imipramine and bupropion. Other studies, using the rat as an animal model, noted that fetuses exposed to imipramine and amitriptyline *in utero* had an increase in skeletal defects and a decrease in weight and growth rate (DiCarlo and Pagnini, 1971; Simpkins *et al.*, 1985).

Gilani (1975) exposed chick embryos to imipramine and produced micromelia and hydrocephalia. Studies by Guram *et al.* (1980, 1982), in which pregnant hamsters were dosed with imipramine, amitriplyline, or chlordiazepoxide (antianxiety agent), reported an increase in the gross defects, exencephaly, cranioschisis, microcephaly, and lower body atrophy in fetal animals.

Other studies using animal models showed no correlation between antidepressants and the production of malformations (Oberholzer, 1964; Jelinek *et al.*, 1967; Hendrickx, 1975).

Sedatives

Thalidomide, a proven human teratogen (Lenz, 1961; McBride, 1961) that was withdrawn from the market in 1962, is a classic example of the causal relationship between drugs and congenital malformations. Unlike other therapeutic agents that have been discussed in this chapter, researchers working with thalidomide could not reproduce the defects that characterized the human abnormality (amelia, phocomelia, radial reduction) in the common laboratory rat or mouse (DiPaolo, 1963; Fickentscher and Kohler, 1974). These defects have, however, been produced in several other species, e.g., rabbit, guinea pig, cat, and primate (Weidman *et al.*, 1963; Homburger *et al.*, 1965; Nudlenian and Traville, 1971; Jonsson, 1972; Tanimura, 1972; Wilson, 1972; Hendrickx and Newman, 1973; Khera, 1975; McBride, 1976).

Considerable controversy has surrounded the use of another drug in this group, Bendectin, during pregnancy. Most epidemiological studies have reported a lack of association between Bendectin and human birth defects (Brent, 1981; Mitchell *et al.*, 1981; Morelock *et al.*, 1982). Some reports have indicated an association between Bendectin and congenital malformations, particularly limb reduction deformities (Menzies, 1978; Rothman *et al.*, 1979; Correy and Newman, 1981). Summaries of available data, however, indicate that Bendectin does not meet the criteria for a teratogenic agent (Holmes 1983; Brent, 1983). The majority of animal teratology studies of this drug have been negative (Gibson *et al.*, 1968; Khera, 1975; Rochelle *et al.*, 1988).

The other major group of sedative drugs, barbiturates, have been included for discussion in the section on anticonvulsant drugs. The majority of studies have concentrated on barbital sodium and pentobarbital. It appears that none of the many other barbiturates have been studied, in particular, in laboratory animals. The evidence indicates that this class of drugs in use today has no teratogenic potential, in particular to skeletal or bone growth, in the human.

Vitamins

There are extensive data regarding the teratogenicity of hyper- and hypovitaminosis in experimental animals. Little research, however, has been done on the possible effect(s) to the human fetus of hypervitaminosis and/ or therapeutic use of these drugs in the pregnant woman.

The introduction of the drug Accutane, in the mid 1980s for the treatment of cystic acne, is the most recent therapeutic agent to meet all the criteria for recognition as a new teratogenic agent in the human. (Wilson, 1977; PDR, 1987). Chemically, Accutane is composed of isotretinoin (13 *cis*-retinoic acid) and is related to both retinoic acid and retinol (vitamin A). Growth and development of bone and the ossification of the skeletal system, however, do not appear to be affected by this drug. The most frequently reported defects associated with *in utero* exposure to Accutane are of the craniofacial region and cardiovascular system.

Vitamins A, B_1, and D, however, show a positive correlation between administration of these therapeutic agents to pregnant animals and the production of fetal malformations. Excessive vitamin A administration, as either retinol, retinyl esters, or retinoic acid, has produced a variety of bone and skeletal abnormalities. In the rat (1) retarded ossification; (2) abnormal chondrogenesis and osteogenesis of limbs and axial skeleton; inhibited somite and limb bud formation; (3) reduction deformities; and (4) decreased fetal growth have been found in rat pups exposed to excess vitamin A or its metabolites *in utero* (Nolen, 1972, 1989; Geelen, 1973; Kistler, 1981; Frazee et al., 1982; Steele et al., 1983; Alles and Sulik, 1989). The same spectra of defects have been found in the fetal mouse (Kochhar, 1973; Nakamura, 1975, 1977; Cusic and Dagg, 1985; Yasuda et al., 1986; Kwasigroch et al., 1986; Pillans, 1988; Sulik and Debhart, 1988); fetal hamster (Shenefelt, 1972; Fraser and Travill, 1978; Wiley, 1983; Wiley et al., 1983; Irving et al., 1986; Howard et al., 1987); fetal monkey (Fantel, 1977; Newell-Morris et al., 1980; Yip et al., 1980; Hendrickx et al., 1980); and chick embryo (Larsen and Janners, 1987; Ballard and Edwards, 1987; Campbell et al., 1987).

Several mechanisms have been proposed to account for the teratogenic action of the retinoids, including influences on cell membrane stability, cell proliferation, and cell death. Review articles by Kochhar (1977, 1985) have suggested that retinoid-induced mesomelia, which is similar to that produced by thalidomide, is a result of the specificity of retinoids for the chondrogenic cells. He observed that retinoids induced cell necrosis in the precartilaginous

Summary of the Teratogenic Effects of Therapeutic Drugs on Bone Growth

Defects	Analgesics	Anesthetics	Anticonvulsants	Anti-infective	Chemotherapeutic	Diuretics	Psychotropics	Vitamin
				Therapeutic Agents				
Appendicular skeleton								
Long bones	Hmor	H	HmR	cmo	cHmrR	mr	H	cMmr
Phalanges	Hmor	m	HmR	cHMmRo	cHMmRro	mr	H	
Axial skeleton								
Skull		mrR	H	cHr	cHMmor		Hmo	
Vertebral column	Mmor	r	Hm	MmoRr	mor		H	
Cartilage delay					mr			cMmr
Decreased fetal weight	HMmr	m	mR	Hm	c	m	mor	cMmr
Delayed ossification	mor	mr	HmR	cMmr	Hor		r	cMmr
Growth retardation		c	HMm	Hmr	cHr	mR	o	
Abortion/resorption	HMmor	cHmRr		H R	mRr r	m	mr	
Ossification centers missing								
Thoracic	mor	HmRr	mR	MmRr	cmor	mr	r	

Abbreviations: c = chick; H = human; M = monkey; m = mouse; o = other (dog, cat, hamster, sheep, etc.); R = rabbit; r = rat.

mesenchymal core of the limbs. Kochhar did not correlate this with programmed cell death as did Alles and Sulick (1989).

Adenine (B_4) is the only one of the B vitamins that has been labeled teratogenic, and this only in rodents. In rat and mouse studies (Fujii, 1970; Fujii and Nishimura, 1972; Jaffe and Johnson, 1973), adenine produced multiple defects of the limbs, mainly on the left side. Vitamin D has been shown to affect limb development only in the rat (Yukioka, 1959; Ornoy, 1971).

Some vitamins have been shown to be highly toxic to bone and skeletal development in animal studies. The therapeutic use of vitamins or hypervitaminosis in the human has not been proven deleterious to the development of the fetus with the exception of the drug Accutane.

Summary

The interaction between therapeutic drugs and the developing skeletal system has been reviewed. The toxic effects of a drug on the fetal development may manifest itself not only in terms of gross anatomical malformations, but also on a cellular level in terms of delayed chondrogenesis and osteogenesis. The skeletal system is probably the most sensitive indicator of teratogenic potential as shown by the wide range of defects that have been described in each section. Evaluation of the stage of ossification attained by the fetus is therefore important in teratogenic studies.

One generalization that readily emerges is that these drugs show species differences in their effect on the skeletal system (e.g., phenytoin, valproic acid, thalidomide).

A second general statment may be made about the wide range of skeletal defects that occur. It is clear that there are several critical periods in the development of bone and the skeletal system. It also appears that these critical periods are distributed throughout pregnancy.

Third, in animal studies, growth retardation is the most consistent toxic effect that therapeutic drugs have in common; however, catch-up growth can occur. This effect has led investigators to equate body weight and degree of ossification of the skeleton and use these as indices of fetal growth in experimental animal studies.

Finally, abnormal ossification is generally attributed to defects in the cartilaginous precursors of skeletal elements. Cell cultures of developing bone, which have quantifiable end points, may be an ideal system in which to screen therapeutic agents for teratogenic potential.

References

Aarskog, D. (1975). Association between maternal intake of diazepam and oral clefts. *Lancet*, **2**: 921.

Abramovici, A., Abramovici, I., Kalman, G., and Liban, E. (1981). Teratogenic effect of chlorimipramine in a young human embryo. *Teratology*, **24**: 42A.

Abramovici, A., Shaklai, M., and Pinkhas, J. (1978). Myeloschisis in a six weeks embryo of a leukemic woman treated by busulfan. *Teratology*, **18**: 241–246.

Agnish, N. D. and Kochhar, D. M. (1976). Direct exposure of postimplantation mouse embryos to 5-bromodeoxyuridine *in vitro* and its effect on subsequent chondrogenesis in the limbs. *J. Embryol. Exp. Morphol.*, **36**: 623–638.

Alford, C. A. and Pass, R. F. (1981). Epidemiology of chronic congenital and perinatal infections of man. *Clin. Perinat.*, **8**: 397–414.

Alles, A. J. and Sulik, K. K. (1989). Retinoic-acid-induced limb-reduction defects: perturbation of zones of programmed cell death as a pathogenetic mechanism. *Teratology*, **40**: 163–171.

Amemiya, K., Hurley, L. S., and Keen, C. L. (1989). Effect of 6-mercaptopurine on ^{65}Zn distribution in the pregnant rat. *Teratology*, **39**: 387–393.

Amemiya, K., Keen, C. L., and Hurley, L. S. (1986). 6-mercaptopurine-induced alterations in mineral metabolism and teratogenesis in the rat. *Teratology*, **34**: 321–334.

Amstey, M. S., Ed., *Virus Infection in Pregnancy*. Grune & Stratton, New York. (1984).

Andre, T. (1956). Studies on the distribution of tritium-labeled dihydrostreptomycin and tetracyclin in the body. *Acta Radiol.*, **142** (suppl.): 52–73.

Appli, L. (1969). Teratologische studien mit imiparmin auf ratte und kaninchen. *Arzneimittel-forschung*, **19**: 1617–1640.

Ashby, R., Davis, L., Dewhurst, B. B., Espinal, R., Penn, R. M., and Upshall, D. G. (1976). Aspects of the teratology of cyclophosphamide (NSC-26271). *Cancer Treat. Rep.*, **60**: 477–482.

Australian Drug Evaluation Committee (1973). Tricyclic antidepressants and limb reduction deformities. *Med. J. Aust.*, **1**: 768–769.

Ballard, R. and Edwards, H. M., Jr. (1988). Effects of dietary zeolite and vitamin A on tibial dyschondroplasia in chickens. *Poult. Sci.*, **67**: 113–119.

Balog, B. and Skinner, S. R. (1984). Unilateral duplication of the femur associated with myelomeningocele. *J. Pediatr. Orthop.*, **4**: 488–490.

Banister, P., Dafoe, C., Smith, E., and Miller, J. (1972). Letter: possible teratogenicity of tricyctic antidepressants. *Lancet*, **1**: 838–839.

Bannigan, J. and Langman, J. (1979). The cellular effect of 5-bromodeoxyuridine on the mammalian embryo. *J. Embryol. Exp. Morphol.*, **50**: 123–135.

Barnhart, E. R. (1987). In: *Physicians Desk Reference*. Medical Economics Co., Oradell, NJ, 1641–1642.

Barr, M., Jr. (1973). The teratogenicity of cadmium chloride in two stocks of Wistar rats. *Teratology*, **7**: 237–242.

Barry, R. M., Diamond, H. D., and Craver, L. F. (1962). Influence of pregnancy on the course of Hodgkin's Disease. *Am. J. Obstet. Gynecol.*, **84**: 445–454.

Barson, A. J. (1972). Malformed infant. *Br. Med. J.*, **2**: 45.

Basford, A. B. and Fink, B. R. (1968). The teratogenicity of halothane in the rat. *Anesthesiology*, **29**: 1167–1173.

Beall, J. R. (1972). Study of the teratogenic potential of diazepam and SCH 12041. *Can. Med. Assoc. J.*, **106**: 1061.

Beall, J. R. (1972). A teratogenic study of chlorpromazine, orphenedrine, perphenazine, and LSD-25 in rats. *Toxicol. Appl. Pharmacol.*, **21**: 230–236.

Beall, J. R. and Klein, M. F. (1977). Enhancement of aspirin-induced teratogenicity by food restriction in rats. *Toxicol. Appl. Pharmacol.*, **39**: 489–495.

Beaudoin, A. R. (1972). Teratogenic action of 2-amino-1,3,4-thiadiazole (ATDA) in rats. *Teratology*, **5**: 250A.

Beaudoin, A. R. (1973). Teratogenic activity of 2-amino-1,3,4-thiadiazole hydrochloride in Wistar rats and the protection afforded by nicotinamide. *Teratology*, **7**: 65–71.

Beaudoin, A. R. (1974). Teratogenicity of sodium arsenate in rats. *Teratology*, **10**: 153–158.

Beck, S. L. (1983). Assessment of adult skeletons to detect prenatal exposure to acetazolamide in mice. *Teratology*, **28**: 45–66.

Beck, S. L. (1989). Prenatal ossification as an indicator of exposure to toxic agents. *Teratology*, **40**: 365–374.

Belafsky, H. A., Breslow, S., Hirsch, L. M., Shangold, J. E., and Stahl, M. B. (1969). Meprobamate during pregnancy. *Obstet. Gynecol.*, **34**: 378–386.

Bennett, I. C., Proffit, W. R., and Norton. L. A. (1967). Determination of growth inhibitory concentrations of tetracycline for bone in organ culture. *Nature*, 216: 176–177.

Bergman, U., Boethius, G., Swartling, P. G., Isacson, D., and Smedby, B. (1990). Teratogenic effects of benzodiazepine use during pregnancy (letter) *J. Pediatr.*, **16**: 490–492.

Berry, C. L. (1971). Transient inhibition of DNA synthesis by methotrexate, in the rat embryo and foetus. *J. Embryol. Exp. Morphol.*, **26**: 469–474.

Béthenod, M. and Frédérich, A. (1975). Les enfants des antiépileptiques. *Pediatrie*, **30**: 227–248.

Bevelander, G. (1964). The effect of tetracycline on mineralization and growth. *Adv. Oral Biol.*, 1: 205–223.

Bevelander, G. and Cohlan, S. Q. (1962). The effect on the rat fetus of transplacentally acquired tetracycline. *Biol Neonat.*, **4**: 365–370.

Bevelander, G., Rolle, G. K., and Cohlan, S. Q. (1961). The effect of the administration of tetracycline on the development of teeth. *J. Dent. Res.*, **40**: 1020–1024.

Beyer, B. K., Guram, M. S., and Geber, W. F. (1984). Incidence and potentiation of external and internal fetal anomalies resulting from chlordiazepoxide and amitriptyline alone and in combination. *Teratology*, **30**: 39–45.

Biddle, F. G. (1975). Teratogenesis of acetazolamide in the CBA/J and SWV strains of mice. *Teratology*, **11**: 31–36.

Biddle, F. G. (1988). Genetic differences in the frequency of acetazolamide-induced ectrodactyly in the mouse exhibit directional dominance of relative embryonic resistance. *Teratology*, **37**: 375–388.

Bieber, S., Nigrelli, R. F., and Hitchings, G. H. (1952). Effects of purine and pyramidine analogues on development of *Rana pipiens*. *Proc. Soc. Exp. Biol. Med.*, **79**: 430–432.

Bjerkedal, T., Czeizel, A., Goujard, J., Kallen, B., Mastroiacova, P., Nevin, N., Oakley, G., and Robert, E. (1982). Valproic acid and spina bifida (letter) *Lancet*, **2**: 1096.

Boland, J. (1951). Reticuloses: clinical experience with nitrogen mustard in Hodgkin's disease. *Br. J. Radiol.*, **24**: 513–515.

Bracken, M. B. and Holford, T. R. (1981). Exposure to prescribed drugs in pregnancy and association with congenital malformations. *Obstet. Gynecol.*, **58**: 336–344.

Brent, R. L. (1981). Drugs as teratogens. The Bendectin saga: another American tragedy. *Teratology*, **23**: 28A.

Brent, R. L. (1983). Editorial. The Bendectin saga: another American tragedy. *Teratology*, 27: 283–286.

Brewton, R. G. and MacCabe, J. A. (1990). Studies of methotrexate-induced limb dysplasias utilizing a ^{51}chromium release assay. *Teratology*, **41**: 211–221.

Bro-Rasmussen, Fr., Jensen, B., Hansen, O. M., and Østergaard, A. H. (1971). Fluorodeoxyuridine-induced malformations in mice. *Acta Pathol. Microbiol. Scand.*, **79**: 55–60.

Brown, N. A., Hoyle, C. I., McCarthy, A., and Wolpert, L. (1989). The development of asymmetry: the sidedness of drug-induced limb abnormalities is reversed in situs inversus mice. *Development*, **107**: 637–642.

Brown, N. A., Shull, G., and Fabro, S. (1979). Assessment of the teratogenic potential of trimethadione in the CD-1 mouse. *Toxicol. Appl. Pharmacol.*, **51**: 59–71.

Brown, N. A., Kao, J., and Fabro, S. (1980). Teratogenic potential of valproic acid. (letter) *Lancet*, **1**: 660–661.

Bruckner, A., Lee, Y. J., O'Shea, K. S., and Henneberry, R. C. (1983). Teratogenic effects of valproic acid and diphenylhydantoin on mouse embryos in culture. *Teratology*, **27**: 29–42.

Brummett, E. S. and Johnson, E. M. (1979a). Morphological alterations in the developing fetal rat limb due to maternal injection of chlorambucil. *Teratology*, **20**: 279–288.

Brummett, E. S. and Johnson, E. M. (1979b). Phosphatase activity and ion levels associated with normal and abnormal skeletogenesis in the fetal rat. *J. Embryol. Exp. Morph.*, **53**: 203–211.

Brunaud, M. (1975). Effect of the meprobamate acepromethazine combination on pregnancy, fetal morphology and postnatal development. *Bull. Chim. Farm.*, **108**: 560–575.

Buttar, H. S. (1980). The effects of the combined administration of ethanol and chlordiazepoxide on the prenatal and postnatal development of rats. *Neurobehav. Toxicol.*, **2**: 270–225.

Buttar, H. S., Dupuis, I., and Khera, K. S. (1976). Fetotoxicity of trimethadione and paramethadione in rats. *Toxicol Appl. Pharmacol.*, **37**: 126.

Buttar, H. S., Dupuis, I., and Khera, K. S. (1978). Dimethadione-induced fetotoxicity in rats. *Toxicology*, **9**: 155–164.

Buttar, H. S., Dupuis, I., and Moffatt, J. H. (1979). Prenatal and postnatal effects of chlordiazepoxide (Librium) in rats. *Toxicol. Appl. Pharmacol.*, **48**: A120.

Buttar, H. S. and Moffatt, J. H. (1983). Pre- and postnatal exposure to propoxyphene and chlordiazepoxide. *Neurobehav. Toxicol. Teratol.*, **5**: 549–556.

Campbell, M., Horton, W., and Keeler, R. (1987). Comparative effects of retinoic acid and jervine on chondrocyte differentiation. *Teratology*, **36**: 235–243.

Canadian Department of National Health and Welfare, Food and Drug Directorate. Lettre of notification to Canadian physicians. Ottawa. December 7, 1962.

Carter, M. P. and Wilson, F. (1962). Tetracycline and congenital limb anomalies. *Lancet*, **2**: 407–408.

Carter, M. P. and Wilson, F. (1963). Antibiotics and congenital malformations. *Lancet*, **1**: 1267.

Castro-Correia, J., Sousa-Nunes, A., and Silva-Bacelar, A. (1974). Teratogenic action of Acetazolamide in mice. *Teratology*, **10**: 221–226.

Center for Disease Control: Valproic acid and spina bifida: a preliminary report. (1982). *Morbid. Mortal. Weekly Rep.*, **32**: 565–566.

Chamberlain, J. G. and Goldyne, M. E. (1970). Intra-amniotic injection of pyridine nucleotides or adenosine triphosphate as countertherapy for 6-aminonicotinamide (6-AN) teratogenesis. *Teratology*, **3**: 229–236.

Chan, A. W. (1984). Effect of combined alcohol and benzodiazepine: a review. *Drug Alcohol Depend.*, **13**: 315–341.

Chapman, W. S. (1989). Lithium use during pregnancy. *J. Fla. Med. Assoc.*, **76**: 454–456.

Chatot, C. L., Klein, H. W., Clapper, M. L., Resor, S. R., Singer, W. D., Russman, B. S., Holmes, G. L., Mattson, R. H., and Cramer, J. A. (1984). Human serum teratogenicity studied by rat embryo culture: epilepsy, anticonvulsant drugs, and nutrition. *Epilepsia*, **25**: 205–216.

Chaube, S., Kury, G., and Murphy, M. L. (1967). Teratogenic effects of cyclophosphamide (NSC-26271) in the rat. *Cancer Chemother. Rep.*, **51**: 363.

Chaube, S. and Murphy, M. L. (1965). The teratogenic effects of cytosine arabinoside (CA) on the rat fetus. *Proc. Am. Assoc. Cancer Res.*, **6**: 11.

Chaube, S. and Murphy, M. L. (1966). The effects of hydroxyurea and related compounds on the rat fetus. *Cancer Res.*, **20**: 1448–1457.

Chaube, S. and Murphy, M. L. (1968). The teratogenic effects of the recent drugs active in cancer chemotherapy. *Adv. Teratol.*, **3**: 181–237.

Chaube, S. and Murphy, M. L. (1973). Protective effect of deoxycytidylic acid (CdMP) on hydroxyurea-induced malformations in rats. *Teratology*, **7**: 79–88.

Chepenik, K. P., Johnson, E. M., and Kaplan, S. (1970). Effects of transitory maternal pteroylglutamic acid (PGA) deficiency on levels of adenosine phosphate in developing rat embryos. *Teratology*, **3**: 229–235.

Christley, J. and Webster, W. S. (1983). Cadmium uptake and distribution in mouse embryos following maternal exposure during the organogenic period: a scintillation and autoradiographic study. *Teratology*, **27**: 305–312.

Ciociola, A. A. and Gautieri, R. F. (1983). Evaluation of the teratogenicity of morphine sulfate administered via a miniature implantable pump. *J. Pharm. Sci.*, **72**: 742–745.

Claussen, U., Krengel, H. G., and Schrors, H. J. (1980). The embryotoxic effects of cyclophosphamide in rabbits tested *in vivo* by I.V. injection and by yolk sac method. *Arzneimitteisforschungschung*, **30**: 1585–1588.

Coakley, M. E. and Brown, N. A. (1986). Valproic acid teratogenicity in whole embryo culture is not prevented by zinc supplementation. *Biochem. Pharmacol.*, **35**: 1052–1055.

Cohen, E. N. (chairman). (1974). Occupational disease among operating room personnel: a national study. Report of an Ad Hoc Committee. *Anesthesiology*, **41**: 321–340.

Cohen, E. N., Bellville, J. W., and Brown, B. W., Jr. (1971). Anesthesia, pregnancy, and miscarriage: a study of operating room nurses and anesthetists. *Anesthesiology*, **35**: 343–347.

Cohen, L. S. (1989). Psychotropic drug use in pregnancy. *Hosp. Community Psychiatry*, **40**: 566–567.

Cohen, L. S., Heller, V. L., and Rosenbaum, J. F. (1989). Treatment guidelines for psychotropic drug use in pregnancy. *Psychosomatics*, **30**: 25–33.

Cohlan, S. Q., Bevelander, G., and Tiamsic, T. (1963). Growth inhibition of prematures receiving tetracycline. A clinical and laboratory investigation of tetracycline-induced bone fluorescence. *Am. J. Dis. Child.*, **105**: 453–461.

Collins, E. (1981). Maternal and fetal effects of acetaminophen and salicylates in pregnancy. *Obstet. Gynecol.*, **58** (suppl.): 57–62.

Collins, M. D., Fradkin, R., and Scott, W. J., Jr. (1989). Induction of postaxial forelimb ectrodactyly with anticonvulsant agents in A/J mice. *Teratology*, **41**: 61–70.

Committee on Drugs: American Academy of Pediatrics. (1979). Anticonvulsants and pregnancy. *Pediatrics*, **63**: 331–333.

Corbett, T. H. (1972). Anesthetics as a cause of abortion. *Fertil. Steril.*, **23**: 866–869.

Corbett, T. H., Cornell, R. G., Endres, J. L., and Lieding, K. (1974). Birth defects among children of nurse-anesthetists. *Anesthesiology*, **41**: 341–344.

Corner, B. D. (1962). Congenital malformations: clinical considerations. *Med. J. South West*, **77**: 46–52.

Corwin, H. and DeMeyer, W. (1980). Failure of clorazepate to cause malformations or fetal wastage in the rat. *Arch. Neural.*, **37**: 347–349.

Crombie, D. L., Pinsent, R. J., and Fleming, D. (1972). Letter: Imipramine in pregnancy. *Br. Med. J.*, **1**: 745.

Crombie, D. L., Pinsent, R. J., Fleming, D. J., Rouquette, C. R., Gonjard, J., and Huel, G. (1975). Fetal effects of tranquilizers in pregnancy. *N. Engl. J. Med.*, **293**: 198–199.

Culbertson, C. (1974). Monistat: a new fungicide for treatment of vulvovaginal candidiasis. *Am. J. Obstet Gynecol.*, **120**: 973–976.

Cusic, A. M. and Dagg, C. P. (1985). Spontaneous and retinoic acid-induced postaxial polydactyly in mice. *Teratology*, **31**: 49–59.

Czeizel, A. (1976). Diazepam, phenytoin, and aetiology of cleft lip and/or cleft palate. *Lancet*, **1**: 810.

Dagg, C. P. (1960). Sensitive stages for the production of developmental abnormalities in mice with 5-fluorouracil. *Am. J. Anat.*, **106**: 89–96.

Dagg, C. P. and Kallio, E. (1962). Teratogenic interaction of fluorodeoxyuridine and thymidine. *Anat. Rec.*, **142**: 301–302.

Danforth, C. H. and Center, E. (1954). Nitrogen mustard as a teratogenic agent in the mouse. *Soc. Exp. Biol. Med.*, **86**: 705–707.

Datu, A. R., Nakamura, H., and Yasuda, M. (1985). Pathogenesis of the mouse forelimb deformity induced by acetazolamide: an electron microscopic study. *Teratology*, **31**: 253–263.

Daube, J. R. and Chou, S. M. (1966). Lissencephaly: two cases. *Neurology*, **16**: 179–191.

DeLaney, A. G. (1983). Anesthesia in the pregnant woman. *Clin. Obstet. Gynecol.*, **26**: 795–800.

Demers, P., Fraser, D., Goldbloom, R. B., Haworth, J. C., LaRochelle, J., MacLean, R., and Murray, T. K. (1968). Effects of tetracyclines on skeletal growth and dentition. *Can. M. Assoc. J.*, **99**: 849–854.

Dennis, L. S. and Stein, S. (1965). Busulfan in pregancy. Report of a case. *JAMA*, **192**: 715–716.

DeSesso, J. M. (1981a). Comparative ultrastructural alterations in rabbit limb-buds after a teratogenic dose of either hydroxyurea or methotrexate. *Teratology*, **23**: 197–215.

DeSesso, J. M. (1981b). Amelioration of teratogenesis. I. Modification of hydroxyurea-induced teratogenesis by the antioxidant propyl gallate. *Teratology*, **24**: 19–35.

DeSesso, J. M. and Jordan, R. L. (1977). Drug-induced limb dysplasias in fetal rabbits. *Teratology*, **15**: 199–212.

Diamond, I., Anderson, M. M., and McCreadie, S. R. (1960). Transplacental transmission of busulfan (Myleran) in a mother with leukemia: production of fetal malformations and cytomegaly. *Pediatrics*, **25**: 85–90.

DiCarlo, R. and Pagnini, G. (1971). Comparative action of amitriptyline and butriptyline on skeletal development in the rat embryo. *Teratology*, **4**: 486.

Didcock, K., Jackson, D., and Robson, J. M. (1956). The action of some nucleotoxic substances on pregnancy. *Br. J. Pharmacol.*, **11**: 437–441.

Dieulangard, P. and Coignet, J. (1966). Sur un cas d'ectrophocomelie peutêtre d'origine medicamenteuse. *Bull. Fed. Soc. Gynec. Obstet. Fr.*, **18**: 85–87.

DiLiberti, H., Farndon, A., Dennis, R., and Curry, C. J. (1984). The fetal valproate syndrome. *Am. J. Med. Genet.*, **19**: 473–481.

Dinsmore, C. E. and Maren, T. H. (1986). Acetazolamide does not disrupt limb regenerate morphogenesis in the salamander, *Plethodon cinereus*. *Teratology*, **33**: 85–91.

DiPaolo, J. A. (1963). Congenital malformation in strain A mice: its experimental production by thalidomide. *JAMA*, **183**: 139–141.

DiPaolo, J. A. (1964). Polydactylism in the offspring of mice injected with 5-bromodeoxyuridine. *Science*, **145**: 501–503.

Dolnick, E. H., Lindahl, I. L., and Terrill, C. E. (1970). Treatment of pregnant ewes with cyclophosphamide. *J. Anim. Sci.*, **31**: 944–946.

Druga, A., Nyitray, M., and Szaszovszky, E. (1980). Experimental teratogenicity of structurally similar compounds with or without piperazine-ring: a preliminary report. *Pol. J. Pharmacol. Pharm.*, **32**: 199–204.

Duncan, W. A. M. and Lemon, P. G. (1974). The effects of methyl-5(6)-butyl-2-benzimidazole carbamate (parbendazole) on reproduction in sheep and other animals. *Cornell Vet.*, **64** (suppl.): 97–103.

Duncan, W. A. M., Lemon, P. G., and Palmer, A. K. (1974). The effects of methyl-5(6)-butyl-2-benzimidazole carbamate (parbendazole) on reproduction in sheep and other animals. *Cornell Vet.*, **64** (suppl. 4): 104–108.

Earl, F. L., Miller, E., and Van Loon, E. J. (1973). Teratogenic research in beagle dogs and miniature swine. Lab. Anim. Drug Test. *Symp. Int. Comm. Lab. Anim. 5th*, Fischer, Stuttgart, 233–247.

Edlund, M. J. and Craig, T. J. (1984). Antipsychotic drug use and birth defects: an epidemiologic reassessment. *Comp. Psychiatry*, **25**: 32–37.

Elia, J., Katz, I. R., and Simpson, G. M. (1987). Teratogenicity of psychotherapeutic medications. *Psychopharmacol. Bull.*, **23**: 531–586.

Elmazar, M. M. A. and Sullivan, F. M. (1981). Effects of prenatal phenytoin administration on postnatal development of the rat. A behavioral teratology study. *Teratology*, **24**: 115–124.

Eluma, F. O., Sucheston, M. E., Hayes, T. G., and Paulson, R. B. (1981). The teratogenic effects of carbamazepine (CMZ) in the CD-1 mouse fetus. *Teratology*, **23**: 33A.

Eluma, F. O., Sucheston, M. E., Hayes, T. G., and Paulson, R. B. (1984). Teratogenic effects of dosage levels and time of administration of carbamazepine, sodium valproate, and diphenylhydantoin on craniofacial development in the CD-1 mouse fetus. *J. Craniofacial. Genet. Dev. Biol.*, **4**: 191–210.

Emerson, D. J. (1962). Congenital malformations due to attempted abortion with aminopterin. *Am. J. Obstet. Gynecol.*, **84**: 356–357.

Engesaeter, L. B. and Skar, A. G. (1978). Effects of oxytetracycline on the mechanical properties of bone and skin in young rats. *Acta Orthop. Scand.*, **49**: 529–534.

Eriksson, M., Catz, C. S., and Yaffe, S. J. (1973). Drugs and pregnancy. Clin. *Obstet. Gynecol.*, **16**: 199–224.

Esaki, K.,Tanioka, Y., Ogata, T., Koizumi, B., and Koizumi, H. (1975). Influence of sodium dipropylacetate (DPA) on the fetuses of the Rhesus monkey. *CIEA Preclin. Rep.*, **1**: 157–164.

Fahim, M. S., Hall, D. G., Jones, T. M., Fahim, Z., and Whitt, F. D. (1970). Drug-steroid interaction in the pregnant rat, fetus, and neonate. *Am. J. Obstet. Gynecol.*, **107**: 1250–1258.

Fantel, A. G., Shepard, T. H., Newell-Morris, L. L., and Moffett, B. C. (1977). Teratogenic effects of retinoic acid in pigtail monkeys (*Macaca nemestrina*). I. General features. *Teratology*, **15**: 65–72.

Faustman, E. M., Kirby, A., Gage, D., and Varnum, M. (1989). *In vitro* developmental toxicity of five direct-acting alkylating agents in rodent embryos: structure-activity patterns. *Teratology*, **40**: 199–210.

Fergurson, M. W. J. (1978). The teratogenic effects of 5-fluoro-2-desoxyuridine (F.U.D.R.) on the Eistan rat fetus, with particular reference to cleft palate. *J. Anat.*, **126**: 37–49.

Fergurson, M. W. J. (1985). Reproductive biology and embryology of the crocodilians. In: *Biology of the Reptilia*. Vol. 14, Gans, C., Billett, F., Maderson, P. F. A., Eds., John Wiley & Sons, New York, 329–492.

Ferm, V. H. (1965) Teratogenic activity of hydroxyurea. *Lancet*, **1**: 1338–1339.

Ferm, V. H. (1966). Severe developmental malformations: malformations induced by urethane and hydroxyurea in the hamster. *Arch. Pathol.* 81: 174–177.

Ferm, V. H. (1972). The teratogenic effects of metals on mammalian embryos. *Adv. Teratol.*, **5**: 51–75.

Ferm, V. H. and Carpenter, S. J. (1968). The relationship of cadmium and zinc in experimental mammalian teratogenesis. *Lab. Invest.*, **18**: 429–432.

Ferm, V. H., Willhite, C., and Kilham, L. (1978). Teratogenic effects of ribavirin on hamster and rat embryos. *Teratology*, **17**: 93–102.

Feuston, M. H. and Scott, W. J., Jr. (1985). Cadmium-induced forelimb ectrodactyly: a proposed mechanism of teratogenesis. *Teratology*, 32: 407–419.

Fickentscher, K. and Kohler, F. (1974). Teratogenicity and embryotoxicity of thalidomide and 3-aza-thalidomide in mice. *Pharmacology*, 11: 193–198.

Fink, B. R., Shepard, T. H., and Blandau, R.J. (1967).Teratogenic activity of nitrous oxide. *Nature*, **214**: 146–148.

Finnell, R. H. (1981). Phenytoin-induced teratogenesis: a mouse model. *Science*, **211**: 483–484.

Finnell, R. H., Shields, H. E. and Chernoff, G. F. (1987). Variable patterns in anticonvulsant drug-induced malformations in mice: comparisons of phenytoin and phenobarbital. *Teratogen. Carcinogen. Mutagen.*, **7**: 541–549.

Finnell, R. H., Shields, H. E., Taylor, S. M., and Chernoff, G. F. (1987). Strain differences in phenobarbital-induced teratogenesis in mice. *Teratology*, **35**: 177–185.

Forbes, S. B. (1940). The etiology of nerve deafness with particular reference to quinine. *South. Med. J.*, **33**: 613–621.

Forsthoefel, P. F. (1972). The effects on mouse development on interactions of 5-fluorouracil with Strong's luxoid gene and its plus and minus modifiers. *Teratology*, **6**: 5–18.

Fraser, B. A. and Travill, A. A. (1978). The effect of retinoic acid on chondrogenesis in the fetal hamster tibia *in vivo*. *J. Embryol. Exp. Morphol.*, **48**: 23–35.

Frazee, W. J., Mallek, H. M., and Nakamoto, T. (1982). The effects of retinoic acid on the growth of mandible and long bone in fetal rats. *Arch. Oral Biol.*, **27**: 561–565.

Freeman, R. (1972). Limb deformities: possible association with drugs. *Med. J. Aust.*, **1**: 606–607.

Fritz, H. and Hess, R. (1970). Ossification of the rat and mouse skeleton in the perinatal period. *Teratology*, **3**: 331–338.

Fritz, H. and Hess, R. (1971). Effects of cyclophosphamide on embryonic development in the rabbit. *Agents Actions*, **2**: 83–86.

Fritz, H., Mueller, H. F., and Hess, R. (1976). Comparative study of the teratogenicity of phenobarbitone, diphenylhydantoin and carbamazepine in mice. *Toxicology*, **6**: 139 (1976).

Fujii, T. (1970). Relation between embryotoxicity of adenine in mice and day of treatment. *Teratology*, **3**: 299–310.

Fujii, T. and Nishimura, H. (1972). Teratogenicity of adenine in the rat embryo. *Okajimas Folia Anat. Jpn.*, **49**: 47–53.

Fujinaga, M., Baden, J. M., and Mazze, R. I. (1989). Susceptible period of nitrous oxide teratogenicity in Sprague-Dawley rats. *Teratology*, **40**: 439–444.

Fujinaga, M. and Mazze, R. I. (1988). Teratogenic and postnatal developmental studies of morphine in Sprague-Dawley rats. *Teratology*, **38**: 401–410.

Gabrielsson, J. and Larsson, K. S. (1987). The use of physiological pharmacokinetic models in studies on the disposition of salicylic acid in pregnancy. In: *Pharmacokinetics in Teratogenesis II*. Nau, H., Scott, W. J., Jr., Eds., CRC Press, Boca Raton, FL, 13–26.

Gal, P. and Sharpless, M. K. (1984). Fetal drug exposure-behavioral teratogenesis. *Drug Intell. Clin. Pharm.*, **18**: 186–201.

Garrett, M. J. (1974). Letter: teratogenic effects of combination chemotherapy. *Ann. Int. Med.*, **80**: 667.

Gebhardt, D. O. E. (1970). The embryolethal and teratogenic effects of cyclophosphamide on mouse embryos. *Teratology*, **3**: 273–277.

Geelen, J. A. G. (1973). Skullbase malformations in rat fetuses with hypervitaminosis A-induced exencephaly. *Teratology*, **7**: 49–56.

Gelenberg, A. J. (1988). Lithium efficacy and adverse effects. *J. Clin. Psychiatry*, **49** (suppl.): 8–11.

Gellis, S. S. and Feingold, M. (1979). Aminopterin embryopathy syndrome. *Am. J. Dis. Child.*, **133**: 1189–1190.

Gerlinger, P. (1964). Action du cyclophosphamide injecté à la mère sur la rélisation de la forme du corps de embryons de lapin. *C.R. Soc. Biol. (Paris)*, **158**: 2154–2157.

German, J., Kowal, A., and Ehlers, K. H. (1970). Trimethadione and human teratogenesis. *Teratology*, **3**: 349–361.

Gibson, J. E. and Becker, B. A. (1968a). Teratologic effects of diphenylhydantoin on Swiss-Webster and A/J mice. *Proc. Soc. Exp. Biol. Med.*, **128**: 905–909.

Gibson, J. E. and Becker, B. A. (1968b). The teratogenicity of cyclophosphamide in mice. *Cancer Res.*, 28: 475–480.

Gibson, J. P., Staples, R. E., Larson, E. J., Kuhn, W. L., Holtkamp, D. E., and Newberne, J. W. (1968). Teratology and reproduction studies with an antinauseant. *Toxicol. Appl. Pharmacol.*, **13**: 439–447.

Gilani, S. H. (1975). The effect of imipramine on the development of the chick embryo. *Teratology*, **11**: 8A.

Gill, T. S., Guram, M. S., and Geber, W. F. (1981). Comparative study of the teratogenic effects of chlordiazepoxide and diazepam in the fetal hamster. *Life Sci.*, **29**: 2141–2147.

Gill, T. S., Guram, M. S., and Geber, W. F. (1982). Haloperidol teratogenicity in the fetal hamster. *Dev. Pharmacol. Ther.*, **4**: 1–5.

Gillick, A. and Bulmer, W. S. (1972). Griseofulvin, a possible teratogen. *Can. Vet. J.*, **13**: 244.

Gilliland, J. and Weinstein, L. (1983). The effect of cancer chemotherapeutic agents on the developing fetus. *Obstet. Gynecol. Surv.*, **38**: 6–13.

Golden, S. and Perman, K. (1980). Bilateral clinical anopthalmia: drugs as potential factors. *South Med. J.*, **73**: 1404–1407.

Goldfield, M. and Weinstein, M. (1973). Lithium in obstetrics: guidelines for clinical use. *Am. J. Obstet. Gynecol.*, **116**: 15–22.

Gottschewski, G. H. M. (1964). Mammalian blastopathies due to drugs. *Nature*, **201**: 1232–1233.

Green, M. C., Azar, C. A., and Maren, T. H. (1973). Strain differences in susceptibility to the teratogenic effect of acetazolamide in mice. *Teratology*, 8: 143–146.

Greenberg, L. H. and Tanaka, K. R. (1964). Congenital anomalies probably induced by cyclophosphamide. *JAMA*, **188**: 423–426.

Gregg, N. M. (1941). Congenital cataract following german measles in the mother. *Trans. Ophthalmol. Soc. Aust.*, **3**: 35–46.

Grubb, R. B. and Montiegel, E. C. (1975). The teratogenic effects of 6-mercaptopurine on chick embryos *in ovo. Teratology*, **11**: 179–186.

Guerriero, F. J. and Fox, K. A. (1977). Benzodiazepines and development of Swiss-Webster mice. *Pharmacol. Res. Commun.*, **9**: 187–196.

Guram, M. S., Gill, T. S., and Gerber, W. F. (1980). Teratogenicity of imipramine and amitriptyline in fetal hamsters. *Res. Commun, Psychol. Psychiatry Behav.*, **5**: 275–282.

Guram, M. S., Gill, T. S., and Gerber, W. F. (1982). Comparative teratogenicity of chlordiazepoxide, amitriptyline, and a combination of the compounds in the fetal hamster. *Neurotoxicology*, **3**: 83–90.

Guy, J. F. and Sucheston, M. E. (1986). Teratogenic effects on the CD-1 mouse embryo exposed to concurrent doses of ethanol and aspirin. *Teratology*, **34**: 249–261.

Hackman, R. M. and Hurley, L. S. (1983). Interaction of dietary zinc, genetic strain, and acetazolamide in teratogenesis in mice. *Teratology*, **28**: 355–368.

Halbreich, U. and Carson, S. W. (1989). Drug studies in women of childbearing age: ethical and methodological considerations. *J. Clin. Psychopharmacol.*, **9**: 328–333.

Hales, B. F. and Jain, R. (1986). Differential effects of 4-hydroperoxycyclophosphamide on limb development *in vitro. Teratology*, **34**: 303–311.

Hales, B. F., Ludeman, S. M., and Boyd, V. L. (1989). Embryotoxicity of phenyl ketone analogs of cyclophosphamide. *Teratology*, **39**: 31–37.

Hall, B. K. (1987). Development of the mandibular skeleton in the embryonic chick as evaluated using the DNA-inhibiting agent 5-fluoro-2'-deoxyuridine. *J. Craniofac. Genet. Dev. Biol.*, **7**: 145–159.

Hall, E. K. (1953). Developmental anomalies in the eye of the rat after various experimental procedures. *Anat. Rec.*, **116**: 383–394.

Hall, G. (1963). A case of phocomelia of the upper limbs. *Med. J. Aust.*, **1**: 449–450.

Hallesy, D. W. and Layton, W. M., Jr. (1967). Forelimb deformity of offspring of rats given dichlorphenamide during pregnancy. *Proc. Soc. Exp. Biol. Med.*, **126**: 6–8.

Hancock, N. A. and Poulter, D. A. L. (1974). The effects of methyl-5(6)-butyl-2-benzimidazole carbamate (parbendazole) on reproduction in sheep and other animals. *Cornell Vet.*, **64** (suppl. 4): 92–96.

Hansen, D. K., Walker, R. C., and Grafton, T. F. (1990). Effect of lithium carbonate on mouse and rat embryos *in vitro. Teratology*, **41**: 155–160.

Hanson, J. W. and Smith, D. W. (1975). The fetal hydantoin syndrome. *J. Pediatr.*, **87**: 285–290.

Hanson, J. W., Ardinger, H., DiLiberti, J., Hughes, E., Harrod, J., Schinzel, A., Clarren, S., and Blackston, D. (1984). Effects of valproic acid on the fetus. *Pediatr. Res.*, **118**: 306A.

Hansson, L. I. (1967). Daily growth in length of diaphysis measured by oxytetracycline in rabbit normally and after medullary plugging. *Acta Orthop. Scand.*, **101** (suppl.): 1–199.

Hansson, L. I., Stenstrom, A., and Thorngren, K.-G. (1968). Skeletal deposition and toxicity of methacycline. *Nature*, **219**: 624–625.

Harbison, R. D. and Becker, B. A. (1969). Relationship of dosage and time of administration of diphenylhydantoin to its teratogenic effect in mice. *Teratology*, **2**: 305–312.

Harbison, R. D. and Becker, B. A. (1972). Diphenylhydantoin teratogenicity in rats. *Toxicol. Appl. Pharmacol.*, **22**: 193–200.

Harper, K. H., Palmer, A. K., and Davies, R. E. (1984). Effect of imipramine upon the pregnancy of laboratory animals. *Arzneimittelforschung*, **15**: 1218–1221.

Harris, R. E. (1966). Coccidioidomycosis complicating pregnancy. Report of three cases and review of the literature. *Obstet. Gynecol.*, **28**: 401–405.

Hart, C. W. and Naunton, R. F. (1964). The ototoxicity of chloroquin phosphate. *Arch. Otolaryngol.*, **80**: 407–412.

Hartz, S. C., Heinonen, O. P., Shapiro, S., Siskind, V., and Slone, D. (1975). Antenatal exposure to meprobamate and chlordiazepoxide in relation to malformations, mental development and childhood mortality. *N. Engl. J. Med.*, **292**: 726–728.

Haskin, D. (1948). Some effects of nitrogen mustard on the development of external body form in the fetal rat. *Anat. Rec.*, **102**: 493–511.

Hendrickx, A. G. (1975). Teratologic evaluation of imipramine hydrochloride in bonnet (*Macaca radiata*), and rhesus monkeys (*Macaca mulatta*). *Teratology*, **11**: 219–222.

Hendrickx, A. G. and Newman, L. (1973). Appendicular skeletal and visceral malformations induced by thalidomide in Bonnet monkeys. *Teratology*, **7**: 151–159.

Hendrickx, A. G., Silverman, S., Pellegrini, M., and Steffek, A. J. (1980). Teratological and radiocephalometric analysis of craniofacial malformations induced with retinoic acid in rhesus monkeys (*Macaca mulatta*). *Teratology*, **22**: 13–22.

Hengst, P. (1972). Teratogenicity of daraprim (pyrimethamine) in man. *Zentralbl. Gynaekol.*, **94**: 551–555.

Herbst, A. L., Ulfelder, H., and Poskanzer, D. C. (1971). Adenocarcinoma of the vagina. Association of maternal stilbestrol therapy with tumor appearance in young women. *N. Eng. J. Med.*, **284**: 878–881.

Hiilesmaa, V. K., Teramo, K., Granstrom, M.-L., and Bardy, A. H. (1981). Fetal head growth retardation associated with maternal antiepileptic drugs. *Lancet*, **2**: 165–167.

Hill, R. M., Veriaud, W. M., Horning, M. G., McCulley, L. B., and Morgan, N. F. (1974). Infants exposed *in utero* to antileptic drugs. A prospective study. *Am. J. Dis. Child.*, **127**: 645–653.

Ho, C.-K., Kaufman, R., and McAlister, W. (1975). Congenital malformations. *Am. J. Dis. Child.*, **129**: 714–716.

Holmes, L. B., Kawanishi, H., and Munoz, A. (1988). Acetazolamide: maternal toxicity, pattern of malformations and litter effect. *Teratology*, **37**: 335–342.

Holmes, L. B. and Trelstad, R. L. (1979). The early limb deformity caused by acetazolamide. *Teratology*, **20**: 289–296.

Holmes, L. S. (1983). Teratogen update: bendectin. *Teratology*, **27**: 277–281.

Holt, D. and Webb, M. (1987). Teratogenicity of ionic cadimum in the Wistar rat. *Arch. Toxicol.*, **59**: 443–447.

Homburger, F., Chaube, S., Eppenberger, M., Bogdanoff, P. D., and Nixon, C. W. (1965). Susceptibility of certain inbred strains of hamsters to teratogenic effects of thalidomide. *Toxicol. Appl. Pharmacol.*, **7**: 686–693.

Hood, R. D. and Bishop, S. L. (1972). Teratogenic effects of sodium arsenate in mice. *Arch. Environ. Health*, **24**: 62–65.

Hood, R. D. and Pike, C. T. (1972). BAL alleviation of arsenate-induced teratogenesis in mice. *Teratology*, **6**: 235–238.

Howard, W. B., Willhite, C. C., and Sharma, R. P. (1987). Structure-toxicity relationships of the tetramethylated tetralin and indane analogs of retinoic acid. *Teratology*, **36**: 303–311.

Huch, A. (1984). The impact of antimitotic and immunosupressive treatment on pregnancy outcome. In: *Drugs and Pregnancy*. Krauer, B., Krauer, F., Hytten, F. E., and del Pozo, E., Eds., Academic Press, London. 215–233.

Idänpään-Heikkilä, J. and Saxén, L. (1973). Possible teratogenicity of imipramine/chloropyramine. *Lancet*, **2**: 282–283.

Inouye, M. and Murakami, U. (1978). Teratogenic effect of N-methy-N'-nitro-N-nitrosoguanidine in mice. *Teratology*, **18**: 263–267.

Irving, D. W., Willhite, C. C., and Burk, D. T. (1986). Morphogenesis of isotretinoin-induced microcephaly and micrognathia studied by scanning electron microscopy. *Teratology*, **34**: 141–153.

Istvan, E. J. (1970). Drug-associated congenital abnormalities. *Canadian Med. Assoc. J.*, **103**: 1394.

Itoi, M., Gefter, J. W., Kaneko, N., Ishii, Y., Ramer, R. M., and Gasset, A. R. (1975). Teratogenicities of ophthalmic drugs. I. Antiviral ophthalmic drugs. *Arch. Ophthalmol.*, **93**: 46–51.

Jacobs, C., Donaldson, S. A., Rosenberg, S. A,. and Kaplan, H. S. (1981). Management of the pregnant patient with Hodgkin's disease. *Ann. Intern. Med.*, **95**: 669–675.

Jaffe, N. R. and Johnson, E. M. (1973). Alterations in the ontogeny and specific activity of phosphomonoesterases associated with abnormal chondrogenesis and osteogenesis in the limbs of fetuses from folic acid-deficient pregnant rats. *Teratology*, **8**: 33–50.

James, L. F. and Keeler, R. F. (1968). Teratogenic effects of aminopterin in sheep. *Teratology*, **1**: 407–412.

Janz, D. (1982). Antiepileptic drugs and pregnancy: altered utilization patterns and teratogenesis. *Epilepsia*, **23** (suppl. 1): 533–563.

Jaskoll, T. F. and Maderson, P. F. A. (1978). A histological study of the development of the avian middle ear and tympanum. *Anat. Rec.*, **190**: 177–200.

Jeavons, P. M. (1984). Sodium valproate and neural tube defects. *Lancet*, **2**: 1282.

Jelinek, V., Zikmund, E., and Reichlova, R. (1967). L'influence de quelques medicaments psychotropes sur le développement du foetus chez le rat. *Therapie*, **22**: 1429–1433.

Jick, H., Holmes, L., Hunter, J., Madsen, S., and Stergachis, A. (1981). First-trimester drug use and congenital disorders. *JAMA*, **246**: 343–346.

Johnson, F. D. (1972). Pregnancy and concurrent chronic myelogenous leukemia. *Am. J. Obstet. Gynecol.*, **112**: 640–644.

Johnson, R. K., Zee-Chung, R. K. Y., Lee, W. W., Acton, E. M., Henry, D. W., and Cheng, C. C. (1979). Experimental antitumor activity of aminoanthraquinones. *Cancer Treat. Rep.*, **63**: 425–439.

Jonsson, B. G. (1972). Thalidomide teratology in swine: a preparatory study. *Acta Pharmacol. Toxicol.*, **31**: 24–26.

Jordan, R. L., Terapane, J. F., and Schumacher, H. J. (1970). Studies on the teratogenicity of methotrexate in rabbits. *Teratology*, **3**: 203A.

Jordan, R. L., Wilson, J. G., and Schumacher, H. J. (1977). Embryotoxicity of the folate antagonist methotrexate in rats and rabbits. *Teratology*, **15**: 73–80.

Jurand, A. (1961). Further investigations on the cytotoxic and morphogenetic effects of some nitrogen mustard derivatives. *J. Embryol. Exp. Morphol.*, **9**: 492–506.

Jurand, A. (1988). Teratogenic activity of lithium carbonate: an experimental update. *Teratology*, **38**: 101–111.

Jurand, A. and Martin, L. V. H. (1990). Teratogenic potential of two neurotropic drugs, haloperidol and dextromoramide, tested on mouse embryos. *Teratology*, **42**: 45–54.

Kallen, B. and Tandberg, A. (1983). Lithium and pregnancy. A cohort study on manic-depressive women. *Acta Psychiatr. Scand.*, **68**: 134–139.

Kameyama, Y., Hoshino, K., and Hayasaka, I. (1974). Morphogenesis of 5-fluorouracil induced polydactylism in mice. Epithelial-mesenchymal interactions in the formation of polydactylism. *Annu. Rep. Environ. Med. Nagoya Univ.*, **21**: 59–66.

Kao, J., Brown, N. A., Schmidt, B., Goulding, E. H., and Fabro, S., (1981). Teratogenicity of valproic acid: *in vivo* and *in vitro* investigation. *Teratogen. Carcinogen. Mutagen.* **1**: 367–382.

Karnofsky, D. A. (1960). Influences of antimetabolites inhibiting nucleic acid metabolism on embryonic development. *Trans. Assoc. Amer. Physicians*, **73**: 334–347.

Karnofsky, D. A. and Lacon, C. R. (1964). Effects of drugs on the skeletal development of the chick embryo. *Clin. Orthop.*, **33**: 59–70.

Karnofsky, D. A., Patterson, P. A., and Ridgeway, L. P. (1949). Effects of folic acid '4-amino' folic acids and related substances on the growth of the chick embryo. *Proc. Soc. Exp. Biol. Med.*, **71**: 447–454.

Katz, R. A. (1988). Effect of diazepam on the embryonic development of the palate in the rat. *J. Craniofac. Genet. Dev. Biol.*, **8**: 155–166.

Keino, H. and Yamamura, H. (1974). Effects of cadmium salt administered to pregnant mice on postnatal development of the offspring. *Teratology*, **10**: 87A.

Kellogg, C. K. (1985). Drugs and chamicals that act on the central nervous system: interpretation of experimental evidence. *Prog. Clin. Biol. Res.* **163C**: 147–153.

Kernis, M. M. (1972). Cysteine interference with chlorambucil-induced teratogenesis in the rat. *Soc. Exp. Biol. Med.*, **139**: 62–65.

Khan, I. and Azam, A. (1969). Teratogenic activity of trifluoperazine, amitriptyline, ethionamide, and thalidomide in pregnant rabbits and mice. *Proc. Eur. Soc. Study Drug Toxic.*, **10**: 235–242.

Khera, K. S. (1975). Effects of methotrexate and acetylsalicylic acid on cat fetal development. *Teratology*, **11**: 25A.

Khera, K. S. (1975). Fetal cardiovascular and other defects induced by thalidomide in cats. *Teratology*, **11**: 65–72.

Khera, K. S. (1975). Teratogenicity study in rats given high doses of pyridoxine (Vitamin B_6) during organogenesis. *Experientia*, **31**: 469–470.

Kimmel, C. A. and Wilson, J. G. (1973). Skeletal deviations in rats: malformations or variations? *Teratology*, 8: 309–316.

Kimmel, C. A., Wilson, J. G., and Schumacher, H. J. (1971). Studies on metabolism and identification of the causative agent in aspirin teratogenesis in rats. *Teratology*, **4**: 15–24.

Kistler, A. (1981). Teratogenesis of retinoic acid in rats: susceptible stages and suppression of retinoic acid-induced limb malformations by cycloheximide. *Teratology*, 23: 25–31.

Kitchin, K. T., Schmid, B. P., and Sanyal, M. K. (1981). Teratogenicity of cyclophosphamide in a coupled microsomal activating/embryo culture system. *Biochem. Pharmacol.*, **30**: 59–64.

Klein, K. L., Scott, W. J., and Wilson, J. G. (1981). Aspirin-induced teratogenesis: a unique pattern of cell death and subsequent polydactyly in the rat. *J. Exp. Zool.*, **216**: 107–112.

Kleinebrecht, J., Degenhardt, K.-H., Franz, J., and Schneider, G. (1972). Variability of limb malformations induced by 5-fluoro-2′-deoxycytidine in mice. *Teratology*, **5**: 295–302.

Kleinebrecht, J., Franz, J., and Degenhardt, K.-H. (1974). Supernumerary distal limb elements induced by 5-fluoro-2′-deoxycytidine in mice. *Teratology*, **9**: 5–10.

Kline, A. H., Blattner, R. J., and Lunin, M. (1964). Transplacental effect of tetracyclines on teeth. *JAMA*, **188**: 178–180.

Knight, E. and Roe, D. A. (1978). Effects of salicylamide and protein restriction on the skeletal development of the rat fetus. *Teratology*, **18**: 17–22.

Knudsen, T. B. and Kochhar, D. M. (1981). Limb development in mouse embryos. III. Cellular events underlying the determination of altered skeletal patterns following treatment with 5′fluoro-2-deoxyuridine. *Teratology*, **23**: 241–251.

Koch, S., Jager-Roman, E., Rating, D., and Helge, H. (1983). Possible teratogenic effect of valproate during pregnancy. *J. Pediatr.*, **103**: 1007–1008.

Kochhar, D. M. (1973). Limb development in mouse embryos. I. Analysis of teratogenic effects of retinoic acid. *Teratology*, 7: 289–298.

Kochhar, D. M. (1977). Cellular basis of congenital limb deformity induced in mice by vitamin A. *Birth Defects*, 13: 111–154.

Kochhar, D. M. (1985). Skeletal morphoge comparative effects of a mutant gene and a teratogen. In: *Developmental Mechanisms: Normal and Abnormal.* Lash, J. W. and Saxen, L., Eds., Alan R. Liss, New York, 259–271.

Kochhar, D. M., Penner, J. D., and McDay, J. A. (1978). Limb development in mouse embryos. II. Reduction defects, cytotoxicity and inhibition of DNA synthesis produced by cytosine arabinoside. *Teratology*, **18**: 71–92.

Kollar, E. J. (1976). The use of organ cultures of embryonic tooth germs for teratological studies. In: *Tests of Teratogenecity In Vitro.* North Holland-American, Amsterdam, 303–334.

Kopelman, A. E., McCullar, F. W., and Heggeness, L. (1975). Limb malformations following maternal use of haloperidol. *JAMA*, **231**: 62–64.

Kris, E. B. (1965). Children of mothers maintained on pharmacotherapy during pregnancy and postpartum. *Curr. Ther. Res.*, **7**: 785–789.

Kromka, M. and Hoar, R. M. (1973). Use of guinea pigs in teratological investigations. *Teratology*, **7**: A–21.

Kuczuk, M. H. and Scott, W. J., Jr., (1984). Potentiation of acetazolamide induced ectrodactyly in SWV and C57BL/6J mice by cadmium sulfate. *Teratology*, **29**: 427–435.

Kury, G., Chaube, S., and Murphy, M. L. (1968). Teratogenic effects of some purine analogues on fetal rats. *Arch. Pathol.*, **86**: 395–402.

Kwasigroch, T. E., Vannoy, J. F., Church, J. K., and Skalko, R. G. (1986). Retinoic acid enhances and depresses *in vitro* development of cartilaginous bone analgen in embryonic mouse limbs. *In Vitro Cell. Dev. Biol.*, **22**: 150–156.

Laegreid, L., Olegard, R., Wahlstrom, J., and Conradi, N. (1987). Abnormalities in children exposed to benzodiazepines *in utero*. *Lancet*, **1**: 108–109.

Landauer, W. (1957). Niacin antagonists and chick development. *J. Exp. Zool.*, **136**: 509–530.

Landauer, W. and Wakasugi, N. (1967). Problems of acetazolamide and N-ethylnicotinamide as teratogens. *J. Exp. Zool.*, **164**: 499–516.

LaPointe, R. and Harvey, E. B. (1964). Salicylamide-induced anomalies in hamster embryos. *J. Exp. Zool.*, **156**: 197–199.

Larsen, H. L. and Janners, M. Y. (1987). Teratogenic effects of retinoic acid and dimethylsulfoxide on embryonic chick wing and somite. *Teratology*, 36: 313–320.

Larsson, K. S. and Bostrom, H. (1965). Teratogenic action of salicylates related to the inhibition of mucopolysaccharide synthesis. *Acta Paediat. Scand.*, **54**: 43–48.

Larsson, K. S., Bostrom, H., and Ericson, B. (1963). Salicylate-induced malformations in mouse embryos. *Acta Paediat. Scand.*, **52**: 36–40.

Layton, W. M., Jr. (1971). Teratogenic action of acetazolamide in golden hamsters. *Teratology*, **4**: 95–102.

Layton, W. M., Jr. and Ferm, V. H. (1980). Protection against cadmium-induced limb malformations by pretreatment with cadmium or mercury. *Teratology*, **21**: 357–360.

Layton, W. M., Jr. and Hallesy, D. W. (1965). Deformity of forelimb in rats; association with high doses of acetazolamide. *Science*, **149**: 306–308.

Lee, H. Y., Keresztury, M. F., Kosciuk, M. C., Nagele, R. G., and Roisen, F. J. (1984). Diazepam inhibits neuralation through its action on myosin-containing microfilaments in early chick embryos. *Comp. Biochem. Physiol.*, **77**: 331–334.

Lejour-Jeanty, M. (1966). Becs-de-lièvre provoqués chez le rat par un dérivé de la pénicilline l'hadacidine. *J. Embryol. Exp. Morphol.*, **15**: 193–211.

Lemon, P. G. and Hancock, N. A. (1974). The effects of methyl-5(6)-butyl-2-benzimidazole carbamate (parbendazole) on reproduction in sheep and other animals. *Cornell Vet.*, **64** (suppl. 4): 77–84.

Lenz, W. (1961). Kindliche Mmssbildungen nach Medikamente-Einnahme wahrend der Gravididat? *Dtsch. Med. Wochenschr.*, **86**: 2555–2556.

Linden, S. and Rich, C.L. (1983). The use of lithium during pregnancy and lactation. *J. Clin. Psychiatry*, **44**: 358–361.

Lindhout, D. and Meinardi, H. (1984). Spina bifida and *in utero* exposure to valproate. *Lancet*, **2**: 396.

Lindhout, D., Rene, J., Hoppener, E. A., and Meinardi, H. (1984). Teratogenicity of antiepileptic drug combinations with special emphasis on epoxidation (of carbamazepine). *Epilepsia*, **25**: 77–83.

Lorente, C. A., Tassinari, M. S., and Keith, D. A. (1981). The effects of phenytoin on rat development: an animal model system for fetal hydantoin syndrome. *Teratology*, **24**: 169–180.

Lowe, C. R. (1973). Congenital malformations among infants born to epileptic women. *Lancet*, **1**: 9–10.

McBride, W. G. (1961). Thalidomide and congenital abnormalities. *Lancet*, **2**: 1358.

McBride, W. G. (1972). Letter: limb deformities associated with iminodibenzyl hydrochloride. *Med. J. Aust.*, **1**: 492.

McBride, W. G. (1976). Studies of the etiology of thalidomide dysmorphogenesis. *Teratology*, **14**: 71–87.

McClain, R. M. and Dammers, K. D. (1981). Toxicologic evaluation of bumetanide, potent diuretic agent. *J. Clin. Pharmacol.*, **21**: 543–554.

McClain, R. M. and Langhoff, L. (1980). Teratogenicity of diphenylhydantoin in the New Zealand white rabbit. *Teratology*, **21**: 371–379.

McClure, H. M., Wilk, A. L., Horigan, E. A., and Pratt, R. M. (1979). Induction of craniofacial malformations in rhesus monkeys (*Macaca mulatta*) with cyclophosphamide. *Cleft Palate J.*, **16**: 248–256.

McColl, J. D., Globus, M., and Robinson, S. (1965). Effect of some therapeutic agents on the developing rat fetus. *Toxicol. Appl. Pharmacol.*, **7**: 409–417.

McKinna, A. J. (1966). Quinine-induced hypoplasia of the optic nerve. *Can. J. Ophthalmol.*, **1**: 261–266.

McNiel, J. R. (1973). The possible teratogenic effect of salicylates on the developing foetus. *Clin. Pediat.*, **12**: 347–350.

Machado, J. P. (1968). Accao mutagenica do busulfan no ratinho (nota previa). *Medico (Porto)*, **49**: 281.

Maier, W. (1964). Unser derzeitiges wissen über äussere schädigende einflüsse auf den embryo und angeborene Missbildungen. *Dtsch. Z. Ges. Gerichtl. Med.*, **55**: 156–172.

Manson, J. M. and Smith, C. C. (1977). Influence of cyclophosphamide and 4-ketocyclophosphamide on mouse limb development. *Teratology*, **15**: 291–299.

Marks, T. A. and Poppe, S. M. (1988). Developmental toxicity of bropirimine in rats after oral administration. *Teratology*, **38**: 7–14.

Martin, J. C. (1984). Perinatal psychoactive drug use: effects on gender, development and function in offspring. *Nebr. Symp. Motiv.*, **32**: 227–266.

Mazze, R. I., Wilson, A. I., Rice, S. A., and Baden, J. M. (1982). Reproduction and fetal development in mice chronically exposed to nitrous oxide. *Teratology*, **26**: 11–16.

Mazze, R. I., Wilson, A. I., Rice, S. A., and Baden, J. M. (1984). Reproduction and fetal development in rats exposed to nitrous oxide. *Teratology*, **30**: 259–265.

Mazze, R. I., Wilson, A. I., Rice, S. A., and Baden, J. M. (1985). Fetal development in mice exposed to isoflurane. *Teratology*, **32**: 339–345.

Mazze, R. I., Fujinaga, M., Rice, S. A., Harris, S. B., and Baden, J. M. (1986). Reproductive and teratogenic effects of nitrous oxide, halothane, isoflurane, and enflurane in Sprague-Dawley rats. *Anesthesiology*, **64**: 339–344.

Massey, K. M. (1966). Teratogenic effects of diphenylhydantoin sodium. *J. Oral Ther.*, **2**: 380–385.

Meadow, S. R. (1968). Anticonvulsant drugs and congenital malformations. *Lancet*, **2**: 1296.

Meltzer, H. J. (1956). Congenital anomalies due to attempted abortion with 4-aminopteroyl-glutamic acid. *JAMA*, **161**: 1263.

Mennie, A. T. (1962). Tetracycline and congenital limb anomalies. *Lancet*, **2**: 480.

Mennuti, M. T., Shepard, T. H., and Mellman, W. J. (1975). Fetal renal malformation following treatment of Hodgkin's disease during pregnancy. *Obstet. Gynecol.*, **46**: 194–196.

Mericer-Parot, L. and Tuchmann-Duplessis, H. (1974). The dysmorphogenic potential of phenytoin: experimental observations. *Drugs*, **8**: 340–353.

Merker, H. J., Pospisil, M., and Murphy, M. L. (1975). The cytotoxic effect of 6-mercapto-purine on the limb bud blastema cells of rat embryos. *Teratology*, **11**: 199–218.

Messerle, K. and Webster, W. S. (1982). The classification and development of cadmium-induced limb defects in mice. *Teratology*, **25**: 61–70.

Middleton, H. D., Plant, J. W., Walker, C. E., Dixon, R. T., and Johns, D. R. (1974). The effects of methyl-5(6)-butyl-2-benzimidazole carbamate (parbendazole) on reproduction in sheep and other animals. *Cornell Vet.*, **64** (suppl. 4): 56–68.

Milaire, J. (1985). Histological changes induced in developing limb buds of C57BL mouse embryos submitted in utero to the combined influence of acetazolamide and cadmium sulfate. *Teratology*, **32**: 433–451.

Milch, R. A., Rall, D. P., and Tobie, J. E. (1958). Fluorescence of tetracycline antibiotics in bone. *J. Bone Jt. Surg.*, **40A**: 897.

Milkovich, L. and van den Berg, B. J. (1974). Effects of prenatal meprobamate and chlordi-azepoxide hydrochloride on human embryonic and fetal development. *N. Engl. J. Med.*, **291**: 1268–1271.

Milkovich, L. and van den Berg, B. J. (1976). An evaluation of teratogenicity of certain anti-nauseant drugs. *Am. J. Obstet. Gynecol.*, **125**: 244–248.

Miller, C. R., Szabo, K. T., and Scott, G. C. (1974). The effects of methyl-5(6)-butyl-2-ben-zimidazole carbamate (parbendazole) on reproduction in sheep and other animals. *Cornell Vet.*, **64** (suppl. 4): 85–91.

Miller, R. P. and Becker, B. A. (1971). Teratogenic effects of diazepam in the Swiss-Webster mouse. *Pharmacologist*, **13**: A274.

Miller, R. P. and Becker, B. A. (1973). The teratogenicity of diazepam metabolites in Swiss-Webster mice. *Toxicol. Appl. Pharmacol.*, **25**: A453.

Miller, R. P. and Becker, B. A. (1975). Teratogenicity of oral diazepam and diphenylhydantoin in mice. *Toxicol. Appl. Pharmacol.*, **32**: 53–61.

Millicovsky, G. and DeSesso, J. M. (1980). Cardiovascular alterations in rabbit embryos in situ after a teratogenic dose of hydroxyurea: an in vivo microscopic study. *Teratology*, **22**: 115–124.

Milunsky, A., Graef, J. W., and Gaynor, M. F., Jr. (1968). Methotrexate-induced congenital malformations. *J. Pediatr.*, **72**: 790–795.

Mirkes, P. E. (1985). Cyclophosphamide teratogenesis: a review. *Teratogen. Carcinogen. Mutagen.*, **5**: 75–88.

Mirkes, P. E., Fantel, A. G., Greenaway, J. C., and Shepard, T. H. (1981). Teratogenicity of cyclophosphamide metabolites: phosphormide mustard, acrolein and 4-ketocyclophos-phamide in rat embryos cultured in vitro. *Toxicol. Appl. Pharmacol.*, **58**: 322–330.

Mitala, J. J., Boardman, J. P., Carrano, R. A., and Iuliucci, J. D. (1984). Novel accessory skull bone in fetal rats after exposure to aspirin. *Teratology*, **30**: 95–98.

Mitchell, A. A., Rosenberg, L., Sharpio, J., and Slone, D. (1981). Birth defects related to Bendectin use in pregnancy. I. Oral clefts and cardiac defects. *JAMA*, **245**: 2311–2314.

Morelock, S., Hingson, R., Kayne, H., Dooling, E., Zuckerman, B., Day, N., Alpert, J. J. and Flowerdew, G. (1982). Bendectin and fetal development, a study of Boston city hospitals. *Am. J. Obstet. Gynecol.*, **142**: 209–213.

Moriarity, A. J. (1963). Trifluoperazine and congenital malformations. *Can. Med. Assoc. J.*, **88**: 97.

Moriarity, A. J. and Nance, M. R. (1963). Trifluoperazine and pregnancy. *Can. Med. Assoc. J.*, **88**: 375–376.

Mortola, J. F. (1989). The use of psychotropic agents in pregnancy and lactation. *Psychiatr. Clin. North Am.*, **12**: 69–87.

Murphy, M. L. (1962). Teratogenic effects in rats of growth-inhibiting chemicals, including studies on thalidomide. *Clin. Proc. Child. Hosp.*, **18**: 307–322.

Murphy, M. L. (1965). Factors influencing teratogenic response to drugs. In: *Teratology: Principles and Techniques*. Wilson, J. G., Warkany, J., Eds., University of Chicago Press, Chicago, chap. 7.

Murphy, M. L. and Chaube, S. (1962). Teratogenic effects of abnormal purines and their ribosides in the rat. *Proc. Am. Assoc. Cancer Res.*, **3**: 347A.

Murphy, M. L. and Chaube, S. (1964). Preliminary survey of hydroxyurea (NSC-32065) as a teratogen. *Cancer Chemother.*, **Rep. 40**: 1–7.

Murphy, M. L., Dagg, C. P., and Karnofsky, D. A. (1957). Comparison of teratogenic chemicals in the rat and chick embryos. *Pediatrics*, **19**: 701–714.

Murphy, M. L., Moro, A. D., and Lacon, C. (1958). The comparative effects of five polyfunctional alkylating agents on the rat fetus with additional notes on the chick embryo. *Ann. N.Y. Acad. Sci.*, **68**: 762–782.

Muther, T. F., Jones, J. C., and Smoak, N. S. (1977). Potentiation by the injection vehicle of the teratological action of acetazolamide in rats. *Teratology*, **15**: 253–260.

Nagele, R. G., Peitrolungo, J. F., Lee, H., and Roisen, F. J. (1981). Diazepam-induced neural tube closure defects in explanted early chick embryos. *Teratology*, **23**: 343–349.

Nakamura, H. (1975). Analysis of limb anomalies induced *in vitro* by vitamin A (retinol) in mice. *Teratology*, **12**: 61–70.

Nakamura, H. (1977). Digital anomalies in the embryonic mouse limb cultured in the presence of excess vitamin A. *Teratology*, **16**: 195–202.

Nakatsuka, T. (1988). Role of myometrial constriction in the induction of wavy ribs in rat fetuses. *Teratology*, **37**: 329–334.

Naruse, I., Collins, M. D., and Scott, W. J., Jr. (1988). Strain differences in the teratogenicity induced by valproic acid in cultured mouse embryos. *Teratology*, **38**: 87–96.

Naruse, I. and Hayashi, Y. (1989). Amelioration of the teratogenicity of cadmium by the metallothionein induced by bismuth nitrate. *Teratology*, **40**: 459–465.

Naruse, I. and Kameyama, Y. (1986). Prevention of polydactyly manifestation in polydactyly Nagoya (Pdn) mice by administration of cytosine arabinoside during pregnancy. *Teratology*, **34**: 283–289.

Nau, H., Zierer, R., Spielmann, H., Neubert, D., and Gansau, C. (1981). A new model for embryotoxicity testing: teratogenicity and pharmacokinetics of valproic acid following constant-rate administration in the mouse with human therapeutic drug and metabolite concentrations. *Life Sci.*, **29**: 2803–2814.

Nau, H., Merker, H. J., Brendel, K., Gansau, C., Hauser, I., and Wittfoht, W. (1984). Disposition, embryotoxicity and teratogenicity of valproic acid in the mouse as related to man. In: *Metabolism of Antiepileptic Drugs*. Levy, R. H., Pitlick, W. H., Eichelbaum, M., and Meijer, J., Eds., Raven Press, New York, 367–372.

Nau, H. and Scott, W. J., Jr. (1987). Teratogenicity of valproic acid and related substances in the mouse: drug accumulation and pH_i in the embryo during organogenesis and structure-activity considerations. *Arch. Toxicol.* **11** (suppl.): 128–139.

Nelson, M. M. and Forfar, J. O. (1971). Associations between drugs administered during pregnancy and congenital abnormalities of the fetus. *Br. Med. J.*, **1**: 523–527.

Newell-Morris, L., Sirianni, J. E., Shepard, T. H., Fantel, A. G., and Moffett, B. C. (1980). Teratogenic effects of retinoic acid in pigtail monkeys (*Macaca nemestrina*). II. Craniofacial features. *Teratology*, 22: 87–101.

Nicholson, H. O. (1968). Cytotoxic drugs in pregnancy. Review of reported cases. *J. Obstet. Gynecol. Br. Cwlth.*, 75: 307–312.

Nolen, G. A. (1972). The effects of various levels of dietary protein on retinoic acid-induced teratogenicity in rats. *Teratology*, 5: 143–152.

Nolen, G. A. (1989). Effect of a high systemic background level of vitamin A on the teratogenicity of all-trans-retinoic acid given either acutely or subacutely. *Teratology*, 39: 333–339.

Nora, J. J., Nora, A. H., and Toews, W. H. (1974). Lithium, Ebstein's anomaly, and other congenital heart defects. *Lancet*, 2: 594–595.

Norton, L. A., Proffit, W. R., and Bennett, I. C. (1968). Effects of tetracycline on bone growth in organ culture. *Growth*, 32: 113–124.

Nudelman, K. L. and Travill, A. A. (1971). A morphological and histochemical study of thalidomide-induced upper limb malformations in rabbit fetuses. *Teratology*, 4: 409–425.

Nurnberg, H. G. (1989). An overview of somatic treatment of psychosis during pregnancy and postpartum. *Gen. Hosp. Psychiatry*, 11: 328–338.

Nurnberg, H. G. and Prudic, J. (1984). Guidelines for treatment of psychosis during pregnancy. *Hosp. Community Psychiatry*, 35: 67–71.

Oberholzer, R. J. H. (1964). Contribution a l'etude d'une action teratogene eventuelle de l'imipramine. *Med. Hyg.*, 22: 557.

Ogura, T., Hatanao, M., Imamura, T., and Shimizu, G. (1973). A study on the safety of adriamycin HCL. Report No. 4: Deformity-inducing (teratological) experiment. *Medicinal Treatment*, 6: 1152–1164.

O'Leary, J. L. and O'Leary, J. A. (1964). Nonthalidomide ectromelia. *Obstet. Gynecol.*, 23: 17–20.

Ornoy, A. (1971). The effects of maternal hypercortisonism and hypervitaminosis D_2 on fetal osteogenesis and ossification in rats. *Teratology*, 4: 383–394.

Owen, G., Smith, T., and Agersborg, H. (1970). Toxicity of some benzodiazepine compounds with CNS activity. *Toxicol. Appl. Pharmacol.*, 16: 556–570.

Padmanabhan, R. and Hameed, M. S. (1986). Exencephaly and axial skeletal dysmorphogenesis induced by maternal exposure to cadmium in the mouse. *J. Craniofacial Genet. Dev. Biol.*, 6: 245–258.

Pap, A. G. and Tarakhovsky, M. L. (1967). Influence of certain drugs on the fetus. *Akush. Ginekol. Moscow*, 43: 10–15.

Patel, D. A. and Patel, A. R. (1980). Clorazepate and congenital malformations. *JAMA*, 244: 135–136.

Patel, V. R. (1973). Natamycin in the treatment of vaginal candidiasis in pregnancy. *Practitioner*, 210: 701–703.

Paulson, R. B., Sucheston, M. E., Hayes, T. G., and Paulson, G. W. (1985). Teratogenic effects of valproate in the CD-1 mouse fetus. *Arch. Neurol.*, 42: 980–983.

Paulson, R. B., Sucheston, M. E., Hayes, T. G., Weiss, H. S., Sachs, L. A., Oca, M., Kernan, B., and Weiss, S. (1988). Effects of sodium valproate and oxygen on the CD-1 mouse fetus. *J. Craniofacial Genet. Dev. Biol.*, 8: 35–45.

Paulson, R. B., Sucheston, M. E., Hayes, T. G., and Weiss, H. S. (1989). Effects of sodium valproate on the craniofacial skeletal pattern in the CD-1 mouse embryo. *J. Craniofacial Genet. Dev. Biol.*, 9: 339–348.

Persaud, T. V. N., Chudley, E. A., and Skalko, R. G. (1985). In: *Basic Concepts in Teratology.* Alan R. Liss, New York, 28, 75–79.

Petrere, J. A., Anderson, J. A., Sakowski, R., Fitzgerald, J. E., and De La Iglesia, F. A. (1986). Teratogenesis of calcium valproate in rabbits. *Teratology*, 34: 263–269.

Petrere, J. A., Kim, S.-A., Anderson, J. A., Fitzgerald, J. E., De La Iglesia, F. A., and Schardein, J. L. (1986). Teratology studies of ametantrone acetate in rats and rabbits. *Teratology*, **34**: 271–278.

Pillans, P. I., Folb, P. I., and Ponzi, S. F. (1988). The effects of *in vivo* administration of teratogenic doses of vitamin A during the preimplantation period in the mouse. *Teratology*, 37: 7–11.

Pinsky, L. and Fraser, F. C. (1959). Production of skeletal malformations in the offspring of pregnant mice treated with 6-aminonicotinamide. *Biol. Neonate*, **1**: 106–112.

Pitts, F. N. (1983). Lithium and pregnancy. *J. Clin. Psychiatry*, **44**: 357.

Pizzuto, J., Aviles, A., Noriega, L., Niz, J., Morales, M., and Romero, F., (1980). Treatment of acute leukemia during pregnancy: presentation of nine cases. *Cancer Treat. Rep.*, 64: 679–683.

Plotkin, S. A. (1984). Prevention of cytomegalovirus infection. (Editorial). *J. Roy. Soc. Med.*, **77**: 94–95.

Poswillo, D. E. (1972). Tridione and paradione as suspected teratogens. An investigation in subhuman primates. *Ann. R. Coll. Surg. Engl.*, **50**: 367–370.

Powell, H.R. and Ekert, H. (1971). Methotrexate-induced congenital malformations. *Med. J. Aust.*, **2**: 1076–1077.

Rachelefsky, G. S., Flynt, J. W., Ebbin, A. J., and Wilson, M. G. (1972). Letter: possible teratogenicity of tricyclic antidepressants. *Lancet*, **1**: 838–839.

Rafla, N. (1987). Limb deformities associated with prochlorperazine. *Am. J. Obstet. Gynecol.*, **156**: 1557.

Ramamurthy, S. V. and Chaudhry, A.P. (1979). Valium (diazepam) — its effects on hamster intrauterine fetal growth. *J. Dent. Res.*, **58**: 2011.

Rathbun, K. C. (1983). Congenital syphilis. *Sex Transm. Dis.*, **10**: 93–99.

Rating, D., Jager-Roman, E., Koch, S., Deichl, A., Hartmann, H., Jakob, S., Beck-Mannagetta, G., Nau, H., and Helge, H. (1987). Major malformations and minor anomalies in the offspring of epileptic parents. In: *Pharmacokinetics in Teratogenesis*. **Vol. 1,** Nau, H. and Scott, W. J., Jr., Eds., CRC Press, Boca Raton, FL, 205–223.

Ravid, R. and Toaff, R. (1972). On the possible teratogenicity of antibiotic drugs administered during pregnancy — a prospective study. In: *Drugs and Fetal Development*. Klingberg, M. A., Abramovici, A., and Chemke, J., Eds., Plenum Press, New York, 505–510.

Reed, H., Briggs, J. N., and Martin, J. K. (1955). Congenital glaucoma, deafness, mental deficiency, and cardiac anomaly following attempted abortion. *J. Pediatr.*, **46**: 182–185.

Reider, R. O., Rosenthal, D., Wender, P., and Blumenthal, H. (1975). The offspring of schizophrenics. Fetal and neonatal deaths. *Arch. Gen. Psychiatry*, **32**: 200–211.

Reiners, J. Wittfoht, W., Nau, H., Vogel, R., Tenschert, B., and Spielmann, H. (1987). Teratogenesis and pharmacokinetics of cyclophosphamide after drug infusion as compared to injection in the mouse during day 10 of gestation. In:*Pharmacokinetics in Teratogenesis*. Vol. 2, Nau, H. and Scott, W. J., Jr., Eds., CRC Press, Boca Raton, FL, 41–48.

Remington, J. S. and Klein, J. O., Eds., (1983). In: *Infectious Diseases of the Fetus and Newborn Infant*. W.B. Saunders, Philadelphia.

Rendle-Short, T. J. (1962). Tetracycline in teeth and bone. *Lancet*, **1**: 1188.

Rifkind, A. B. (1974). Teratogenic effects of trimethadione and dimethadione in the chick embryo. *Toxicol. Appl. Pharmacol.*, **30**: 452–457.

Ringrose, C. A. D. (1972). The hazard of neurotropic drugs in the fertile years. *Can. Med. Assoc. J.*, **106**: 1058.

Ritter, E. J., Scott, W. J., Jr., Randall, J. L., and Ritter, J. M. (1987). Teratogenicity of di(2-ethylhexyl)phthalate, 2-ethylhexanol, 2-ethylhexanoic acid, and valproic acid, and potentiation by caffeine. *Teratology*, **35**: 41–46.

Ritter, E. J., Scott, W. J., and Wilson, J. G. (1973). Relationship of temporal patterns of cell death and development to malformations in the rat limb. Possible mechanisms of teratogenesis with inhibitors of DNA synthesis. *Teratology*, **7**: 219–226.

Ritter, E. J., Scott, W. J., and Wilson, J. G. (1975). Inhibition of ATP synthesis associated with 6-aminonicotinamide (6-AN) teratogenesis in rat embryos. *Teratology*, **12**: 233–238.

Ritter, E. J., Scott, W. J., Jr., Wilson, J. G., Mathinos, P. R., and Randall, J. L. (1982). Potentiative interactions between caffeine and various teratogenic agents. *Teratology*, **25**: 95–100.

Robens, J. T. (1969). Teratologic studies of carbaryl, diazinon, norea, disulfiram and thiram in small laboratory animals. *Toxicol. Appl. Pharmacol.*, **15**: 152–163.

Robert, E. and Guibaud, P. (1982). Maternal valproic acid and congenital neural tube defects. *Lancet*, **2**: 937.

Robert, E. and Rosa, F. (1983). Valproate and birth defects. *Lancet*, **2**: 1142.

Robertson, R. T., Allen, H. L., and Bokelman, D. L. (1979). Aspirin: teratogenic evaluation in the dog. *Teratology*, **20**: 313–320.

Robertson, R. T., Minsker, D. H., Bokelman, D. L., Durand, G., and Conquet, P. (1981). Potassium loss as a causative factor for skeletal malformations in rats produced by indacrinone: a new investigational loop diuretic. *Toxicol. Appl. Pharmacol.*, **60**: 142–150.

Robinson, G. E., Stewart, D. E., and Flak, E. (1986). The rational use of psychotropic drugs in pregnancy and postpartum. *Can. J. Psychiatry*, **31**: 183–190.

Robson, J. M. and Sullivan, F. M. (1963). The production of foetal abnormalities in rabbits by imipramine. *Lancet*, **1**: 638–639.

Rochelle, W. T., Price, C. J., Marr, M. C., and Kimmel, C. A. (1988). Developmental toxicity evaluation of Bendectin in CD rats. *Teratology*, **37**: 539–552.

Rodriquez, M. D. and Friman, M. (1985). Teratogenic effect of trifluoperazine in rats and mice. *Acta Biol. Hung.*, **36**: 233–237.

Roetz, R. and Michels, G. (1977). Quantitative aspekete der Teratogenen Wirkung von 5-Brom-2'-Desoxyuridin (BUdR) an der Fetalen Mauseextremitat. *Verh. Anat. Ges.*, **71**: 629–634.

Rohovsky, M. W., Newberne, J. W., and Gibson, J. P. (1971). Preclinical toxicity studies with tilorone hydrochloride, an oral interferon inducer. *Toxicol. Appl. Pharmacol.*, **19**: 415A.

Roizin, L., Lazar, M., and Gold, G. (1966). Prenatal effects of phenothiazines. *Fed. Proc.*, **25**: 353.

Roll, R. (1971). Teratologic studies with thiram (TMTD) on two strains of mice. *Arch. Toxicol. (Berlin)*, **27**: 173–186.

Rolle, G. K. and Bevelander, G. (1966). Further studies on the effect of tetracyclines on the developing skeleton of the chick embryo. *J. Morphol.*, **118**: 317–330.

Rosenberg, L., Mitchell, A. A., Parsells, J. L., Pashayan, H., Louik, C., and Shapiro, S. (1983). Lack of relation of oral clefts to diazepam use during pregnancy. *N. Engl. J. Med.*, **309**: 1282–1285.

Rosenberg, P. and Kirves, A. (1973). Miscarriages among operating theatre staff. *Acta Anaesthesiol. Scand.*, **53** (suppl): 37–42.

Rosi, D., Peruzzotti, G., Dennis, E. W., Berberian, D. A., Freele, H., and Archer, S. (1965). A new active metabolite of "Miracil D". *Nature*, **208**: 1005–1006.

Roux, C. and Horvath, C. (1971). Teratogenic effect of hadacidin in mice and hamsters. *C.R. Soc. Biol.*, **164**: 2171–2175.

Rudd, N. L. and Freedom, R. M. (1979). A possible primidone embryopathy. *J. Pediatr.*, **94**: 835.

Ruffolo, P. and Ferm, V. (1965). The embryocidal and teratogenic effects of 5-bromodeoxyuridine in the pregnant hamster. *Lab. Invest.*, **14**: 1547–1553.

Rumeau-Rouquette, C., Goujard, J., and Huel, G. (1977). Possible teratogenic effect of phenothiazines in human beings. *Teratology*, **15**: 57–64.

Sadler, T. W. and Kochhar, D. M. (1975). Teratogenic effects of chlorabucil on *in vivo* and *in vitro* organogenesis in mice. *Teratology*, **12**: 71–78.

Safra, M. J. and Oakley, G. P. (1975). Association between cleft lip with or without cleft palate and prenatal exposure to diazepam. *Lancet*, **2**: 478–480.

Saito, H., Kobayashi, H., Takeno, S., and Sakai, T. (1984). Fetal toxicity of benzodiazepines in rats. *Res. Commun. Chem. Pathol. Pharmacol.*, **46**: 437–447.

Sanyal, M. K., Kitchin, K. T., and Dixon, R. L. (1981). Rat conceptus development *in vitro*: comparative effects of alkylating agents. *Toxicol. Appl. Pharmacol.*, **57**: 14–19.

Satish, J., Pratt, B. M., and Sanyal, M. K. (1985). Differential dysmorphogenesis induced by microinjection of an alkylating agent into rat conceptuses cultured *in vitro*. *Teratology*, **31**: 61–72.

Saunders, L. Z., Shone, D. K., Philip, J. R., and Birkhead, H. A. (1974). The effects of methyl-5(6)-butyl-2-benzimidazole carbamate (parbendazole) on reproduction in sheep and other animals. *Cornell Vet.*, **64** (suppl. 4): 7–40.

Saxén, I. (1975). Associations between oral clefts and drugs taken during pregnancy. *Int. J. Epidemiol.*, **4**: 37–44.

Saxén, I. and Saxén, L. (1975). Association between maternal intake of diazepam and oral clefts. *Lancet*, **2**: 498.

Saxén, L. (1965). Tetracycline: effect on osteogenesis *in vitro*. *Science*, **149**: 870–872.

Sayli, B. S. (1966). Consanguinity, aspirin and phocomelia. *Lancet*, **1**: 876.

Schardein, J. L. (1976). In: *Drugs as Teratogens*. CRC Press, Cleveland, 57–66, 113–122.

Schardein, J. L. (1985). Cancer chemotherapeutic agents. In: *Chemically Induced Birth Defects*. Marcel Dekker, New York, 467–520.

Schardein, J. L., Hentz, D. L., Petrere, J. A., Fitzgerald, J. E., and Kurtz, S. M. (1977). The effect of vidarabine on the development of the offspring of rats, rabbits, and monkeys. *Teratology*, **15**: 231–242.

Schmid, B. P., Goulding, E., Kitchin, K. T., and Sanyal, M. K. (1981). Assessment of the teratogenic potential of acrolein and cyclophosphamide in a rat embryo culture system. *Toxicology*, **22**: 235–243.

Schmidt, R. R., Abbott, P. K., and Cotler, J. M. (1982). *In vitro* effects of the teratogen and folic acid antagonist, 9-methyl pteroylglutamic acid, on glycosaminoglycan accumulation in fetal rat limbs. *Teratology*, **26**: 53–57.

Schmidt, R. R., Chepenik, K. P., and Paynton, B. V. (1977). Effects of the teratogenic folic acid antagonist, 9-methyl pteroylglutamic acid, on hydroxyproline levels in fetal rat limbs. *J. Embryol. Exp. Morphol.*, **41**: 289–294.

Schoji, R. and Ohzu, E. (1965). Effect of endoxan on developing mouse embryos. *J. Fac. Sc. Hokkaido Univ.*, **15**: 662–665.

Schreiner, C. M., Hirsch, K. S., and Scott, W. J., Jr., (1981). Carbonicanhydrase distribution in rodent embryos and its relationship to acetazolamide teratogenesis. *J. Histochem. Cytochem.*, **29**: 1213–1218.

Scott, W. J., Jr. (1970). Effects of intrauterine administration of acetazolamide in rats. *Teratology*, **3**: 261–268.

Scott, W. J., Jr., (1979). Physiological cell death in normal and abnormal rodent limb development. In: *Advances in the Study of Birth Defects*. Persaud, T. V. N., Ed., University Park Press, Baltimore, 135–142.

Scott, W. J., Jr., (1981). Pathogenesis of bromodeoxyuridine-induced polydactyly. *Teratology*, 23: 383–389.

Scott, W. J., Jr., Butcher, R. E., Kindt, C. W., and Wilson, J. G. (1972). Greater sensitivity of female than male rat embryos to acetazolamide teratogenicity. *Teratology*, **6**: 239–240.

Scott, W. J., Jr., Hirsch, J. M., DeSesso, J. M., and Wilson, J. G. (1981). Comparative studies on acetazolamide teratogenesis in pregnant rats, rabbits, and rhesus monkeys. *Teratology*, **24**: 37–42.

Scott, W. J., Ritter, E. J., and Wilson, J. G. (1977). Delayed appearance of ectodermal cell death as a mechanism of polydactyly induction. *J. Embryol. Exp. Morphol.*, **42**: 93–104.

Scott, W. J., Ritter, E. J., and Wilson, J. G. (1980). Ectodermal and mesodermal cell death patterns in 6-mercaptopurine riboside-induced digital deformities. *Teratology*, **21**: 271–279.

Scott, E., Ritter, E., Wilson, J., and Schreiner, C. (1978). A second mechanism of polydactyly induction. *Teratology*, **17**: 37A–38A.

Scott, W. J., Wilson, J. G., and Ritter, E. J. (1972). The teratogenic, biochemical and histological effects of aminothiadiazole (ATD) and their reversibility of nicotinamide. *Teratology*, **5**: 266A.

Seip, M. (1976). Growth retardation, dysmorphic facies and minor malformations following massive exposure to phenobarbital *in utero*. *Acta Pediatr. Scand.*, **65**: 617–621.

Sfetsos, M. (1970). Panmyelopathy due to Daraprim® used in treatment of toxoplasmosis. *Med. Klin.*, **65**: 1039–1042.

Shah, R. M. (1977). Effects of prenatal administration of hadacidin, a cancer chemotherapeutic agent, on the development of hamster fetuses. *J. Embryol. Exp. Morph.*, **39**: 203–220.

Sharma, A. and Rawat, A. K. (1986). Teratogenic effects of lithium and ethanol in the developing fetus. *Alcohol*, **3**: 101–106.

Shaw, E. B. (1972). Fetal damage due to maternal aminopterin injection. Follow-up at age 9 years. *Am. J. Dis. Child.*, **124**: 93–94.

Shenefelt, R. E. (1972). Morphogenesis of malformations in hamsters caused by retinoic acid: relation to dose and stage at treatment. *Teratology*, **5**: 103–118.

Sherry, C. J. (1977). Chlorpromazine: a potential physiological teratogen. *Experientia*, **33**: 493–494.

Sieber, S. M., Whang-Peng, J., and Adamson, R. H. (1974). Teratogenic and cytogenetic effects of hycanthone in mice and rabbits. *Teratology*, **10**: 227–236.

Sieber, S. M., Whang-Peng, J., Botkin, C., and Knutsen, T. (1978). Teratogenic and cytogenetic effects of some plant-derived antitumor agents (vincristine, colchicine, maytansine, VP-16-213 and VM-26) in mice. *Teratology*, **18**: 31–48.

Simpkins, J. W., Field, F. P., Torosian, G., and Soltis, E. E. (1985). Effects of prenatal exposure to tricyclic antidepressants on adrenergic responses in progeny. *Dev. Pharmacol. Ther.*, **8**: 17–33.

Sinclair, J. G. (1950). A specific tranplacental effect of urethane in mice. *Tex. Rep. Biol. Med.*, **8**: 623–632.

Singh, M. and Shah, G. L. (1989). Teratogenic effects of phenytoin on chick embryos. *Teratology*, **40**: 453–458.

Singh, S. (1971). The teratogenicity of cyclophosphamide (endoxan-asta) in rats. *Indian J. Med. Res.*, **59**: 1128–1135.

Singh, S. and Padmamabhan, R. (1979). Effect of chlorpromazine on skeletalogenesis. *Acta Orthop. Scand.*, **50**: 151–159.

Singh, S. and Sanyal, A. K. (1974). Abnormal patterns of ossification in the hands of foetuses produced by cyclophosphamide administration to pregnant rats. *Acta Anat.*, **89**: 121–133.

Skalko, R. G. and Gold, M. P. (1974). Teratogenicity of methotrexate in mice. *Teratology*, **9**: 159–164.

Skalko, R. G. and Packard, D. S., Jr., (1973). The teratogenic response of the mouse embryo to 5-iododeoxyuridine. *Experientia*, **29**: 198–200.

Skalko, R. G., Packard, D. S., Jr., Schwendimann, R. N. and Raggio, J. F. (1971). The teratogenic response of mouse embryos to 5-bromodeoxyuridine. *Teratology*, 4: 87–93.

Slone, D., Siskind, V., Heinone, O., Monson, R., Kaufman, D., and Shapiro, S. (1977). Antenatal exposure to the phenothiazines in relation to congenital malformations, perinatal mortality rate, birth weight, and intelligence quotient score. *Am. J. Obstet. Gynecol.*, **128**: 486–488.

Slonitskaya, N. N. (1969). Teratogenic effect of griseofulvin-forte on rat fetus. *Antibiotiki.*, **14**: 44–48.

Smith, B. E. (1968). Teratogenic capabilities of surgical anaesthesia. *Adv. Teratol.*, **3**: 127–179.

Smith, B. E. (1974). Teratology in anesthesia. *Clin. Obstet. Gynecol.*, **17**: 145–163.

Smith, D. J. and Joffe, J. M. (1975). Increased neonatal mortality in offspring of male rats treated with methadone or morphine before mating. *Nature*, **253**: 202–203.

Sobel, D. E. (1961). Infant mortality and malformations in children of schizophrenic women. *Psychiatr. Q.*, **35**: 60–64.

Sobrian, S. K. (1977). Prenatal morphine administration alters behavioral development in the rat. *Pharmacol. Biochem. Behav.*, **7**: 285–288.

Speidel, B. D. and Meadow, S. R. (1974). Epilepsy, anticonvulsants and congenital malformations. *Drugs*, **8**: 354–356.

Spence, A. A., Knill-Jones, R. P., and Newman, B. J. (1974). Studies of morbidity in anaesthetists with special reference to obstetric history. *Proc. R. Soc. Med.*, **67**: 989–990.

Spielvogel, A. and Wile, J. (1986). Treatment of the psychotic pregnant patient. *Psychosomatics*, **27**: 487–492.

Starreveld-Zimmerman, A. A. E., Van Der Kolk, W. J., Meinardi, H., and Elshove, J. (1973). Are anticonvulsants teratogenic? *Lancet*, **2**: 48–49.

Steele, C. E., Trasler, D. G., and New, D. A. T. (1983). An *in vivo/in vitro* evaluation of the teratogenic action of excess vitamin A. *Teratology*, **28**: 209–214.

Stenchever, M. A. and Parks, K. J. (1975). Some effects of diazepam on pregnancy in the Balb/c mouse. *Am. J. Obstet. Gynecol.*, **121**: 765–770.

Sucheston, M. E., Hayes, T. G., Paulson, R. B., and King, J. E. (1979). Fetal malformations in valproate sodium treated CD-1 mice. *Teratology*, **19**: 49A.

Sucheston, M. E., Hayes, T. G., and Eluma, F. O. (1986). Relationship between ossification and body weight of the CD-1 mouse fetus exposed *in utero* to anticonvulsant drugs. *Teratogen. Carcinogen. Mutagen.*, **6**: 537–546.

Sugrue, S. P. and DeSesso, J. M. (1982). Altered glycosaminoglycan composition of rat forelimb-buds during hydroxyurea teratogenesis: an indication of repair. *Teratology*, **26**: 71–83.

Sulik, K. K. and Dehart, D. B. (1988). Retinoic-acid-induced limb malformations resulting from apical ectodermal ridge cell death. *Teratology*, **37**: 527–537.

Sulik, K. K., Johnson, M. C., Ambrose, L. J. H., and Dorgan, D. (1979). Phenytoin (dilantin)-induced cleft lip and palate in A/J mice: a scanning and transmission electron microscopic study. *Anat. Rec.*, **195**: 243–255.

Sullivan, F. M. and McElhatton, P. R. (1975). Teratogenic activity of the antiepileptic drugs phenobarbitone, phenytoin, and primidone in mice. *Toxicol. Appl. Pharmacol.*, **34**: 271–282.

Sullivan, F. M. and McElhatton, P. R. (1977). A comparison of the teratogenic activity of the antiepileptic drugs carbamazepine, clonazepam, ethosuximide, phenobarbital, phenytoin and primidone in mice. *Toxicol. Appl. Pharmacol.*, **40**: 365–378.

Swartz, W. J. (1980). Response of early chick embryo to busulfan. *Teratology*, **21**: 1–8.

Szabo, K. T. (1970). Teratogenic effect of lithium carbonate in the foetal mouse. *Nature*, **225**: 73–75.

Szabo, K. T. and Brent, R. (1974). Species differences in experimental teratogenesis by tranquilizing agents. *Lancet*, **1**: 565.

Szabo, K. T. and Kang, J. Y. (1969). Comparitive teratogenic studies with various therapeutic agents in mice and rabbits. *Teratology*, **2**: 270.

Szabo, K. T., Miller, C. R., and Scott, G. C. (1974). The effects of methyl-5(6)-butyl-2-benzimidazole carbamate (parbendazole) on reproduction in sheep and other animals. *Cornell Vet.*, **64** (suppl. 4): 41–55.

Tanimura, T. (1961). Developmental disturbances in the offspring induced by administration of mitomycin C to mice during pregnancy. *Acta. Anat.*, **36**: 354.

Tanimura, T. (1972). Effects on macaque embryos of drugs reported or suspected to be teratogenic to humans. *Acta Endocrinol.*, **166** (suppl. 71): 293–308.

Tanimura, T. and Lee, S. (1972). Discussions on the suspected teratogenicity of quinine to humans. *Teratology*, **6**: 122.

Tanimura, T., Owaki, Y., and Nishimura, H. (1967). Effect of administration of thiopental sodium to pregnant mice upon development of their offspring. *Okajimas Fol Anat. Jpn.*, **43**: 219–226.

Taylor, H. M. (1937). Prenatal medication and its relation to the fetal ear. *Surg. Gynecol. Obstet.*, **64**: 542–546.

Tein, I. and MacGregor, D. L. (1985). Possible valproate teratogenicity. *Arch. Neurol.*, **42**: 291–293.

Tellone, C. I., Baldwin, J. K., and Sofia, R. D. (1980). Teratogenic activity in the mouse after oral administration of acetazolamide. *Drug Chem. Toxicol.*, **3**: 83–98.

Theisen, C. T., Fradkin, R., and Wilson, J. G. (1973). Teratogenicity of hydroxyurea in rhesus monkey. *Teratology*, **7**: A29.

Thiersch, J. B. (1952). Therapeutic abortions with a folic acid antagonist, 4-aminopteroylglutamic acid (4-amino P.G.A.) administered by the oral route. *Am. J. Obstet. Gynecol.*, **63**: 1298–1304.

Thiersch, J. B. (1954). Effect of certain 2,4-diamopyrimidine antagonists of folic acid on pregnancy and rat fetus. *Proc. Soc. Exp. Biol. Med.*, **87**: 571–577.

Thiersch, J. B. (1956). The control of reproduction in rats with the aid of antimetabolites, and early experiences with antimetabolites as abortifacient agents in man. *Acta Endocrinol.*, **28** (suppl.): 37–45.

Thiersch, J. B. and Philips, F. S. (1950). Effects of 4-aminopteroylglutamic acid (aminopterin) on early pregnancy (17885). *Soc. Exp. Biol. Med. Proc.*, **74**: 204–208.

Thompson, D. J., Dyke, I. L., Lower, C. E., Molello, J. A., and LeBeau, J. E. (1981). Effects of L-alanosine (NSC-153353) on reproduction and prenatal development in Sprague-Dawley rats. *Toxicologist*, **1**: 28.

Thompson, D. J., Molello, J. A., Strebing, R. J., and Dyke, I. L. (1978). Teratogenicity of adriamycin and daunomycin in the rat and rabbit. *Teratology*, **17**: 151–158.

Thompson, D. J., Warner, S. D., and Robinson, V. B. (1974). Teratology studies on orally administrated chloroform in the rat and rabbit. *Toxicol. Appl. Pharmacol.*, **29**: 348–357.

Toaff, R. and Ravid, R. (1966). Tetracyclines and the teeth. *Lancet*, **2**: 281–282.

Toledo, T. M., Harper, R. C., and Moser, R. H. (1971). Fetal effects during cyclophosphamide and irradiation therapy. *Ann. Intern. Med.*, **74**: 87–91.

Trasler, D. G. (1965). Aspirin-induced cleft lip and other malformations in mice. *Lancet*, **1**: 606–607.

Tuchmann-Duplessis, H. (1984). Drugs and other xenobiotics as teratogens. *Pharmacol. Ther.*, **26**: 273–344.

Tucker, W. (1983). Preclinical toxicology of bupropion: an overview. *J. Clin. Psychiatry*, **44**: 60–62.

Turner, G. and Collins, E. (1975). Fetal effects of regular salicylate ingestion in pregnancy. *Lancet*, **2**: 338–339.

Turner, S., Sucheston, M. E., DePhilip, R. M., and Paulson, R. B. (1989). Teratogenic effects on the neuroepithelium of the CD-1 mouse embryo exposed *in utero* to sodium valproate. *Teratology*, **41**: 421–442.

Ugen, K. E. and Scott, W. J., Jr., (1985). Potentiation of acetazolamide induced ectrodactyly in Wistar rats by vasoactive agents and physical clamping of the uterus. *Teratology*, **31**: 273–278.

Ungvary, G., Tatrai, E., Lorincz, M., and Barcza, G. (1983). Combined embryotoxic action of toluene, a widely used industrial chemical, and acetylsalicylic acid (aspirin). *Teratology*, **27**: 261–269.

U.S. Department of Health and Human Services (1983). Toxoplasmosis. *NIH Publ.*, No. 83–308.

Van Waes, A. and Van de Velde, E. (1969). Safety evaluation of haloperidol in the treatment of hyperemesis gravidarum. *J. Clin. Pharmacol.*, **9**: 224–227.

Vartiainen, E. and Tervila, L. (1970). The use of candeptin for treatment of moniliasis. *Acta Obstet. Gynecol. Scand.*, **2** (suppl.): 21–24.

Vessey, M. P. and Nunn, J. F. (1980). Occupational hazards of anaesthesia (editorial). *Br. Med. J.*, **281**: 696–698.

Vevera, J. and Zatloukal, F. (1964). Pripad vrozenych malformaci zpusobenych pravdepodobne atebrinem, podaranym vranem tehotenstvi. *Cesk. Pediatr.*, 19: 211–212.

Von Kreybig, T. (1965). Die Teratogene wirkung Cyclophosphamide Waarend der Embryonalen Entwicklungsphase bei der Ratte. *Naunyn-Schmeidebergs. Arch. Pharmakol.*, **252**: 173–195.

Vorhees, C. V. (1983). Fetal anticonvulsant syndrome in rats: dose- and period-response relationships of prenatal diphenylhydantoin, trimethadione and phenobarbital exposure on the structural and functional development of the offspring. *J. Pharmacol. Exp. Ther.*, **227**: 274–287.

Vorhees, C. V. (1987). Teratogenicity and developmental toxicity of valproic acid in rats. *Teratology*, **35**: 195–202.

Walford, P. A. (1963). Antibiotics and congenital malformations. *Lancet*, **2**: 298–299.

Walker, B. E. and Patterson, A. (1974). Induction of cleft palate in mice by tranquilizers and barbiturates. *Teratology*, **10**: 159–164.

Wallman, I. S. and Hilton, H. B. (1962). Teeth pigmented by tetracycline. *Lancet*, **1**: 827–829.

Warkany, J. (1981). Teratogenicity of folic acid antagonists. *Cancer Bull.*, **33**: 76–77.

Warkany, J. (1988). Teratology update: lithium. *Teratology*, **38**: 593–597.

Warkany, J., Beaudry, P. H., and Hornstein, S. (1959). Attempted abortion with alminopterin (4-amino-pteroylglutamic acid). Malformations of the child. *Am. J. Dis. Child.*, 97: 274–281.

Warkany, J. and Takacs, E. (1959). Experimental production of congenital malformations in rats by salicylate poisoning. *Am. J. Pathol.*, **35**: 315–320.

Weidman, W. H., Young, H. H., and Zollman, P. E. (1963). The effect of thalidomide on the unborn puppy. *Proc. Staff Meet. Mayo Clin.*, **38**: 518–522.

Weingarten, P. L., Ream, J. R., Jr., and Pappas, A. M. (1971). Teratogenicity of myleran against musculoskeletal tissue in the rat. *Clin. Orthop.*, **75**: 236.

Wharton, R. S., Wilson, A. I., Mazze, R. I., Baden, J. M., and Rice, S. A. (1979). Fetal morphology in mice exposed to halothane. *Anesthesiology*, **51**: 532–537.

Wharton, R. S., Sievenpiper, T. S., and Mazze, R. I. (1980). Developmental toxicity of methoxyflurane in mice. *Anesth. Analg.*, **59**: 421–425.

Wharton, R. S., Mazze, R. I., and Wilson, A. I. (1981). Reproduction and fetal development in mice chronically exposed to enflurane. *Anesthesiology*, **54**: 505–510.

White, T. E., Baggs, R. B., and Miller, R. K. (1986). Cadmium-induced hydrocephalus in the rat fetus following direct fetal injections. *Teratology*, **33**: 65C.

Whittle, B.A. (1976).Pre-clinical teratological studies on sodium valproate (Epilim) and other anticonvulsants. In: *Clinical and Pharmacological Aspects of Sodium Valproate (Epilim) in the Treatment of Epilepsy*. Legg, N. J., Ed., Turnbridge Wells, England, 105–111.

World Health Organization. (1972). Reports on schistosomicidal drugs. *Bol. Ofic. Sanit. Panamer.*, **6**: 82.

Wiger, R., Trygg, B., and Holme, J.A. (1989). Toxic effects of cyclophosphamide in differentiating chicken limb bud cell culture using rat liver 9,000g supernatant or an *in vitro* short-term test for proteratogens. *Teratology*, **40**: 603–613.

Wiley, M. J. (1983). The pathogenesis of retinoic acid-induced vertebral abnormalities in golden Syrian hamster fetuses. *Teratology*, 28: 341–353.

Wiley, M. J., Cauwenbergs, P., and Taylor, I. M. (1983). Effects of retinoic acid on the development of the facial skeleton in hamsters: early changes involving cranial neural crest cells. *Acta Anat.*, **116**: 180–192.

Williams, K. A. B., Scott, J. M., Macfarlane, D. E., Williamson, J. M. W., Elias-Jones, T. F., and Williams, H. (1981). Congenital toxoplasmosis: a prospective survey in the west of Scotland. *J. Infect.*, 3: 219.

Wilson, F. (1962). Congenital defects in the newborn. *Lancet*, **2**: 2

Wilson, J. G. (1964). Teratogenic interaction of chemical agents in the rat. *J. Pharm. Exp. Ther.*, **144**: 429–436.

Wilson, J. G. (1971). Use of rhesus monkeys in teratological studies. *Fed. Proc.*, **30**: 104–109.

Wilson, J. G. (1972). Present status of drugs as teratogens in man. *Teratology*, **7**: 3–16.

Wilson, J. G. (1972). Abnormalities of intrauterine development in non-human primates. *Acta Endrocrinol.*, **166** (suppl. 71): 261–292.

Wilson, J. G. (1977). Embryotoxicity of drugs in man. In: *Handbook of Teratology*. Wilson, J. G. and Fraser, F. C., Eds., Plenum Press, New York, 308–355.

Wilson, J. G., Maren, T. H., Takano, K., and Ellison, A. (1968). Teratogenic action of carbonic anhydrase inhibitors in the rat. *Teratology*, **1**: 51–69.

Wilson, J. G., Ritter, E. J., Scott, W. J., and Fradkin, R. (1977). Comparative distribution and embryotoxicity of acetylsalicylic acid in pregnant rats and rhesus monkeys. *Toxicol. Appl. Pharmacol.*, **41**: 67–68.

Woo, D. C., McClain, R. M., and Hoar, R. M. (1978). Potentiation of methotrexate embryolethality by aspirin in rats. *Teratology*, **17**: 37–42. (1978).

Wotring, G. E. and Beaudoin, A. R. (1980). A study of cartilaginous fusions, DNA synthesis, and protein synthesis in embryonic rat limbs after injection of aminothiadiazole. *Teratology*, **21**: 381–396.

Wray, S. D., Hassell, T. M., Phillips, C., and Johnston, C. M. (1982). Preliminary study of the effects of carbamazepine in congenital orofacial defects in offspring of A/J mice. *Epilepsia*, **23**: 101–110.

Wright, H. N. (1967). Chronic toxicity studies of analgesic and antipyretic drugs and congeners. *Toxicol. Appl. Pharmacol.*, **11**: 280–292.

Yanoff, M., Allman, M. I., and Fine, B. S. (1982). Congenital herpes simplex virus, type 2, bilateral endophthalmitis. *Metab. Pediatr. Syst. Ophthalmol.*, **6**: 287.

Yasuda, Y. (1977). Digital anomalies of mouse limbs induced by treatment with urethan *in vitro*. *Teratology*, **15**: 89–96.

Yasuda, Y., Okamoto, M., Konishi, H., Matsuo, T., Kihara, T., and Tanimura, T. (1986). Developmental anomalies induced by all-trans retinoic acid in fetal mice. I. Macroscopic findings. *Teratology*, 34: 37–49.

Yen, P.K.-J. and Shaw, J.H. (1972). Preliminary study of inhibitory effects of tetracyclines on membraneous bone growth in rhesus monkeys. *J. Dent. Res.*, **51**: 1651–1657.

Yip, J. E., Kokich, V. G., and Shepard, T. H. (1980). The effect of high doses of retinoic acid on prenatal craniofacial development in *Macaca nemestrina*. *Teratology*, **21**: 29–38.

Yu, J. F., Yang, Y. S., Wang, W. Y., Xiong, G. X., and Chen, M. S. (1988). Mutagenicity and teratogenicity of chlorpromazine and scopolamine. *Chin. Med. J.*, **101**: 339–345.

Yukioka, K., Yamamoto, Y., Tonoike, H., Inaba, T., Miyoshi, T., and Akena, G. (1959). Experimental studies on the effect of D-hypervitaminosis on rat fetuses. *J. Osaka City Med. Cent.*, **8**: 34–38.

Zackai, E. H., Mellman, W. J., Neiderer, B., and Hanson, J. W. (1975). The fetal trimethadione syndrome. *J. Pediatr.*, **87**: 280–284.

Zagon, I. S. and McLaughlin, P. J. (1977). Effects of chronic morphine administration in the rat. *Pharmacology*, **15**: 302–310.

Zbinden, G. R. E., Bagdon, R. E., Keith, E. F., Phillips, R. D., and Randall, L. O. (1961). Experimental and clinical toxicology of chlordiazepoxide. *Toxicol. Appl. Pharmacol.*, **3**: 619–637.

Zengel, A. L., Keith, D. A., and Tassinari, M. S. (1989). Prenatal exposure to phenytoin and its effect on postnatal growth and craniofacial proportion in the rat. *J. Craniofacial Genet. Dev. Biol.*, **9**: 147–160.

Zolcinski, A., Heimroth, T., and Ujec, M. (1966). Quinine as the cause of dysplasia of the fetus. *Zentralbl. Gynaekol.*, 88: 99–104.

9

Bone and Individual Aging

J. CASTANET, H. FRANCILLON-VIEILLOT, F. J. MEUNIER, and A. DE RICQLES

URA CNRS 1137
Equipe de Recherche "Formations squelettiques"
Laboratoire d'Anatomie Comparée
Université Paris 7
Paris, France

Introduction

Time and its measurement have long attracted the interest of humanity. Aging individuals, i.e., determining the time elapsed between birth and a moment of life (between birth and death, time corresponds to longevity) is a necessity in many fields of research involving biological systems and organisms.

To date several methods have been proposed to assess the age of wild animals. The best would be to follow wild animals in nature from birth by the mark-release-recapture technique (e.g., Durham and Benett, 1963) but such a practice is, of course, very labor intensive, requiring a very long time to yield results. In many cases when biotopes are not easily accessible (e.g., swamps, tropical rivers), recapture is highly impractical or unlikely. Moreover, such a method cannot be used with fossil material.

Many other methods use change during life of various morphometric data such as size frequencies (Petersen, 1892; Tanaka, 1956), lens weight (Teska and Pinder, 1986), tooth grinding (Bourlière and Spitz, 1975; Brothwell, 1989), testis lobation (Humphrey, 1922; Lofts, 1984), isotopic ratio, and also the progressive changes of bone and other hard tissue structures. The latter will be considered in the second part of this chapter. However, these methods are more or less accurate and generally allow, at best, the establishment of broad and overlapping age groups or even only the separation of juveniles from adults. Moreover, such methods require the use of specimens of known ages to establish a reference sample to be compared with the wild animals to be aged. Accordingly, as noted by Halliday and Verrell (1988) these methods often "assume what they set out to demonstrate" i.e., age and size are statistically related whatever the population or individual studied. Morphometric criteria imply, in order to be accurate, a great deal of nonvariability or standardization of the biological objects (organisms, populations) dealt with.

Another method available for individual aging uses the natural marks recorded in hard tissues — chiefly the skeleton — of growing animals (Clerc, 1927; Peabody, 1961; Klevezal and Kleinenberg, 1967; Castanet et al., 1977). If these marks are the expression of a rhythm of known periodicity, it is formally clear that they could be used as a chronological tool providing temporal data. Such a method which can deal with invertebrate as well as vertebrate hard tissues, whether they are mineralized (shells, bones, teeth) or not (epidermal scutes, horns), can be given the general name of *sclerochronology* (Jepsen, 1964). When it involves only mineralized skeletal tissues the term *skeletochronology* (Castanet et al., 1977) is currently used. However, more specific terms according to the element or tissues used have been proposed: scalimetry and otolithometry are very old terms used respectively for dermal scales and otoliths of bony fishes (see Meunier, 1988). Osteochronology was proposed for vertebrate bones only (Boet and Le Louarn, 1985). According to the topic of this multivolume series, we will mostly concentrate on the bony tissues of the vertebrates as the main criterion used for individual aging.

In principle, skeletochronology is fundamentally different from technique using morphometric data. Since growth marks (GM) are attuned to an external rhythm their deposition may be largely independent of specific, populational, or individual variations. In that sense, the method does not need a reference system for each study as do morphometric methods and the count of GM since they are demonstrated as periodical structures among many vertebrates, can directly provide, at least in theory, the individual age.

GM have long been recognized in vertebrate bones: e.g., Hederström, 1759, Clerc, 1927, in osteichthyes; Harris, 1927, in mammals; Mattox, 1935, in reptiles: Senning, 1940, in amphibians. However, as the chronological significance of these marks remained largely unknown until recently, their practical use was empirical and contested by many authors. Today, it has been experimentally demonstrated in several species belonging to different vertebrates classes that if these bone marks are basically related to endogenous rhythms, they are mainly synchronized and reinforced by environmental cycles (seasonality). Such a point of view can explain the presence of growth marks in homeothermic animals, as well as among poekilothermic vertebrates living under more or less constant climatic conditions. However, several recent observations show that growth marks are sharpest in organisms living under a strong seasonality (e.g., Esteban-Ruiz, 1990; Castanet and Baez, 1991). Whatever these facts the practical use of bone GM for aging individuals is now largely refined. Moreover, accurate comparative histological studies of bone growth within and between species and populations now appear to be able to provide much additional data; bone skeletochronology documents not only the individual age or longevity but also data such as time of sexual maturity, bone growth rate and morphogenesis, sexual and interpopulational dimorphism, cycles of activity and of reproduction. Moreover, bone growth analysis can provide information about environmental conditions and period of death (e.g., Casteel, 1972, 1976). Therefore, when functionally interpreted, bone tissue appears to be a powerful chronological tool in such diverse fields of research as populations biology, evolutionary mechanics, taxonomy, climatology, and seasonality for both extant and extinct animals.

Skeletochronology

Bone Growth Marks (GM): Fundamental Aspects

Localization

It is now well established that the presence of GM in the skeleton of vertebrates is a general phenomenon. These marks are fundamentally recorded in every part of the primary periosteal compacta of bone tissue, mostly in the lamellar-zonal patterns of bone tissues, less often in the fibrolamellar complex (Ricqlès, 1975). This is because the dense vascularization which characterizes this last group of tissues makes cyclical GM less obvious (e.g., Ricqlès, 1983). When bone GM are absent it is often the consequence of bone remodeling which secondarily removes the earlier primary bone.

According to the growth dynamics of each skeletal element, bone GM can be more or less distinct. In practice one will select the bone with the highest number of marks, with the clearest marks and where their removal by remodeling will be as small as possible.

According to bone morphogenesis and morphology, there are two main ways to observe GM: either directly at the surface of whole elements as in flat bones (bone *in toto*) or inside them, by using sections, as in long bones.

Growth Marks on Bone In Toto.   GM can appear at the surface of more or less compact and bulky bones, observed under reflected light as in the articular faces of vertebrae zygapophyses in amphibians (Willis, 1954) or reptiles (Peabody, 1958, 1961; Warren, 1963; Castanet, 1974; Minakami, 1979), or on the opercular bones, cleithra, or vertebral centra in fishes (see Table 1 in Meunier, 1988). When bones or parts of them are small, flat, thin, and consequently more or less translucent, GM can also be observed by reflected or transmitted light (Fig. 1). Immersion in fluids (water, glycerol, xylol, and various other organic fluids) increases bone transparency or the contrast between different GM. In bony fishes, GM are easily counted on flat bones such as the opercular (e.g., Blake and Blake, 1978; Bardach, 1955; Fagade, 1974; Lecomte *et al.*, 1986) and cleithrum (Casselman, 1974, 1990) using transmitted light. The parasphenoid (Senning, 1940) and the pterygoid (Schroeder and Baskett, 1968; Bruneau and Magnin, 1980) were successfully used for aging amphibians. Among reptiles, snakes especially exhibit bones which are flattened enough to be aged by external observation. Good results were obtained with the ectopterygoid (Bryuzgin, 1939; Petter-Rousseau, 1953) and the supra-angular (Fig. 1) (Saint-Girons, 1965; Castanet, 1974; Nishimura, 1990) but many flat bones of the skull also exhibit GM. In birds or mammals there are, to our knowledge, no observations of GM on bones *in toto* if one excepts Harris's papers (1927, 1931) describing such marks on radiograms of human long bones. Thus, complementary studies remain to be done in this area.

Growth Marks on Bone Sections.   The GM present at the surface of bone always appear in bone sections as local histological variations. These marks can be observed by reflected light on polished surfaces of thick cross sections (e.g., Peabody, 1961; Deelder and Willemse, 1973) but more accurately by transmitted ordinary and/or polarized light through thin sections (10 to 100 μm in thickness) of undemineralized fresh or fossil bones. However, for extant animals, demineralized stained sections frequently provide the best results (Fig. 2).

Among fishes, transverse sections of the lepidotrichia or the spiny fin rays (Figs. 3 and 4) — especially in the Siluroids — are currently used for age determination (Meunier *et al.*, 1979; Beamish, 1981; Lecomte *et al.*, 1985, 1986 and Table 1 in Meunier, 1988). In amphibians and reptiles with poorly vascularized bones, the shaft diaphyses of long bones of the limbs provide the best results for individual aging, although some attempts have been made to use sections of flat bones of the skull in tortoises (Suzuki, 1963)

Table 1.

Structure and Composition of the Skeletal Growth Marks

OBSERVATION TECHNIC	ZONE	ANNULUS	LAG
In toto BONES natural light	- opaque - wide	- translucent - narrow	discontinuity
HISTOLOGICAL SLIDES Ordinary light	- high cellular density - numerous and long cellular extensions	- low cellular density - sparser and shorter cytoplasmic extensions	discontinuity
Polarized light	- isotropic - woven bone, sometimes parallel fibered bone	- anisotropic - lamellar bone, sometimes parallel fibered bone	- very birefringent narrow lines (10 to 15 µm)
Fibers' specific dyes	idem polarized light	idem polarized light	more or less chromophilic
MET	idem polarized light	idem polarized light	more or less electron-lucent (1 to 3 µm)
Hematoxylin dye	lightly chromophilic	slightly more hematoxylinophilic	highly hematoxylinophilic
Toluidin blue	metachromatic	orthochromatic	more or less metachromatic
Microradiography	more or less equally mineralized		lightly hypermineralized

and crocodilians (Buffrénil, 1980) as well. For the limbless species, such as snakes, no sections of bones provide very useful GM (Castanet, 1974), owing to their internal resorption.

Compact cortical bone tissues of long bone shafts in mammals and birds, as well as in marine turtles, can hardly be used for skeletochronology, owing

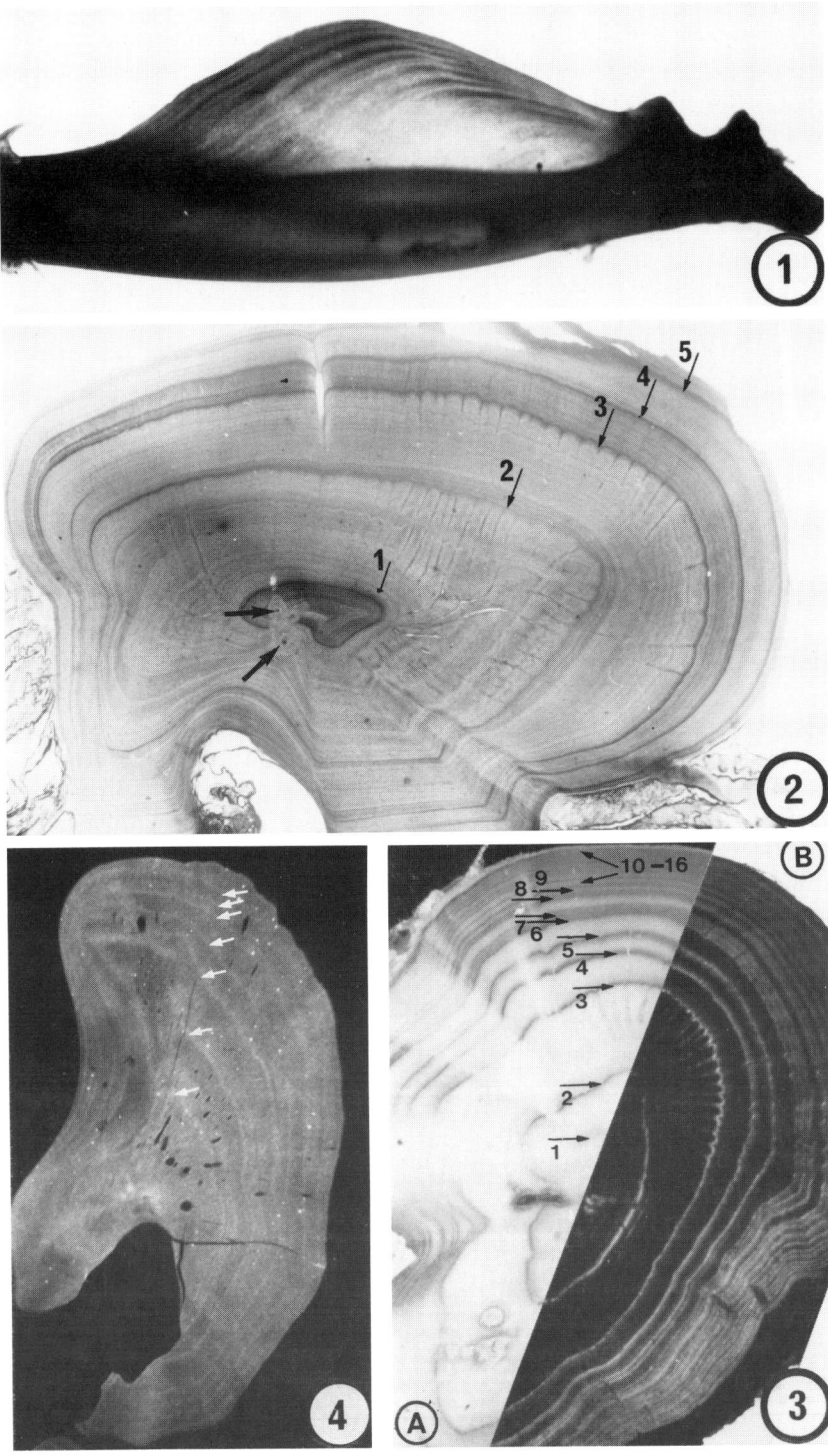

either to their high initial vascularization or to a high remodeling rate later on (Figs. 5 and 6). However, in some mammals, GM are clear and accurate for aging as observed on transverse sections of the dentary (Fig. 12) (lower jaw) (Klevezal and Kleinenberg, 1967; Pascal and Castanet, 1978; Buffrénil, 1982). Among mammals, rest lines in teeth tissues are perhaps more widely used. Dentine may be used for some terrestrial and marine carnivorous mammals (e.g., Perrin and Myrick, 1980) but cementum appears to be the most useful tissue in many other species (e.g., Klevezal and Kleinenberg, 1967; Morris, 1972; Miller, 1974; Grue and Jensen, 1979) including man (e.g., Charles *et al.*, 1986; Condon *et al.*, 1986; Grosskopf, 1990). Only a few studies deal with skeletochronology in birds (Van Soest and Van Utrecht, 1971; Klevezal, 1972; Lewis, 1979; Nelson and Bookhout, 1980; Koubek and Hrabe, 1984) and until now, as far as we know, no bones have been found to give accurate results. However, Koubek and Hrabe (1984) claimed to be able to age the pheasant, *Phasianus colchicus*, counting GM in outer cortical bone of the phalanges.

Terminology and Organization

Since Amprino (1947), organization of the "second order" i.e., histological structures of primary (periosteal) compact bone, is known to be the expression of the rate of local osteogenesis (see Chapter 1, Volume 3 in this series). For the present purposes, we will keep in mind that three main categories of fibrillar organization of bone matrix are classically recognized: (1) woven bone matrix associated with a high rate of osteogenesis, (2) lamellar bone matrix associated with a low rate of osteogenesis, and (3) parallel-fibered bone matrix linked to an intermediary rate of bone deposition. Each category can gradually merge into the other.

Three categories of GM can be recognized: opaque layers (zones), translucent layers (*annuli*), and lines of arrested growth (LAG) (Fig. 5).

Figs. 1. through 4. *Boiga irregularis* (Reptilia, Serpentes, Colubridae). Growth marks on the posterior part of the mandible observed with transmitted light (Fig. 1). Large opaque zones which alternate with narrow translucent annuli are as obvious on this tropical species as on snakes living under temperate climates. (× 12). Preparation from P. Collins.) *Cyprinus carpio* (Pisces, Teleostei, Cyprinidae). Cross-section of a dorsal spiny ray (Ehrlich's hematoxylin) showing five LAG (Fig. 2). The two last LAG being closer can be interpreted as the result of the sexual maturation in the 4th year of life. Arrows indicate two secondary osteones. (× 25.) *Cyprinus carpio* (Pisces, Teleostei, Cyprinidae). Cross-section (ground section) of a dorsal spiny ray showing 16 annuli (Fig. 3). Note the tightening of the annuli after the fourth (indicating the sexual maturity) and then after the tenth with slowing down of growth in the aged carp. (A) reflected light with black ground; (B) transmitted light. (× 12.) *Cyprinus carpio* (Pisces, Teleostei, Cyprinidae). Microradiography of cross-section of a dorsal spiny ray showing hypermineralized annuli (arrows) (Fig. 4). Note the scarceness of vascular canals. (× 11.)

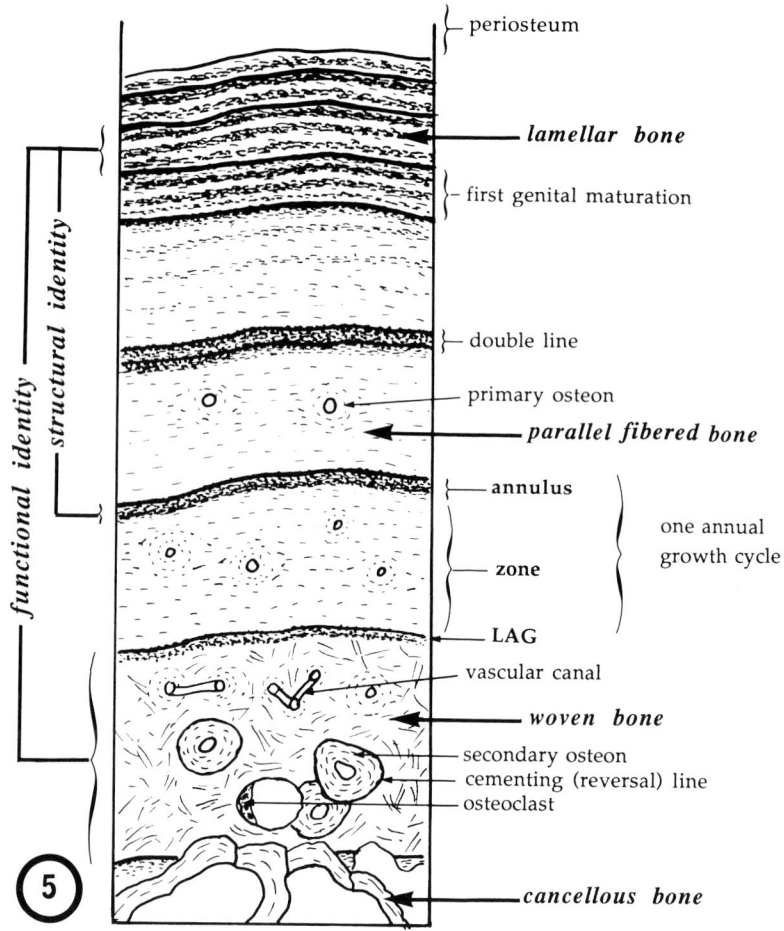

Fig. 5. Diagram of the general organization of bone tissue: cross-section in the cortex of a long bone at the diaphysis level. For detailed comments, see text.

Opaque Layers (Fast-Growing Layers). First termed "zones" by Peabody (1961), these layers correspond to periods of general active osteogenesis. Thus, they are the widest marks (Figs. 1 and 3). Generally, in fast-growing young individuals, opaque layers are made of woven fibered bone with numerous roundish osteocytic lacunae randomly distributed. In adults or locally in a bone when general body growth decreases, the structure of zones changes to parallel-fibered bone matrix or, occasionally to lamellar bone matrix with more flattened, less numerous cell lacunae. Due to their structure, zones are more opaque than other marks. Thus, they appear dark in transmitted light and white in reflected light.

Annuli *(Slow-Growing Layers) (Figs. 1 and 3)*. This name was also pro-posed by Peabody (1961) for bone (it was used earlier with another signif-icance in otholitometry). Because *annuli* correspond to periods of slow osteo-genesis they are always narrower than adjacent zones. Generally being made of lamellar bone matrix, they appear more translucent than the zones: white in transmitted light and opaque in reflected light.

LAG. Lines of arrested growth (rest lines; in French: lignes d'arrêt de croissance: LAC), belong to the "cementing lines" family and are function-ally defined as rest lines (e.g., Castanet, 1981 and Chapter 1, Volume 3). These structures depict temporary arrests of local osteogenesis (about a few weeks, Smirina *et al.*, 1986). They always have a very low thickness (some micrometers). Their histological characteristics are largely described in Chapter 1, Volume 3 in this series. More translucent than other marks, LAG are also the most refringent (Fig. 7) and appear as the brightest bone structures under polarized light. They are also the most chromophilic with dyes such as hematoxylin (e.g., Figs. 2, 8, and 12) and are generally hyper-mineralized (Fig. 4). LAG can appear inside *annuli* or (most often) bordering them, or alone, directly alternating with the zones. Table 1 gives more details about the structures and the composition of the bone growth marks.

Periodicity: Experimental Validation of Skeletochronology

Skeletochronology is based on the observation that skeletal (and overall) growth is often a periodical phenomenon. Together, a zone and an *annulus/* LAG correspond to one complete growth cycle. In many studies of temperate species authors assume that a set of growth marks (e.g., zone + annulus or/and LAG) is laid down each year, and, therefore, that chronological age is accurately reflected by the number of *annuli* or LAG. This hypothesis has to be tested for each ecological study, especially when the local biology of the species is unknown. There are several experimental approaches available to validate skeletochronology (animals of known age, mark-release-recapture and fluorescent labeling) which can be associated with one other, and which will now be discussed.

Known Age Animals. Validity of age estimation by skeletochronology was first checked by Schroeder and Baskett (1968) on 42 bullfrogs (*Rana cates-beiana*) of known age. Transformed frogs of the year and transforming tad-poles were collected and finger and toe clipped for later identification. They were confined in pens for several years. After death, the pterygoids were removed and examined with transmitted light. The posterior part of the bones showed narrow opaque marks alternating with broad translucent bands. Schroeder and Baskett (1968) hypothesized that the narrow marks resulted from periods of arrested growth during winter and that the broad

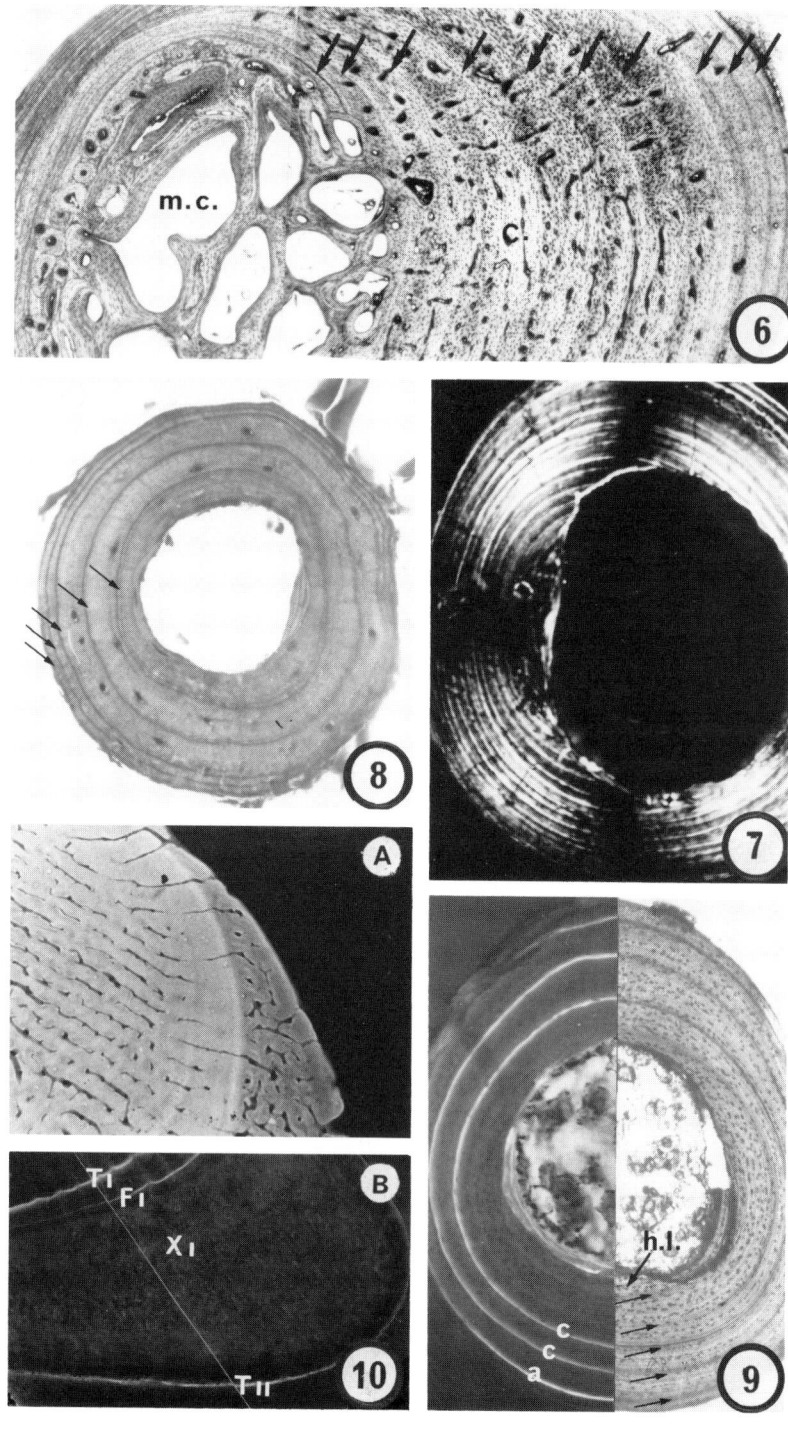

translucent bands represented growth during more favorable periods. Indeed, the position of the "GM" varied with date of capture. Pterygoid bones from frogs captured at the beginning of the growing season (May) had the past winter's mark at the tip. As the growing season progressed, these marks progressively drifted farther from the bone tip. Their assumption about the identity of GM was confirmed by the known-age animals. For instance, frogs with no GM belonged to the age group which had not overwintered since metamorphosis, and frogs with two GM belonged to the age group which had lived through two winters postmetamorphosis. Thus, the technique of age determination by counting GM appeared satisfactory for estimating the age of bullfrogs through the 5th year after metamorphosis.

Similarly, from a study of the cross-sections of the diaphyses of two lizards (*Lacerta lepida*) of known age, respectively 2 and 10 years, Castanet (1978) showed qualitatively that they exhibit an alternation of LAG which were formed each year during the cold season.

Mark-Release-Recapture. Using a mark-release-recapture (MRR) approach, the difference between the number of GM observed in a recaptured individual and the number of GM observed in that individual at the time of first capture was expected to equal the number of winters elapsed between

---

Figs. 6. through 10. *Testudo hermanni* (Reptilia, Chelonia, Testudinae) (Fig. 6). Cross-section of middiaphyseal region of femur stained by Ehrlich's hematoxylin. Evolution of the bone tissue during bone growth in thickness (see Figs. 1 and 3 for comparison). At least ten annual growth cycles can be observed on this bone (arrows). m.c.: medullary cavity with bone trabeculae and secondary osteons. c.: cortex with blood canals and some primary osteons. (× 27.) *Gallotia goliath* (Reptilia, Squamata, Lacertidae) (Fig. 7). Fossil species (Holocene) from Canary Islands. Cross-section (ground section) of middiaphyseal region of femur observed under polarized light. About 14 to 16 clear lines of arrest growth can be counted. (× 21.) *Desmognathus ochrophaeus* (Amphibia, Caudata, Plethodontidae) (Fig. 8). Cross-section of middiaphyseal region of femur stained by Ehrlich's hematoxylin. This bone cortex similar to those of many other caudata is avascular and made of pseudolamellar bone matrix. Scarce and randomly distributed cells are present. 5 LAG (arrows) are evident in this specimen. (× 90.) *Lacerta viridis* (Reptilia, Squamata, Lacertidae) (Fig. 9). Cross-section of middiaphyseal region of femur. This specimen, bred in semi-captivity, was labeled for 3 successive years at the beginning of spring with fluorochrome (c = calcein; a = alizarine). Left: undemineralized slide showing fluorescent labels. Right: same slide after demineralization showing hematoxylinophilic LAG. The situation of experimental and natural marks clearly indicates that LAG are annual and correspond to the winter for this species. 5 LAG (arrows) + hatching line (hl) can be observed on this specimen which consequently was 5 years old. (× 45.) *Hoplosternum littorale* (Pisces, Teleostei, Callichthyidae) (Fig. 10). Cross-section (ground section) in a pectoral spiny ray of a male, showing variations of the vascularization of bone. The fish has been regularly labeled four times with three fluorochromes (2-month period between injections). (T = tetracycline; C = calcein; X = xylenol orange). The deposition rate of bone is about 1 to 3 μm/d between T1 and F1 for the poorly vascularized bone and 23 μm/d for the hypervascularized bone (see Boujard and Meunier, 1991). (A) Microradiography; (B) Fluorescent microscope. (× 40.)

initial capture and recapture. Herewith are some examples in amphibians and reptiles.

Hemelaar and Van Gelder (1980) observed cross-section of toes of the common toad (*Bufo bufo*). From 1975 to 1978, adult toads were caught at spawning sites, marked by toe-clipping and released. Many of the toads were caught in 3 (and some in 4) successive years. Hemelaar and Van Gelder (1980) selected toes clipped in several years from the same toads; a total of 89 toads were available. Cross-section of toes showed broad growth rings separated from each other by LAG. The results of the analysis of all cross-sections was that more than 90% of the recaptured toads showed an increase in the number of growth rings that equaled the difference in years between capture and recapture. These data provide strong evidence that in adult *B. bufo* of the populations studied, one growth ring is formed each year.

Similarly, Bruneau and Magnin (1980) on the pterygoids of bullfrogs and Gibbons and McCarthy (1983) on cross-sections of phalanges, showed that the increase in the number of visible GM exactly reflected the number of years lived by the animals. Similar results were obtained by Kalb and Zug (1990) in a population of *B. americanus* living in a suburban park in northern Virginia.

The development of the number of LAG was also followed by Caetano (1988) for 3 years on the urodeles *Triturus marmoratus* and *T. boscai* kept in captivity under conditions similar to their natural habitat. She showed an addition of one LAG per year in the phalanges of *T. marmoratus* and in the humerus of *T. boscai*.

As far as we know, only two studies have used natural populations of reptiles to determine if a constant number of LAG (e.g., one LAG) is formed per year and in both studies, the results are positive. Warren (1963) obtained four known-age snakes using MRR techiques exhibiting the expected number of GM. Pilorge and Castanet (1981) conducted a thorough study on the lizard *Lacerta vivipara* using simultaneously size-frequency, MRR, and skeletochronology which concurred with each other.

Fluorescent Labeling.   Experimental studies using vital fluorescent labeling of bones, as performed by several authors, is the best experimental approach for age validation, especially if associated with release-recapture. Fluorochromes are incorporated into skeletal tissues at the site of active mineralization where they may be later detected by fluorescent microscopy (Milch *et al.* 1957; Olerud and Lorenzi, 1970; Rahn and Perren, 1971; Suzuki and Mathews, 1966; Boivin and Meunier, 1978). Using several injections of fluorochromes at different times of the year, it is possible to compare the positions of the fluorescent lines and of the various GM, especially hematoxylinophilic lines and *annuli* and so to state precisely the time of GM formation within the year (Figs. 9 and 10).

One of the first experimental studies with fluorescent labeling in lower tetrapods was conducted by Smirina (1972). She injected tetracycline in 1968 to 50 frogs (*Rana temporaria*), then alizarin in 7 frogs recaptured in 1969. Two years later Smirina found 4 frogs with the 1969 mark and showed that 1 cementing line appears each year. Similar demonstrations of the annual deposition of LAG were obtained with another anuran: *R. esculenta* by Francillon and Castanet (1985) and with some urodeles *Triturus cristatus* (Francillon, 1979) *Notophtalmus viridescens, Desmognathus ochrophaeus* (Kazmer, 1986), and *T. marmoratus* (Caetano and Castanet, 1987).

Among reptiles, similar results were obtained in *Lacerta viridis* (Fig. 9) by Castanet (1985), and some experimental data were also published by Castanet and Naulleau (1985) about the annual periodicity of skeletal GM among snakes (*Vipera aspis*) living in their natural environment.

Although such experimental studies are rarer in fishes when age is estimated with bone support (Casselman, 1974; Beamish and McFarlane, 1983; Cass and Beamish, 1983), fluorescent labeling has also been used to validate age estimations. For example, Meunier and Pascal (1981) raised carps for 4 years and showed that LAG appeared in fin rays during each winter. They concluded that counting of LAG is reliable for age determination. The accuracy of this technique in fishes was also emphasized by Beamish and McFarlane (1983) and Casselman (1987). Such techniques have also been used to validate age estimations in sharks and rays, the labeling tissue being calcified cartilage (Holden and Vince, 1973; Beamish and McFarlane, 1983; Smith, 1984).

Functional Significance and Determinism of Growth Marks

According to the functional categories of bone matrix and their organization, GM can be defined as the histological expression of any temporary time-dependent variation in bone growth rate. Thus, GM determinism can be understood through the determinism of growth rate variations. Two main aspects can be dealt with: (1) the formation of the marks and their chronology and (2) the determinism of their spatial organization in bone.

Growth Mark Formation and Chronology. External and internal rhythms. Periodical GM — For poikilothermic species living in temperate climates seasonality is the main factor that directly provides the yearly cyclical growth rhythm of the organism as recorded in its skeleton. Moreover, it has been suggested that many biological rhythms, e.g., reproductive cycle, could also induce cyclical deposition in bone as LAG. However, as noted above, GM also appear in homeothermic animals and in poikilotherms living in more or less constant conditions throughout the year (e.g., Castanet and Gasc, 1986). In these cases, GM are less obviously expressed in bone than for an animal submitted to contrasted seasonality but such observations are nevertheless relevant to whether an internal endogenous growth rhythm is present. Briefly, the current opinion is that bone growth variations and associated GM are ultimately caused by an internal (genetically based) rhythm which under natural conditions becomes synchronized with, and reinforced by, the seasonal cycles (Castanet, 1985, 1986–1987; Castanet and Naulleau, 1985) even if these cycles have a low amplitude (Meunier *et al.*, 1979).

Nonperiodical GM. — Noncyclical events can affect the growth of the organism and generate GM. Hatching (Figs. 9 and 13) (Smirina, 1974; Castanet, 1978, 1985; Lecomte *et al.*, 1985) or metamorphosis (Hemelaar, 1985) which correspond to strong physiological stresses induce LAG. Abnormal climatic variations, diseases, or individual starvation periods can also induce GM occasionally (Storey, 1958) although, in practice, the origin of such occasional (= supplementary) marks is not always easy to understand. Moreover they are difficult to identify because all GM have the same structure, with consequences for the reliability of the estimated age (see above.).

Determinism of the Structure and Spatial Organization of Growth Marks. The external periodic or nonperiodic phenomena which lead to bone growth variations interact with general individual growth processes and locally with those of the different skeletal elements. According to bone morphogenesis, the histological structure and the spatial aspect of GM change from place to place in the same bone and between different bones of the same individual (Fig. 5). Similarly, according to the general evolution of the growth rate throughout life, the structure of GM and their sequence will change from birth to death. Until sexual maturity, when body growth rate is high, annuli or LAG are well separated by wide zones of fast-growing tissues. They will become closer and closer during adulthood and very close to each other with aging (Figs. 2 and 3). Of course, when skeletal growth definitively stops, no more GM are recorded locally. This has practical consequences for age determination if growth stops relatively early during life. Finally, individual and interpopulational skeletal growth variations also lead to differences in the histological expression and spatial organization of bone GM (e.g., Castanet et Naulleau, 1985; Zug *et al.*, 1986; Esteban-Ruiz, 1990; Castanet and Baez, 1991).

Table 2 shows the possible interpretation of periodical GM formation, structural evolution, and spatial organization. Table 3 summarizes the determinism of growth rate variations and their consequences on the skeleton.

Practical Use of Skeletal Growth Marks for Aging Individuals

General

In order to apply skeletochronological methodology to a given species it is necessary to develop an optimal strategy to reduce mistakes and dead

Table 2.
Interpretation of the GM Formation

	HIGH METABOLISM PERIOD (SPRING-SUMMER) ZONES young——adult——old		SLOW METABOLISM PERIOD (WINTER) ANNULI - LAG young——adult——old			VERY SLOW METABOLISM PERIOD (WINTER)
FAST GROWING BONE AND BONY AREAS — Flat bones in their faster growth axis	woven bone	parallel fibered bone	parallel fibered bone		lamellar bone	LAG
INTERMEDIARY GROWING BONE AND BONY AREAS - Thickening of many long bones - Flat bones: transitory regions between fast and slow growing axis	woven bone	parallel fibered bone	Annulus with lamellar bone	LAG	LAG	LAG
SLOW GROWING BONE AND BONY AREAS - Flat bones in their slower growing axis - Thickening of some cylindral bones (ribs)	parallel fibered bone	lamellar bone	LAG	LAG	LAG	LAG

Table 3.
Determination of Formation and Spatiotemporal Organization of the Skeletal Growth Marks

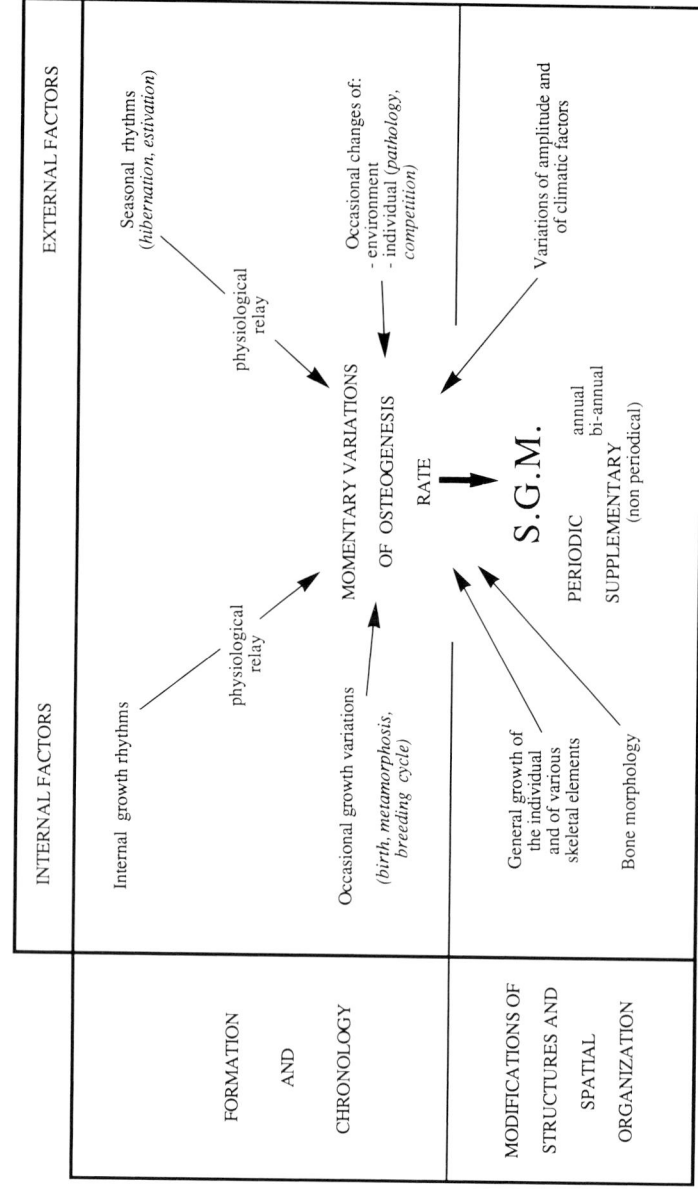

ends, especially when the biology of the species to be studied is little known
or even unknown. In such cases there are no preestablished recipes but
some reasoned and logical steps can yield profitable results for a study of
aging. The technical approach must be chosen according to the scientific
aim and to the available material. Here it is necessary to remember that for
the osteichthyes, beside various bones, the scientist has other supporting
organs available (scales and otoliths) for individual aging. In the same way,
for various mammals tooth cementum or dentine can also be used advan-
tageously for individual aging. These alternatives to bone must be considered
in choosing the technical approach.

In a given species, all bones do not have the same practical value because
the external cycles that modulate animal growth can be recorded quite
differently as GM in the bone tissues, depending on local specific conditions
of growth. Among two relatively close species useful GM can be recorded
by anatomically different nonhomologous bones. Therefore, if one can generally propose specific bones for skeletochronological studies in selected
species, according to the practice of former authors, in the case of taxa never
studied before it is necessary to start by an exploratory screening of the
various skeletal elements. Then the most informative skeletal elements can
be selected for further studies, taking into account the number and consist-
ency of GM and such criteria as the difficulties of preparing the material,
time and economical constraints, and sample size.

Fixation of the material is generally simple because the histological information is recorded in the extracellular mineralized matrices which are much
more forgiving than cells regarding fixation requirements. Frequently, the
work is performed directly on dry bones. Alcohol or congelated preservation
are also appropriate. It is generally not advisable to use acid fixatives
because their decalcifying action can reduce histological information and
preclude the following technical steps. For *in toto* observation, flat bones are
cleaned with hypochlorite, KOH, or, best, digestive enzymes (trypsin, pep-
sin . . .).

Generally the aim of the technical preparation is to enhance the optical
contrast which results from the different physical properties of the GM to
light. Thin sections performed according to petrographic techniques are at
the basis of most skeletochronological works, especially those dealing with
fossil material. However, to show the LAG, histological staining (Ehrlich or
Delafield hematoxylin, for instance) after previous decalcification must be
performed on sections obtained with a freeze microtome (or in case of
nonavailability with the standard paraffin microtome). A survey of bone
tissue with the classical histological techniques will bring much data on, for
example, matrices and cement lines, which will yield additional information
on the structural support of the GM.

As for scalimetry and otolithometry, objective study of the GM must be
preferably performed by at least two observers and requires three steps,
especially in the case of new material (Fig. 11).

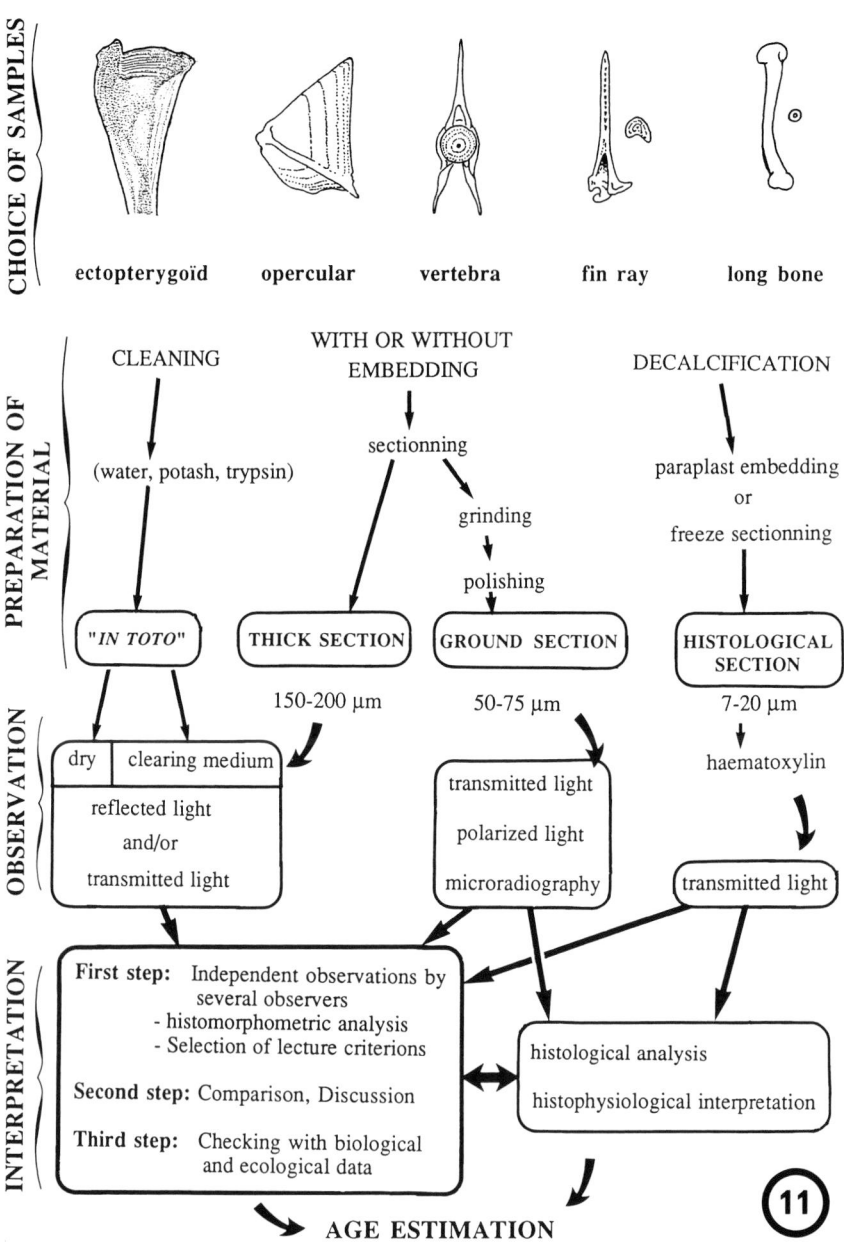

Fig. 11. Diagram summing up the successive steps for age estimation in the vertebrates. See text for more details and the various techniques.

First step. Each observer "reads" alone the preparations, without any knowledge about the biological and ecological data concerning the animals and the date of their capture. This "blind analysis" is necessary to build up an objective analysis of the histological sections or of the bones *in toto* and to decipher the possible significance of cyclical GM and various informative histological characteristics. Such details as "zones", *annuli*, LAG, relative width of each growth zone, their number, the distance between the last *annulus* (or the last LAG), and the margin of the studied skeletal element are especially noteworthy. These data, as histomorphogenetical parameters, provide clues to interpret both temporal and spatial aspects of growth dynamics. A scenario of the local bone growth can thus be attempted. At the end of this step each observer can thus propose a number of growth cycles or even an absolute aging.

Second step. The observers compare their results and, if necessary, study the preparations again in order to match their observations and interpretation. Moreover, they try to understand the reasons of the disagreements — if any — resulting from the first step.

Third step. This includes a comparison of the preliminary skeletochronological results obtained after the two first steps with the various biological parameters of the animals (length, weight, sex . . .) and with all the data available about capture, the physical and/or climatic parameters, etc. This allows a control of the coherence of all the data with the proposed absolute age. At this stage various fine details recorded in the bony tissues will play an important role: osteogenesis rates in the bone, development of vascularization, types of bony tissues, etc., and will start to make sense in the overall interpretation of the animal's growth pattern.

This three-step methodology allows the construction of a growth scenario for the population studied and of some hypotheses on the biology of the animals, especially about growth. If the results look inconsistent (number of *annuli* far too high or too low regarding the size of a given individual for example) the study of the material is started again and the causes of the disagreements analyzed or eventually the sample withdrawn as atypical.

It is necessary to follow a histological approach as precise as possible because the mere counting of GM, as on a flat bone observed *in toto*, leads to incomplete use of the other information potentially available in bone structures. Bone histology when correctly interpreted gives interesting information useful for refining the growth scenario. It is of course necessary to validate this scenario as far as possible before systematic aging of each individual in the sample. If possible, when the material is abundant, the monthly study of the margins of the growing bones gives good and accurate arguments to favor a given growth hypothesis. However, the best validation is provided by experimental studies *in natura* with vital labeling coupled with capture-recapture techniques. In that case, precise dating of each growth mark along the year and the possibility of histological quantification of osteogenic activities give direct and detailed validation for the method of aging (see above).

In some cases, the GM of some bones in an unknown species may be assumed *a priori* to be annual *in natura* whereas others found in other bones of the same individual may not (Hill *et al.*, 1989).

Practical Problems

All the difficulties encountered in practice by the authors cannot be cited here. However, we will report the main ones. They principally deal with the histological appearance and features of the LAG or *annuli* and also their ultimate disappearance from bone. Another main difficulty is the possible presence of supplementary GM (see above).

In some cases, the GM on bone *in toto* (LAG and *annuli*) may show only a weak optical contrast that makes counting difficult. This difficulty can be partly overcome by the use of an appropriate clearing medium (see above).

A gross underestimation of the LAG number may result from the apparent splitting of one thick LAG into numerous thin lines (Fig. 16), as occurs, for example, in phalanges of *Triturus marmoratus* (Francillon-Vieillot *et al.*, 1990) or in spiny rays of *Lethrinus nebulosus* (Meunier *et al.*, 1979). One would be tempted to count only one thick LAG and to discard the numerous thin lines into which the thick LAG resolves. However, when comparing the sections of the phalange and of the femur of the same newt, it has been shown that each thin line must indeed be counted as a true LAG.

Another difficulty is the presence of double LAG, which appear as two very closely adjacent twin lines (Fig. 13). When this pattern is widespread in the whole sample and for several age classes, the question of two growth cycles a year can seriously arise and twin LAG may then be counted as a single one representing 1 year (Fig. 14). This has been clearly observed among populations of *T. marmoratus* from high altitudes in the north of Portugal (Caetano *et al.*, 1985) where they have an estivating and hibernating period each year.

One of the main difficulties in skeletochronological studies is the destruction of bone GM by biological processes. Bone is a living tissue that undergoes many transformations owing to bone modeling and especially to bone remodeling (e.g., bone resorption-reconstruction). This last bone property is generally considered as the consequence of the mechanical constraints and physiological demands through life (Amprino, 1948, 1967; Dhem, 1967; and see Volume 2 in this series). Bone remodeling is histologically represented first by a destruction of bone tissue (osteoclastic activity), then by secondary osteogenesis (osteoblastic activity), the successive processes destroying the primary bone and obviously the cortical GM inside. When bone remodeling is locally restricted, GM can be partly spared (Figs. 12, 13, and 17) and aging remains possible. Conversely, if remodeling is intense as in mammals, birds, and some other vertebrates in connection with a high bone turnover, one or several of the first GM deposited may be completely removed. In that case age will be underestimated. A peculiar aspect of bone remodeling deals with endosteal resorption at the periphery of the medullar cavity (Figs. 13 and 15). If initially formed yearly rings are resorbed by later erosion and remodeling of the bone, individual age also can be underestimated.

For intracortical as for endosteal destruction of GM (Fig. 15), the number of resorbed rings must be determined by back calculation (Castanet and Cheylan, 1979; Hemelaar, 1985; Leclair and Castanet, 1987; Meunier *et al.*, 1979). For that purpose the method of Hemelaar (1985) is based on the comparison of the pattern of year rings and diameter of medullar cavity in a given phalanx of adults with the diameter of this phalanx in 1st year toads before hibernation (thus roughly corresponding to the diameter of the first rest line). Some recent studies suggest that differences in the intensity of perimedullary endosteal bone resorption could be viewed as an informative characteristic. For instance, in *Bufo bufo* Smirina (1983) and Hemelaar (1986) have demonstrated a sexual dimorphism expressed by the different number of rest lines removed by endosteal resorption among males and females in a given population.

Main Results Obtained by Skeletochronology

All the data obtained since the early use of bone skeletochronological methods need not to be reported here; however, some of the main results and prospects may be summarized.

Several Distinct Populations of One Species May Be Studied, Allowing Interpopulational Comparisons. For example the skeletochronological analysis of the phalanges in allopatric populations of the European common toad living under different climatological conditions was conducted by Hemelaar (1986). By studying populations in five countries (Netherlands, Germany, France, Norway, Switzerland), she was able to analyze several demographic parameters such as age structure and size distribution of the spawning populations, annual growth, age and size at first sexual maturity. She found interpopulational differences as follows: toads from populations living at high altitude or northern latitude generally mature later and at larger sizes, may live longer, grow faster at equal sizes, and may reach larger sizes than those living in low land or southern latitudes.

Different Sympatric Species May Be Simultaneously Studied. For example, the skeletochronological method was applied to two closely related species of newts (*Triturus cristatus* and *T. marmoratus*) by Francillon-Vieillot *et al.* (1990). One of the results concerns the age of sexual maturity in the two species. The age at which *T. marmoratus* first matures (4 years) was significantly higher than that of *T. cristatus* (2 to 3 years). Such data are of obvious interest

266 J. Castanet et al.

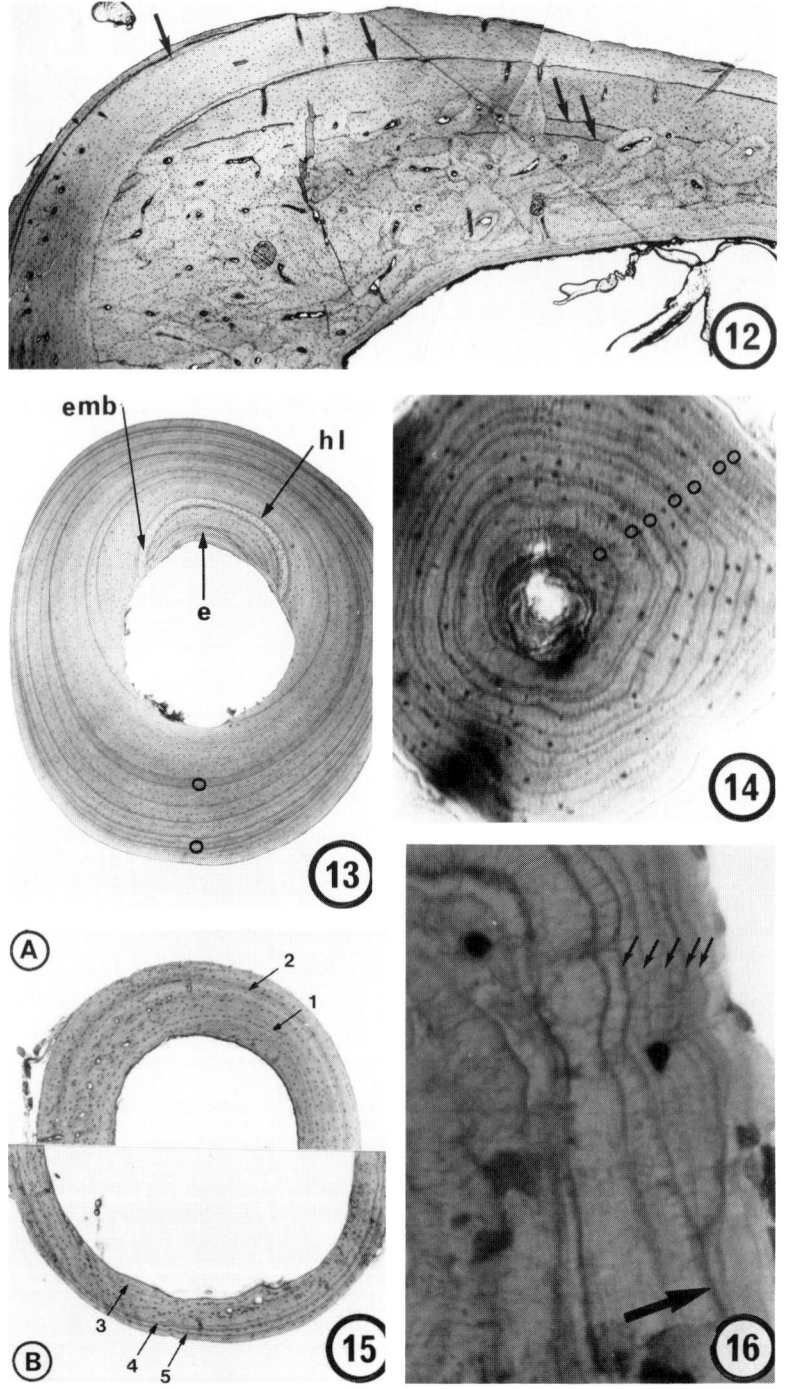

for the ecological and microevolutionary study of sympatric, potentially competing species.

Another Result of the Skeletochronological Method is the Relation Existing between Precise Ecological Conditions and the Fine Patterns of the Lines of Arrested Growth. For example Caetano and Castanet (1987) caught five *T. marmoratus* from a highly elevated station in Portugal and carried them to Paris where they were kept for 4 years under natural external conditions. The change in conditions of life appears to be strongly correlated with the change observed in the fine spatial organization of the LAG. Indeed during the free mountain life two (twin) LAG were deposited each year while in a more equable climate (in Paris) only a simple LAG appeared each winter.

This qualitative observation confirms the comparison between the lowland populations of *T. marmoratus* with single LAG and high altitudes populations with double-twin LAG (Caetano *et al.*, 1985).

Comparisons between Closely Related Extinct and Extant Species Can Provide Valuable Data on Species Specific Growth Strategies, Paleoclimatology, and Micro-evolutionary Process. For example, Castanet and Baez (1991) studying island living lizards of the endemic Canarias genus *Gallotia* demonstrated that the large body size of the fossil species *G. goliath* was the result of a high longevity

---

Figs. 12. through 16. *Cercopithecus nictitans* (Mammalia, Primate, Cercopithecidae) (Fig. 12). Part of a cross-section in the mandible stained by Ehrlich's hematoxylin. LAG are clear in the primary bone (arrows), but these lines are removed by internal remodeling and disappear in the haversian bone. (× 27.) *Gallotia galloti* (Reptilia, Squamata, Lacertidae) (Fig. 13). Femoral shaft diaphysis made of parallel-fibered bone. Cross-section stained by Ehrlich's hematoxylin. Owing to bone drift during ontogenesis the endosteal bone resorption did not completely remove the first steps of the bone growth. About 6 winter LAG can be counted. Some are locally double (o). e: endosteal bone. emb: embryonic bone. hl: hatching line merged with the first winter LAG. This lizard was about 7 years old. (× 25.) *Triturus marmoratus* (Amphibia, Caudata, Salamandridae) (Fig. 14). Humeral shaft diaphysis made of parallel-fibered bone. Cross-section stained by Ehrlich's hematoxylin. In most newts of this population from altitude (1500 m) in the north of Portugal, LAG appear as steps of paired lines (o). Such a sequence was demonstrated to be linked to a double-yearly cycle of activity. Lowland newts which have only one period of activity and inactivity each year only expressed single LAG. This newt was about 10 years old. (× 80.) *Bufo pentoni* (Amphibia, Anura, Bufonidae) (Fig. 15). Cross-section of middiaphyseal region of femur stained with Ehrlich's hematoxylin, 20 μm thick. The two half sections allow comparison between a 3-year-old (A) and a 6-year-old toad (B). The two first lines are present in the younger and they are eroded by endosteal resorption in the older. (× 35.) *Triturus marmoratus* (Amphibia, Caudata, Salamandridae) (Fig. 16). Cross-section of middiaphyseal region of a phalange of the third toe of the hindlimb. A thick LAG (large arrow) splits into numerous ones (little arrows). The comparison of this section with the section of the femur of the same animal allowed each thin LAG to be counted as a true LAG. This newt was 12 years old (see Francillon-Vieillot *et al.*, 1990). (× 400.)

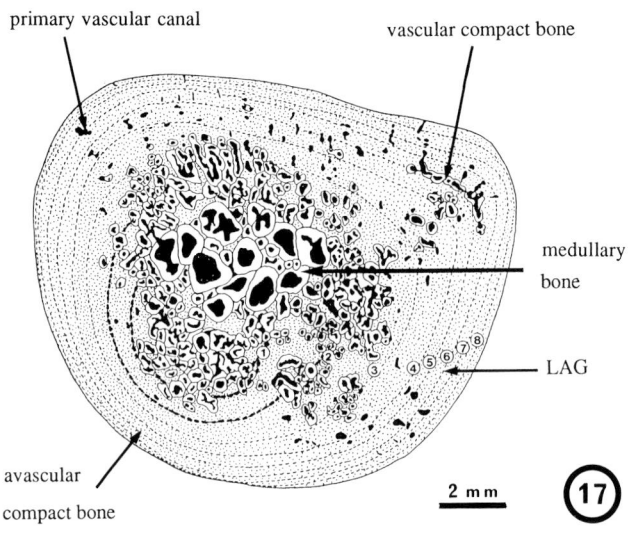

primary vascular canal

vascular compact bone

medullary
bone

LAG

avascular
compact bone

2 m m

17

Fig. 17. General organization of a rib (cross-section) in an undetermined teleostean fish. The center of the section shows a vascularized compacta. LAG 3 to 8 are well visible in the cortical bone whereas in the medullary region they are partly destroyed (1 and 2) by remodeling. (Black = primary and secondary vascular canals; white = secondary bone; dotted area = primary bone).

rather than a high growth rate, which was found to be similar to those of living species of *Gallotia*.

Compared to similar aging methods such as scalimetry or otolithometry, investigations of bony tissues present some specific advantages. The histological functional interpretation of the various patterns of bone tissues allows construction of detailed hypotheses about the growth dynamics of individual bones, whole skeletons, and extrapolation to the complete organism. In turn, if a validation of the growth hypotheses can be obtained, reliable values about individual age will be reached. Valuable data about bone growth rates can be deduced from the actual type of bony tissue and/or from its density of vascularization. Although the technical processing and later analysis of bone is probably longer than with other methods, the richness of potential information on growth provided by bony tissues probably balances in many circumstances this technical handicap.

Other Age Criteria Provided by Bone

It has been emphasized many times that size, shape, structure, and bone composition change throughout the life. If these transformations were demonstrated to be closely age dependent, they could be used as age criterion.

In this way, many techniques, more or less sophisticated, were developed in mammals and especially humans, by archeologists and forensic medicine specialists.

However, it must be kept in mind that all these techniques provide an indirect age assessment and need a reference sample of known age, belonging to the same population, to avoid the consequence of variability. This is already constraining. Moreover, as demonstrated by Masset (1971; see also Bocquet et al., 1978; Masset, 1982, 1989), the results concerning age at death are distorted if the different age groups of the reference population are not numerically homogenous.

Two categories of bony age criteria can be distinguished here: those belonging to gross morphology and microanatomical level of integration (structures of first order *sensu* Petersen, 1930) on the one hand and those from the bone histological level (structures of second order, Petersen, 1930) on the other hand. See also Chapter 1 in Volume 3 of this series.

Morphological and Microanatomical Criteria (Table 4)

Dimensions

Since individual body size is an obvious (but complex and highly variable) function of age, the evaluation of bone dimensions (sizes, weight) from fetal skeletons (Kosa, 1989) throughout life has been proposed as an age criterion for a long time in many works. This makes a field of itself in the plentiful anthropological, veterinary, pathological, and theriological literature. A major critical reevaluation comes from Bouvier (1988) who uses the evolution of the mandibular dimensions in the rhesus monkey. Some older works used the size and weight of the bacculum in mustelids (Walton, 1968) or the size and development of the suspensory tuberosities of the ischiatic arches in squirrels (Colburn, 1986). However, as recognized by Bouvier (1988), "the important point is that unrelated groups of conspecific monkeys, also raised under different environmental conditions, could exhibit considerable variability in absolute skeletal dimensions." That considerably limits the interest of the method which in fact appears only able to separate juveniles from adults and sometimes to demonstrate a sexual dimorphism rather than giving precise individual aging.

Shape, Morphology, and Bone Synostosis

Closely linked to size, the age-dependent evolution of some bone micro-morphological structures was used in some mammals and in several parts of the human skeleton. The use of the surface patterns of the pubic symphysis is summarized by Bocquet et al. (1978). Classically, the authors describe

Table 4.
Some Recent Examples of Age Estimation from Morphological and Microanatomical Criteria

Great categories of variables	Taxa	Material	Authors	Results
Size Size and weight Degree of long bone ossification	Rhesus Macaques Mustelids Squirrels	Mandible Bacculum Ischiatic arches tuberosities	Bouvier, 1988 Walton, 1968 Colburn, 1986	Accuracy in months: m±5; f±7 Distinction juveniles / adults m = male; f = female
Bone surface patterns	Human	Pubic symphysis Articular faces of clavicles	Nemeskeri et al., 1960 Szilvassy et al., 1978-79-80	Five age groups Three age groups
Skull bone sutures	Human		Masset, 1982-1989	Weak correlation between age and sutures synostosis. Error < 10 years only in 50% of cases
Epiphyseal unions	Human Monkey Macaques Monkey Macaques	Long bones Long bones Postcranial skeleton	see Ubalaker, 1989 Cheverud, 1981 Kimura & Hamada, 1990	Accuracy in months: m±4,7; f±5,2 Especially significant until 9 years
Cortical index	Human	Clavicle	Kaur & Jit, 1990	Increases from 15 to 30 years and decreases after.
Cortico diaphyseal index		Femur and humerus midshaft	Dequeker, 1975; Bergot et al., 1976	Usable from 40 to 90 years. Better for females than for males.

For more details and references see *Age Markers in the Human Skeleton*. Iscan, M. Y., Ed., Charles C Thomas, Springfield, IL (1989).

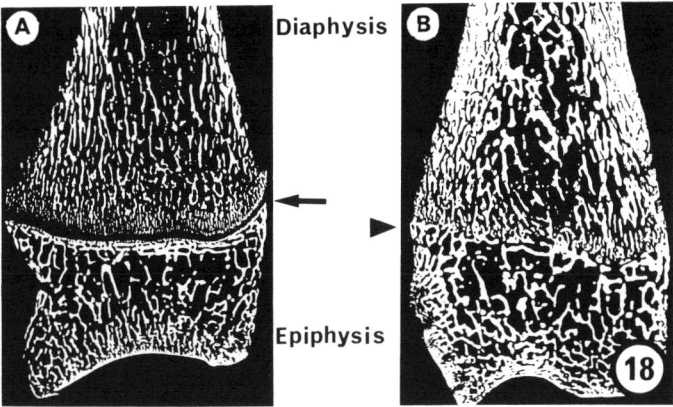

Fig. 18. *Canis canis* (Mammalia, Carnivora, Canidae). Microradiography of a longitudinal section in the distal epiphysis of a radius. (A) Young specimen that shows active longitudinal growth, the unmineralized growth cartilage (arrow) is obvious ($\times$ 3.2). (B) Adult specimen that has stopped its growth: the growth cartilage (arrow head) has disappeared ($\times$ 2.6). (From Dhem, 1967.)

several morphological stages (e.g., five by Nemeskeri *et al.* 1960) and relate them to different age groups. Szilvassy *et al.* (1979) and Szilvassy (1978, 1980) separate three age groups ranging from 18 to 30 years from the sternal articular faces of the clavicula.

The union of skull bones (e.g., Bocquet *et al.*, 1978) and the timing of epiphyseal unions (Fig. 18) of various long bones have been systematically studied to estimate the early age of humans (for previous literature see Ubelaker, 1989 and Kimura and Hamada, 1990). Such a criterion was used in monkeys (e.g., Cheverud, 1981; Kimura and Hamada, 1990). In this last careful and accurate study involving 40 epiphyseal unions from the skeleton of many individuals of two subspecies, Kimura and Hamada (1990) found significant correlations with age before 9 years (more or less the adolescent period) but more inaccurate after. They also claimed that these results obtained on laboratory material cannot be applied directly to wild macaques. Similar studies have been performed on many species of wild and domestic mammals, especially within the frame of veterinary and cynegetic literature. Finally, Kimura and Hamada (1990) admit that "epiphyseal union could allow more precise age estimation than body mass or dental eruption during a certain range of ages." Ubelaker (1989) also underlines the population variability involved in human long bones growth and its importance for aging process.

Microanatomy

The majority of these methods have been devised for humans and deal with the decrease of bone quantity (bone mass) and bone density (e.g., linked to the increase of bone porosity) with aging. They use either thin bone slices of biopsies or radiographic techniques for *in vivo* investigations. Age estimation from variation of cortical thickness (cortical index) has been recently improved on the human clavicle (Kaur and Jit, 1990) but most studies use the cortical thickness of the femur or humerus diaphyseal shaft (e.g., Dequeker, 1975; Bergot and Bocquet, 1976; Thompson, 1980; Bergot, 1983; Gunness-Hey, 1985; Bohr and Schaadt, 1990; Bergot *et al.*, 1990). Briefly, it is now demonstrated that bone volume decreases by (1) decrease in number and thickness of bone trabeculae, (2) decrease in corticodiaphyseal index, and (3) increase of bone porosity in humans — more in females than in males — from about 40 to 90 years (Fig. 19). It must be noticed that during this age range the mean degree of mineralization (= bone mineral density) of healthy bone tissue itself does not change (Bergot et al., 1990).

Nevertheless, such bone tissue loss varies between different skeletal sites and in a given organ from one region to another (Bergot *et al.*, 1990). Moreover, many external (pathology, life conditions, physical activity, feeding . . .) and internal (genetic) factors greatly modulate the bone parameters and induce an individual variability which makes inaccurate a straightforward indexing of the sample of unknown age to the reference population. As noticed by Sorg *et al.* (1989), "the discrepancy between biological and chronological age can be remarkable in some individual resulting in over or underaging remains." Moreover, it is clear that such microanatomical bone variations can be used in aging humans only after 35 or 40 years.

Histological Age Criteria (Table 5)

Only used until today to estimate age of humans, Balthazard and Lebrun (1911; *in* Kurzawski, 1983) were probably the first to propose the possibility of age estimation using bone microstructures. Amprino and Bairati (1936, 1938) provided precise background data and insightful analysis of the subject as did Enlow (1966). However, Kerley (1965) really set up the method which in contrast to previous ones (Bocquet *et al.*, 1978) deals with intracortical bone tissue remodeling, i.e., area, quality, and quantity of primary and secondary blood canals and secondary osteons (Fig. 20). In his first study, Kerley (1965) derived age estimations from the development of the number of intact secondary osteons, parts of them, and of nonhaversian canals. He also estimated the percentage of lamellar bone in the outer third of the cortex in ground sections from the midshaft of the femur, tibia, and fibula. By regression analysis and appropriate charts of these histological

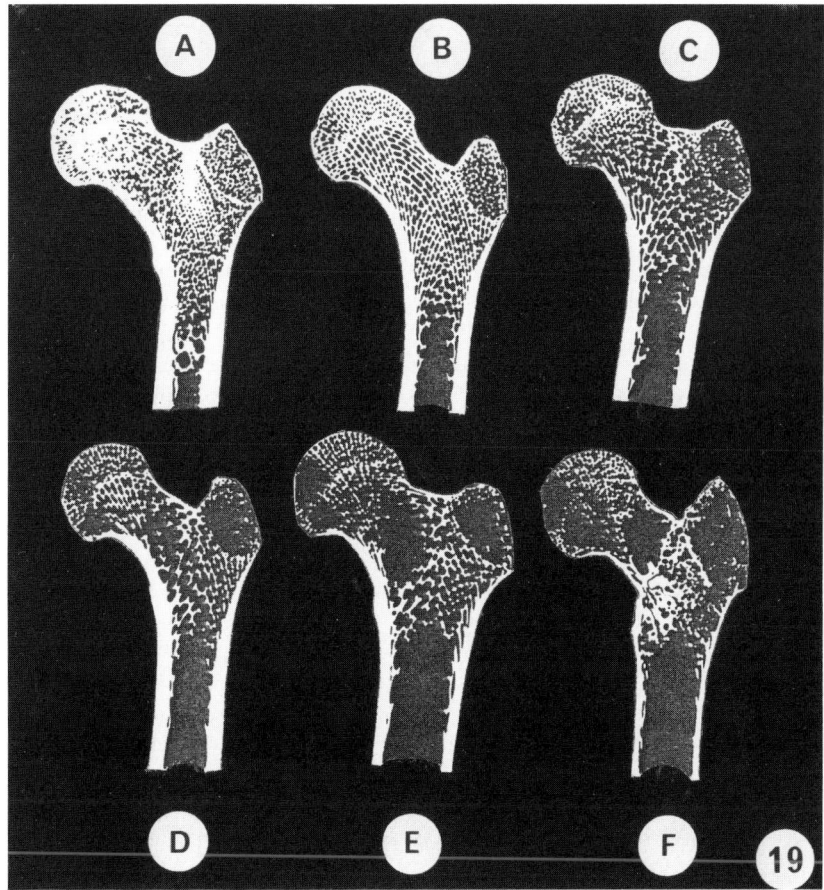

Fig. 19. *Homo sapiens* (Mammalia, Primate, Hominidae). Microradiography of a longitudinal section in the proximal part of a femur in six humans of increasing mean age: A = 31.4; B = 44.0; C = 52.6; D = 56.0; E = 63.3; Fe = 67.8 years. Note the regular thinning of the cortical diaphysis with aging and also the rarefaction of the trabeculae in the epiphyseal spongiosa, two typical features of the decreasing bone mass in the human skeleton after age 30. (Modified from Sorg *et al.*, 1989 after Acsàdi and Nemeskéri, 1970.)

variables, Kerley (1965) has shown the results to be accurate at 85 to 95% within more or less 10 years, from birth to 95 years. After 1965 he refined his method (e.g., Kerley, 1972; Kerley and Ubelaker, 1978). Following Kerley, many authors have used this histological method, each one providing some personal opinion, modification, and explanation (e.g., Alhquist and Damsten, 1969; Singh and Gunberg, 1970; Iwamoto *et al.*, 1978; Fiala, 1980; Hauser *et al.*, 1980; Stout and Gehlert, 1982). The "core technique" of

Table 5.
Some Examples of Age Estimation Mostly from Histological Criteria in Humans

Authors	Material	Variables	Results
Balthazard & Lebrun, 1911	tibia	Haversian canal diameter	
Kerley, 1965 Kerley & Ubelaker, 1978	femur, tibia and fibula cortex	1- II osteons and fragments number 2- % of lamellar bone at periphery 3- Non-Haversian blood vessels	1 : increase with age. 2-3 : decrease with age. "Profile table": 87%:± 5 years; 100%: ±10 years No sexual differences.
Ahlquist & Damsten, 1969	femur	% osteons and part of them	
Singh & Gunberg 1970	femur, tibia, mandible	1- II osteons number 2- Lamellae number by osteon 3- Average diameter of Haversian canals	1-2: increase with age 3: decrease with age
Thompson, 1978, 79, 80	4 cm "cores " diameter removed at the midshaft section of femora, humerus, tibia, ulna.	14 histological variables, e.g.: 1- II osteons number 2- Haversian canals and primary osteons number and area 3- Lamellae number by osteons 5 non histological variables: a- cortical thickness b- cortical bone density	1-2-3: increase with age (males and females) a-b: decrease with age for females; more or less constant for males.
Ericksen, 1991	Complete cross sections of the femoral midshaft	8 histological variables, e.g.: 1- II osteons number and fragments 2- Resorption spaces 3- Non-Haversian canals 4- Unremodeled bone	1: increase with age 2: more or less constant 3-4: decrease with age (especially after forty)

Modified from Kurzawski, 1983.

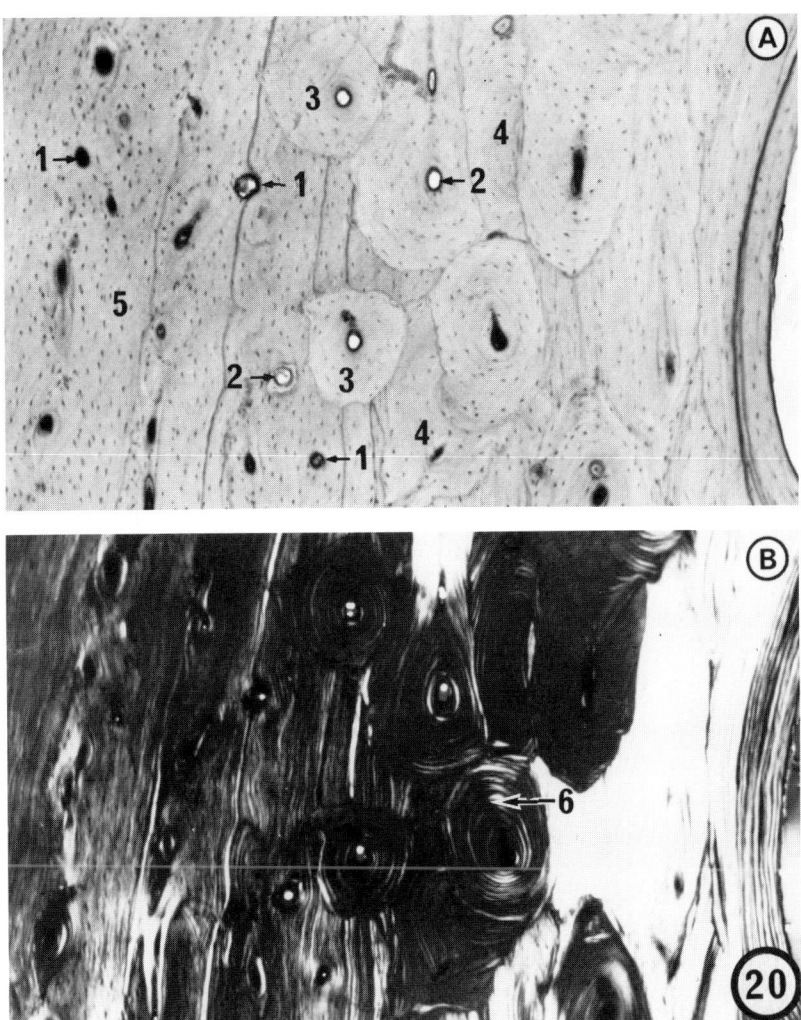

Fig. 20. *Macaca arctoides* (Mammalia, Primate, Cercopithecidae). Part of a cross-section in the mandible. A: stained by Ehrlich's hematoxylin. B: polarized light. Some of the histological variables taken into account for age estimation are 1 — Non-Haversian canals (= primary vascular canals), 2 — Haversian canals, 3 — complete II osteons, 4 — fragment, 5 — unremodeled circumferential bone (= primary bone), 6 — Lamellae. (× 75.)

Thompson (1980), also used by Gunness-Hey (1985), which combines histological and nonhistological variables, also provides reliable age estimation. In general, all the variables studied are age related but most of them are found more significant for females than for males (Thompson, 1980).

Finally, comparisons made between the different studies using Kerley's method and its variations (Bouvier and Ubelaker, 1977; Stout and Gehlert, 1980; Kursawski, 1983; Uytterschaut, 1985) show that they are in fair agreement with each other. The general opinion may be summarized by the conclusion of Stout and Gehlert (1980): "Based upon both accuracy and reliability, averaging age prediction by Kerley's regression formulae appears to be the method of choice for broad application of histological aging." Nevertheless, for osteological characters, populational and individual variability must not be underestimated. Even Stout (1989) emphasizes that "a single section from one bone, therefore, may not be representative of the skeleton as a whole" and that "age prediction based upon a single bone can be highly unreliable."

Clearly all the methods dealing with bone morphology, radiology, and histomorphometry especially because of their high biological variability dependency must be used with much caution. In Iscan's opinion (1989) "their accuracy are very much at the mercy of the individual applying them." That leads Maples (1989) to conclude, by what is for us an overstatement, that age estimation is "an art, not a precise science."

Concluding Remarks

By using bone GM as well as other progressive transformations of bone structures closely related to the time flow, the skeletal tissues now appear as an essential chronological tool in many fields of research. First, in many cases, results provided by bone histology are the most reliable, compared to other techniques of age estimation. Second, if individual age is the key datum which can be extracted from bone structures, many other biological — and nonbiological — parameters can be reached by the histological analysis of skeletal structures. Third, bone — and tooth — tissues remain the unique possibility to obtain data from fossil and subfossil material. Finally, all these unique characteristics confer on those methodologies a high heuristical value, the possibilities of which are probably not yet entirely discovered.

Nevertheless, as for all "biological methods" the use of bone structures for age estimation and related data is not without difficulties and will never provide 100% reliable results. In practice these methods need validation and careful interpretation of the bone growth dynamic as well as error estimation. Thus, such bone methodologies cannot be considered as automatic or "routine". In fact, on the one hand, the determinism and the functional significance of bone structures are only beginning to be known and, on the other, most of the physiological relays controlling bone morphogenesis and its precise spatiotemporal organization also need to be clarified. Then, future basic ecophysiological studies on these topics will undoubtedly increase the reliability and the performances of bone as a tool for chronology.

References

Acsàdi, G. and Nermeskéri, J. (1970). *History of Human Life Span and Mortality*. Akademiai, Kiado, Budapest.

Ahlqvist, J. and Damsten, O. (1969). A modification of Kerley's method for the microscopic determination of age in human bone. *J. Forensic Sci.*, **14**: 205–213.

Amprino, R. (1947). La structure du tissu osseux envisagée comme expression de différences dans la vitesse de l'accroissement. *Arch. Biol.*, **58**: 315–330.

Amprino, R. (1948). A contribution to the functional meaning of the substitution of primary by secondary bone tissue. *Acta Anat.*, **5**: 291–300.

Amprino, R. (1967). Bone histophysiology. *Guy's Hospital Rep.*, **116**: 51–69.

Amprino, R. and Bairati, A. (1936). Processi di ricostuzione e di riassorbimente nella sostanza compatta della ossa dell'uomo. *Z. Zell.*, **24**: 439–511.

Amprino, R. and Bairati, A. (1938). La variazioni nella struttura dell'osso in relazione all eta e la loro importanza medico forenze. *Arch. Antrop. Crim.*, **16**: 61–74.

Balthazard, V. and Lebrun. (1911). Les canaux de Havers aux différents âges. *Ann. Hyg. Publ. Med. Leg.*, **15**: 144–152.

Bardach, J. E. (1955). The opercular bone of the yellow perch, *Perca flavescens*, as a tool for age and growth studies. *Copeia*, **2**: 107–109.

Beamish, R. J. (1981). Use of fin-ray sections to age Walleye Pollock, Pacific cod and albacore, and the importance of this method. *Trans. Am. Fish. Soc.*, **110**: 287–299.

Beamish, R. J. and McFarlane, G. A. (1983). The forgotten requirement for age validation in fisheries biology. *Trans. Am. Fish. Soc.*, **112**: 735–743.

Bergot, C. (1983). Variations du Volume Osseux et de la Densité Minérale au cours du Vieillissement. Thèse Doctorat d'Etat, Université Paris 7, Paris, 321.

Bergot, C. and Bocquet, J. P. (1976). Etude systématique en fonction de l'âge de l'os spongieux et de l'os cortical de l'humérus et du fémur. *Bull. Mem. Soc. Anthrop. Paris*, **13**: 215–242.

Bergot, C., Laval-Jeanet, A. M., Bouysse, S., and Laval-Jeanet, M. (1990). Variations du volume osseux et de la densité minérale au cours du vieillissement chez l'Homme. *Rev. Rhumat.*, **57**: 791–798.

Blake, C. and Blake, B. F. (1978). The use of opercular bones in the study of age and growth in *Labeo senegalensis* from Lake Kainji, Nigeria. *J. Fish Biol.*, **13**: 287–295.

Bocquet, J. P., Maia Neto, M. A., Tavares Da Rocha, M. A., and Xavier De Morais, M. H. (1978). Estimation de l'âge au décès des squelettes d'adultes par régressions multiples. *Contr. Est. Antrop. Port.*, **10**: 107–167.

Boet, P. and Le Louarn, H. (1985). La croissance du poisson. Techniques d'étude. In: *Gestion Piscicole des Lacs et Retenues Artificielles*. Gerdeaux, D. and Billard, R., Eds., 125–142.

Bohr, H. H. and Schaadt, O. P. (1990). Structural changes of the femoral shaft with age measured by dual photon absorptiometry, *Bone Miner.*, **11**: 357–362.

Boivin, G. and Meunier, F. (1978). Bone formation and fluorescent labelling in teleost fishes, Tissus Calcifiés des Poissons, Brest, May 12–13, 1978.

Boujard, T. and Meunier, F. J. (1991). Croissance de l'épine pectorale, histologie osseuse et dimorphisme sexuel chez l'atipa, *Hoplosternum littorale* Hancock, 1828 (Callichthyidae, Siluriforme). *Cybium*, **15**: 55–68.

Bourlière, F. and Spitz, F. (1975). La dynamique des populations de mammifères. In: *Problèmes d'Écologie: la Démographie des Populations de Vertébrés*. Lamotte, M. and Bourlière, F., Eds., Masson, Paris, 77–145.

Bouvier, M. (1988). Age estimation in rhesus macaques (*Macaca mulatta*) based on mandibular dimensions. *Am. J. Primat.*, **15**: 129–142.

Bouvier, M. and Ubelaker, D. H. (1977). A comparison of two methods for the microscopic determination of age at death. *Am. J. Phys. Anthrop.*, **46**: 391–394.

Brothwell, D. R. (1989). The relationship of tooth wear to aging. In: *Age Markers in the Human Skeleton*. Iscan, M. Y., Ed., Charles C Thomas, Springfield, IL, 303–317.

Bruneau, M. and Magnin, E. (1980). Croissance, nutrition et reproduction des Ouaouarons, *Rana catesbeiana* Shaw (*Amphibia, Anura*) des Laurentides au nord de Montréal. *Can. J. Zool.*, **58**: 175–183.

Bryuzgin, V. L. (1939). A procedure for investigating age and growth in Reptillia. *Dokl. Acad. Nauk SSSR*, **23**: 403–405.

Buffrénil, V. de (1980). Mise en évidence de l'incidence des conditions de milieu sur la croissance de *Crocodylus siamensis* (Schneider, 1801) et valeur des marques de croissance squelettiques comme indicateur de l'âge individuel. *Arch. Zool. Exp. Gen.*, **121**: 63–76.

Buffrénil, V. de (1982). Données préliminaires sur la présence de lignes d'arrêt de croissance périostiques dans la mandibule du marsouin commun, *Phocoena phocoena* (L.), et leur utilisation comme indicateur de l'âge. *Can. J. Zool.*, **60**: 2557–2567.

Caetano, M. H. (1988). Estudo Sobre a Biologia das Populacôes Portuguesas de *Triturus marmoratus* (Latreille, 1800) e *Triturus boscai* (Lataste, 1879). Morfologia, Ecologia, Crescimento e Variabilidade. Ph.D. Thesis, Lisbon, 360.

Caetano, M. H. and Castanet, J. (1987). Experimental data on bone growth and age in *Triturus marmoratus* (Amphibia, Urodeles). 4th Meeting of the European Society of Herpetology. Nijmegen (NL) Août 1987, 87–90.

Caetano, M. H., Castanet, J., and Francillon, H. (1985). Détermination de l'âge de *Triturus marmoratus* (Latreille 1800) du Parc National de Peneda Geres (Portugal) par squelettochronologie. *Amphibia-Reptilia*, **6**: 117–132.

Cass, A. J. and Beamish, R. J. (1983). First evidence of validity of the fin-ray method of age determination for marine fishes. *N. Am. J. Fish. Manage.*, **3**: 182–188.

Casselman, J. M. (1974). Analysis of hard tissue of pike *Esox lucius* L. with special reference to age and growth. In: *The Ageing of Fish*, Bagenal, T. B., Ed., Unwin Brothers, Old Woking, Surrey, England, 13–27.

Casselman, J. M. (1987). Determination of age and growth. In: *The Biology of Fish Growth*. Weatherley, A. H. and Gill, H. S., Eds., Academic Press, London, 209–242.

Casselman, J. M. (1990). Growth and relative size of calcified structures of fish. *Trans. Am. Fish. Soc.*, **119**: 673–688.

Castanet, J. (1974). Etude histologique des marques squelettiques de croissance chez *Vipera aspis* L. (*Ophidia, Viperidae*). *Zool. Scripta*, **3**: 137–151.

Castanet, J. (1978). Les marques de croissance osseuse comme indicateurs de l'âge chez les lézards. *Acta Zool.*, **59**: 35–48.

Castanet, J. (1981). Nouvelles données sur les lignes cimentantes de l'os. *Arch. Biol.*, **92**: 1–24.

Castanet, J. (1985). La squelettochronologie chez les reptiles. I. Résultats expérimentaux sur la signification des marques de croissance squelettiques utilisées comme critère d'âge chez les lézards et les tortues. *Ann. Sc. Nat. Zool. Paris*, **7**: 23–40.

Castanet, J. (1986–1987). La squelettochronologie chez les Reptiles. III. Applications. *Ann. Sc. Nat. Zool. Paris*, **8**: 157–172.

Castanet, J. and Baez, M. (1991). Adaptation and evolution in *Gallotia* lizards from the Canary Islands: age, growth, maturity and longevity. *Amphibia-Reptilia*, **12**: 81–102.

Castanet, J. and Cheylan, M. (1979). Les marques de croissance des os et des écailles comme indicateur de l'âge chez *Testudo hermanni* et *Testudo graeca* (Reptilia, Chelonia, Testudinidae), *J. Can. Zool.*, **57**: 1649–1665.

Castanet, J. and Gasc, J. P. (1986). Age individuel, longévité et cycle d'activité chez *Leposoma gulanense*, microtelidé de litière de l'écosystème forestier guyanais. In: *Vertébrés et Forêts Tropicales Humides d'Afrique et d'Amérique*. *Mém. Mus. Nat. Hist. Nat. (Paris)*, **132**: 281–288.

Castanet, J., Meunier, F. J., and Ricqlès, A. de (1977). L'enregistrement de la croissance cyclique par le tissu osseux chez les Vertébrés poikilothermes: données comparatives et essai de synthèse. *Bull. Biol. Fr. Belg.*, **111**: 183–202.

Castanet, J. and Naulleau, G. (1985). La squelettochronologie chez les Reptiles. II. Résultats expérimentaux sur la signification des marques de croissance squelettiques utilisées comme critère d'âge chez les serpents. Remarques sur la croissance et la longévité de la Vipère Aspic. *Ann. Sc. Nat. Zool. Paris*, **7**: 41–62.

Casteel, R. W. (1972). Some archaeological uses of fish remains. *Am. Antiquity*, **37**: 404–419.

Castell, R. W. (1976). *Fish Remains in Archaeology and Paleo-Environmental Studies*. Academic Press, New York, 180.

Charles, D. K., Condon, K., Cheverud, J. M., and Buikstra, J. E. (1986). Cementum annulation and age determination in *Homo sapiens*. I. Tooth variability and observer error. *Am. J. Phys. Anthrop.*, **71**: 311–320.

Cheverud, J. M. (1981). Epiphyseal union and dental eruption in *Macaca mulatta*. *Am. J. Phys. Anthrop.*, **56**: 157–167.

Clerc, W. (1927). Etude de la périodicité de la croissance d'après les plans isodynamiques des os. *Rev. Suisse Zool.*, **34**: 477–496.

Colburn, M. L. (1986). Suspensory tuberosities for aging and sexing squirrels. *J. Wildl. Manage.*, **50**: 456–459.

Condon, H., Charles, D. K., Cheverud, J. M., and Buikstra, J. E. (1986). Cementum annulation and age determination in *Homo sapiens*. II. Estimates and accuracy. *Am. J. Phys. Anthrop.*, **71**: 321–330.

Deelder, C. L. and Willemse, J. J. (1973). Age determination in fresh-water teleosts, based on annular structures in fin-rays. *Aquaculture*, **1**: 365–371.

Dequeker, J. (1975). Bone and ageing. *Ann. Rheum. Dis.*, **34**: 100–115.

Dhem, A. (1967). *Le Remaniement de l'Os Adulte*. Maloine, Paris, 1–118.

Durham, L. and Bennett, G. W. (1963). Age, growth and homing in the bullfrog. *J. Wildl. Manage.*, **27**: 107–123.

Enlow, D. H. (1966). An evaluation of the use of bone histology in forensic medicine and anthropology. In: *IIIe International Congress of Anatomists: Symposium on Joint and Bones*. Evans, G., Eds., Springer, Berlin, 92–112.

Ericksen, M. F. (1991). Histologic estimation of age at death using the anterior cortex of the femur. *Am. J. Phys. Anthrop.*, **84**: 171–179.

Esteban-Ruiz, M. L. (1990). Evolution del Género *Rana* en la Peninsula Iberica: Estudio de la Variabilidad Morphologica y Genetica del Complejo *Rana temporaria* L. Doctoral thesis Universidad Complutense de Madrid, Madrid, 211.

Fagade, S. O. (1974). Age determination in *Tilapia melanoptheron* (Ruppell) in the Lagos Lagoon, Lagos, Nigeria. In: *Ageing of Fish*. Bagenal, T. B., Ed., Unwin Brothers, London, 71–77.

Fiala, P. (1980). Structure of the long limb bones and its significance in determining age in man. *Fol. Morphol.*, **28**: 259–263.

Francillon, H. (1979). Etude expérimentale des marques de croissance sur les humérus et les fémurs de Tritons cretés (*Triturus cristatus cristatus* Laurenti) en relation avec la détermination de l'âge individuel. *Acta Zool.*, **60**: 223–232.

Francillon-Vieillot, H., Arntzen, J. W., and Géraudie, J., (1990). Age, growth and longevity of sympatric *Triturus cristatus*, *T. marmoratus* and their hybrids (Amphibia, Urodela). A squeletochronological comparison. *J. Herpetol.*, **24**: 13–22.

Francillon, H. and Castanet, J. (1985). Mise en évidence expérimentale du caractère annuel des lignes d'arrêt de croissance squelettique chez *Rana esculenta* (Amphibia, Anura). *C.R. Acad. Sci. Paris*, **300**: 327–332.

Gibbons, M. M. and McCarthy, T. K. (1983). Age determination of frogs and toads (Amphibia, Anura) from North-western Europe, *Zool. Scripta*, **12**: 145–151.

Grosskopf, B. (1990). Individual Altersbestimmung mit Hilfe von Zuwachsringen im Zement bodengelagerter menschlicher Zähne. *Z. Rechtsmed.*, **103**: 351–359.

Grue, H. and Jensen, B. (1979). Review of the formation of incremental lines in tooth cementum of terrestrial mammals. *Dan. Rev. Game Biol.*, **11**: 1–48.

Gunness-Hey, M. (1985). Age-related bone loss in a prehistoric Koniag Eskimo population. *Ossa*, **12**: 41–47.

Halliday, T. R. and Verrell, P. A. (1988). Body size and age in amphibians and reptiles, *J. Herpetol.*, **22**: 253–265.

Harris, H. A. (1927). Bony striation of the metaphysis as an indication of cessation of growth in the long bones. In: *Comp. Rond. Assoc. Anat.*, **266**.

Harris, H. A. (1931). Lines of arrested growth in the long bones in childhood: the correlation of histological and radiographic appearances in clinical and experimental conditions. *Br. J. Radiol.*, **4**: 561–622.

Hauser, R., Barres, D., Durigon, M., and Derobert, L. (1980). Identification par l'histomorphométrie du fémur et du tibia. *Acta Med. Leg. et Soc.*, **30**: 91–97.

Hederström, H. (1759). Rönan Fiskars Alder. *Handl. Kungl. Vetensk.*, **20**: 222–229.

Hemelaar, A. (1985). An improved method to estimate the number of year rings resorbed in phalanges of *Bufo bufo* (L.) and its application to populations from different latitudes and altitudes. *Amphibia-Reptilia*, **6**: 323–343.

Hemelaar, A. (1986). Demographic Study on *Bufo bufo* L. (anura, amphibia) from Different Climates, by Means of Skeletochronology. Ph.D. thesis, University of Nijmegen, The Netherlands, 135.

Hemelaar, A. S. M. and Van Gelder, J. J. (1980). Annual growth rings in phalanges of *Bufo bufo* (Anura, Amphibia) from The Netherlands and their use for age determination. *Neth. J. Zool.*, **30**: 129–135.

Hill, K. T., Radtke, R. L., and Caillet, G. M. (1989). A comparative analysis of growth zones in four calcified structures of pacific blue marlin, *Makaira nigricans. Fish. Bull.*, **87**: 829–843.

Holden, M. J. and Vince, M. R. (1973). Age validation studies on the centra of *Raja clavata* using tetracycline. *J. Cons. Explor. Mer.*, **35**: 13–17.

Humphrey, R. R. (1922). The multiple testis in urodeles. *Biol. Bull.*, **43**: 45–67.

Iscan, M. Y. (1989). Assessment of age at death in the human skeleton. In: *Age Markers in the Human Skeleton.* Iscan, M. Y., Ed., Charles C Thomas, Springfield, IL, 5–15.

Iwamoto, S. and Koniki, M. (1978). Study on the age-related changes of the compact bone and the age estimation. II. On the humerus. *Acta Med. Kinki Univ.*, **3**: 203–208.

Jepsen, G. L. (1964). Riddles of the terrible lizards. *Am. Sci.*, **52**: 227–246.

Kalb, H. J. and Zug, G. R. (1990). Age estimates for a population of American toads, *Bufo americanus* (Salientia: Bufonidae), in Northern Virginia. *Brimlevyana*, **16**: 79–86.

Kaur, H. and Jit, I. (1990). Age estimation from cortical index of the human clavicle in Northwest Indians. *Am. J. Phys. Anthrop.*, **83**: 297–305.

Kazmer, D. J. (1986). Determination of Urodele Amphibians by Bone Growth Annuli. M.Sc. thesis, Clemson University, Clemson, SC, 118.

Kerley, E. R. (1965). The microscopic determination of age in human bone. *Am. J. Phys. Anthrop.*, **23**: 149–164.

Kerley, E. R. (1972). Special observations in skeletal identification. *J. For. Sci.*, **17**: 349–357.

Kerley, E. R. and Ubelaker, D. H. (1978). Revisions in the microscopic method of estimating age at death in human cortical bone. *Am. J. Phys. Anthrop.*, **49**: 545–546.

Kimura, T. and Hamada, Y. (1990). Development of epiphyseal union in Japanese macaques of known chronological age. *Primates*, **31**: 79–93.

Klevezal, G. A. (1972). Determination of age in birds by layers in the periostal zone. *Zool. Zh.*, **57**: 917–922.

Klevezal, G. A. and Kleinenberg, S. E. (1967). Age determination of mammals from annual layers in teeth and bones. *Transl. Rus., Israel Progr. Sci. Transl., Jerusalem* 1969, IPST Cat. No. 5433.

Koubek, P. and Hrabe, V. (1984). Estimating the age of male *Phasianus colchicus* by bone histology and spur length. *Folia Zool.*, **33**: 303–313.

Kosa, F. (1989). Age estimation from the fetal skeleton. In: *Age Markers in the Human Skeleton.* Iscan, M. Y., Ed., Charles C Thomas, Springfield, IL, 21–54.

Kurzawski, V. (1983). Mise au point sur les méthodes de détermination de l'âge par voie histologique osseuse. *Bull. Mem. Soc. Anthrop. Paris*, **13**: 413–424.

Leclair, R. and Castanet, J. (1987). A skeletochronological assessment of age and growth in the frog *Rana pipiens* Schreber (Amphibia, Anura) from southwestern Quebec. *Copeia*, **2**: 361–369.

Lecomte, F., Meunier, F. J., and Rojas-Beltran, R. (1985). Mise en évidence d'un double cycle de croissance annuel chez un Silure de Guyane, *Arius couma* (Val., 1839) (Teleostei, Siluriformes, Ariidae) à partir de l'étude squelettochronologique des épines de nageoires. *C.R. Acad. Sci. Paris*, **300**: 181–184.

Lecomte, F., Meunier, F. J., and Rojas-Beltran, R. (1986). Données préliminaires sur la croissance de deux téléostéens de Guyane, *Arius proops* (Ariidae, Siluriformes) et *Leporinus friderici* (Anostomidae, Characoidei). *Cybium*, **10**: 121–134.

Lewis, J. C. (1979). Periosteal layers do not indicate ages of sandhill cranes. *J. Wildl. Manage.*, **43**: 269–271.

Lofts, B. (1984). Amphibians. In: *Marshall's Physiology of Reproduction.* Vol. 1, Lamming, G.-E., Ed., Churchill Livingstone, London, 127–205.

Maples, W. R. (1989). The practical application of age estimation techniques. In: *Age Markers in the Human Skeleton.* Iscan, M. Y., Ed., Charles C Thomas, Springfield, IL, 319–324.

Masset, C. (1971). Erreurs systématiques dans la détermination de l'âge par les sutures crâniennes. *Bull. Mem. Soc. Anthrop. Paris*, **12**: 85–105.

Masset, C. (1982). Estimation de l'Age au Décès par les Sutures Crâniennes. Thèse Doctorat d'Etat Université Paris 7, Paris.

Masset, C. (1989). Age estimation on the basis of cranial structures. In: *Age Markers in the Human Skeleton.* Iscan, M. Y., Ed., Charles C Thomas, Springfield, IL, 71–104.

Mattox, N. T. (1935). Annular rings in the long bones of turtles and their correlation with size. *Trans. Ill. St. Acad. Sci.*, **28**: 255–256.

Meunier, F. J. (1988). Détermination de l'âge individuel chez les Ostéichthyens à l'aide de la squelettochronologie: historique et méthodologie, *Acta Oecologica, Oecol. Gen.*, **9**: 299–329.

Meunier, F J. (1992). L'estimation de l'âge individuel chez les Chondricthyens: revue bibliographique des problèmes méthodologiques. In: *Tissus durs et âge individuel des Vertébrés.* Baglinière, J. L., Castanet, J., Conand, F., and Meunier, F. J., Eds., Colloques et Séminaires, ORSTOM-INRA, 281–297.

Meunier, F. J. and Pascal, M. (1981). Etude expérimentale de la croissance cyclique des rayons de nageoire de la carpe (*Cyprinus carpio* L.). Résultats préliminaires. *Aquaculture*, **26**: 23–40.

Meunier, F. J., Pascal, M., and Loubens, G. (1979). Comparaison de méthodes squelettochronologiques et considérations fonctionnelles sur le tissu osseux acellulaire d'un Ostéichthyen du Lagon NéoCalédonien. *Aquaculture*, **17**: 137–157.

Milch, R. A., Rall, D. P., and Tobie, J. E. (1957). Bone localization of tetracyclines. *J. Natl. Cancer Inst.*, **19**: 87–93.

Miller, F. L. (1974). Biology of the Kaminuriak population of barrenground caribou. II. Dentition as an indicator of age and sex: composition and socialization of the population. *Can. Wildl. Serv. Report Ser.*, **31**: 1–87.

Minakami, K. (1979). An estimation of age and life-span of the genus *Trimeresurus* (Reptilia, Serpentes, Viperidae) on Amami Oshima island, Japan. *J. Herpetol.*, **13**: 147–152.

Morris, P. (1972). A review of mammalian age determination methods. *Mammal Rev.*, **2**: 69–104.

Nelson, R. C. and Bookhout, T. A. (1980). Counts of periosteal layers invalid for aging Canada geese. *J. Wildl. Manage.*, **44**: 518–521.

Nemeskeri, J., Harsanyi, L., and Acsadi, G. (1960). Methoden zur Diagnose des Lebensalters von Skelettfunden. *Anthrop. Anz. Jg.*, **24**: 70–95.

Nishimura, M. (1990). Age estimation of habu, *Trimeresurus flavoviridis* (Viperidae) using growth bands in angulares. *Amphibia-Reptilia*, **11**: 411–418.

Olerud, S. and Lorenzi, G. L. (1970). Triple fluorochrome labelling in bone formation and bone resorption, *J. Bone Jt. Surg.*, **52A**: 274–278.

Pascal, M. and Castanet, J. (1978). Méthodes de détermination de l'âge chez le chat haret des îles Kerguelen. *Terre Vie*, **32**: 529–555.

Peabody, F. E. (1958). A Kansas drought recorded in growth zones of a bullsnake. *Copeia*, **2**: 91–94.

Peabody, F. E. (1961). Annual growth zones in vertebrates (living and fossil). *J. Morphol.*, **108**: 11–62.

Perrin, W. F. and Myrick, A. C. (1980). Age determination of toothed whales and sirenians. In: Int. Whaling Commission Report of the I. W. C., *Special Issue* 3, Perrin, W. F. and Myrick, A. C., Eds., La Jolla, CA, 229.

Petersen, C. G. I. (1892). Fiskenesbiologische forhold i Holboek Fjord, 1890–1891, Beret, *Landbugmimist Dan. Bio. Sta. (Fisheirbant)*, **1**: 121–184.

Petersen, H. (1930). Die Organe des Skelettsystems. In: *Handbuch der mikroskopische Anatomie der Menschen*, Möllendorf, V., Ed., Springer, Berlin, 699.

Petter-Rousseaux, A. (1953). Recherches sur la croissance et le cycle d'activité testiculaires de *Natrix natrix helvetica* (Lacépède). *Terre Vie*, **4**: 175–223.

Pilorge, T. and Casanet, J. (1981). Détermination de l'âge dans une population naturelle du lézard vivipare *Lacerta vivipara*. *Acta Oecologica. Oecol. Gen.*, **2**: 387–397.

Rahn, B. A. and Perren, S. M. (1971). Xylenol orange, a fluorochrome useful in polychrome sequential labelling of calcifying tissues. *Stain Techn.*, **46**: 125–129.

Ricqlès, A. de (1975). Recherches paléohistologiques sur les os longs des Tétrapodes. VII. Sur la classification, la signification fonctionnelle et l'histoire des tissus osseux des Tétrapodes. Ire partie. *An. Paleontol.*, **61**: 51–129.

Ricqlès, A. de (1983). Cyclical growth in the long limb bones of a Sauropod Dinosaur. *Acta Paleont. Polonica*, **28**: 225–232.

Saint-Girons, H. (1965). Les critères d'âge chez les reptiles et leurs applications à l'étude de la structure des populations sauvages. *Terre Vie*, **112**: 342–358.

Schroeder, E. E. and Baskett, T. (1968). Age estimation, growth rates and population structures in Missouri bullfrogs. *Copeia*, **3**: 583–592.

Senning, W. G. (1940). A study of age determination and growth of *Necturus maculosus*, based on the parasphenoid bone. *Am. J. Anat.*, **66**: 483–494.

Singh, I. J. and Gunberg, D. L. (1970). Estimation of age at death in human males from quantitative histology of bone fragments. *Am. J. Phys. Anthrop.*, **33**: 373–382.

Smirina, E. M. (1972). Annual layers in bones of *Rana temporaria*. *Zool. Zh.*, **51**: 1529–1534.

Smirina, E. M. (1974). Prospects of age determination by bone layers in Reptilia. *Zool. Zh.*, **53**: 111–117.

Smirina, E. M. (1983). Age determination and retrospective body size evaluation in the live common toads, *Bufo bufo. Zool. Zh.*, **62**: 437–444.

Smirina, E. M., Klevezal, G. A., and Berger, L. (1986). Experimental investigation of the annual layer formation in bones of Amphibians. *Zool. J.*, **65**: 1526–1534.

Smith, S. E. (1984). Timing of vertebral-band deposition in tetracycline-injected leopard sharks. *Trans. Am. Fish. Soc.*, **113**: 308–313.

Sorg, M. H., Andrews, R. P., and Iscan, M. Y., (1989). Radiographic aging of the adult. In: *Age Markers in the Human Skeleton*. Iscan, M. Y., Ed., Charles C Thomas, Springfield, IL, 169–194.

Storey, E. (1958). The effect of intermittent cortisone administration in the rabbit. *J. Bone Jt. Surg.*, **40**: 103–115.

Stout, S. D. (1989). The use of cortical bone histology to estimate age at death. In: *Age Markers in the Human Skeleton.* Iscan, M. Y., Ed., Charles C Thomas, Springfield, IL, 195–210.

Stout, S. D. and Gehlert, S. J. (1980). The relative accuracy and reliability of histological aging methods. *Forensic Sci. Int.*, **15**: 181–190.

Stout, S. D. and Gehlert, S. J. (1982). Effects of field size when using Kerley's histological method for determination of age at death. *Am. J. Phys. Anthrop.*, **58**: 123–125.

Susuki, H. K. (1963). Studies on the osseous system of the slider turtle. *Ann. N.Y. Acad. Sci.*, **109**: 351–410.

Suzuki, H. K. and Mathews, A. (1966). Two color fluorescent labelling of mineralizing tissues with tetracycline and 2-4-bis (*N-N'*-dicarbomethylaminomethyl) fluorescein. *Stain Techn.*, **41**: 57–60.

Szilvassy, J. (1978). Eine Methode zur Alterbestimmung mit Hilfe der sternalen Gelenksflächen der Sclüsselbeine. *Mitt. Anthrop. Ges. Wien.*, **8**: 166–168.

Szilvassy, J. (1980). Age determination on the sternal articular faces of the clavicula. *J. Hum. Evol.*, **9**: 609–610.

Szilvassy, J., Holler, W., Keck, G., Windischbauer, G., Cabaj, A., and Jahn, J. (1979). Alterbestimmung an den sternalen Gelenksflächen der Sclüsselbeine mit Hilfe der Moiré-Topographie. *Ann. Naturhistor. Mus. Wien.*, **82**: 759–767.

Tanaka, S. (1956). A method of analyzing the polymodal frequency distribution and its application to the length distribution of porgy *Taius tamifrons*. *Bull. Tokai. Reg. Fish. Res. Lab.*, **14**: 1–12.

Teska, W. R. and Pinder, J. E. (1986). Effects of nutrition on age determination using eye lens weights. *Growth*, **50**: 362–370.

Thompson, D. D. (1978). Age Related Changes in Osteon Remodeling and Bone Mineralization. Ph.D. thesis, University of Connecticut, Storrs.

Thompson, D. D. (1979). The core technic in the determination of age at death in skeletons. *J. Forensic. Sci.*, **24**: 902–915.

Thompson, D. D. (1980). Age changes in bone mineralization, cortical thickness and Haversian canal area. *Calcif. Tissue Int.*, **31**: 5–11.

Ubelaker, H. D. (1989). The estimation of age at death from immature human bone. In: *Age Markers in the Human Skeleton*. Iscan, M. Y., Ed., Charles C Thomas, Ed., Springfield, IL, 55–70.

Uytterschaut, H. T. (1985). Determination of skeletal age by histological methods. *Z. Morph. Anthrop.*, **75**: 331–340.

Van Soest, R. W. M. and Van Utrecht, W. L. (1971). The layered structure of bones of birds as a possible indication of age. *Bijdr. Diesk.*, **41**: 61–66.

Walton, K. C. (1968). The baculum as an age indicator in the polecat *Putorius putorius*. *J. Zool.*, **156**: 533–536.

Warren, J. W. (1963). Growth Zones in the Skeleton of Recent and Fossil Vertebrates. Ph.D. thesis, University of California at Los Angeles, Los Angeles, 136.

Willis, Y. L. (1954). Breeding, Transformation and Determination of Age of the Bullfrog (*Rana catesbeiana* Shaw) in Missouri. M.A. thesis, University of Missouri, Columbia.

Zug, G., Wynn, A. H., and Ruckdeschel, C. (1986). Age determination of loggerhead sea turtles. *Caretta caretta*, by incremental growth marks in the skeleton. *Smithson. Contrib. Zool.*, **427**: 1–34.

10

Mechanical Properties of Cortical and Trabecular Bone

TONY M. KEAVENY and WILSON C. HAYES
Orthopaedic Biomechanics Laboratory
Charles A. Dana Research Institute
Beth Israel Hospital and Harvard Medical School
Boston, Massachusetts

Introduction

From an engineering perspective, bone is a unique and remarkable material. As a tissue, it exhibits wide variations in morphology, ranging from

8827-9/93/$0.00 + $.50

the delicate, open-celled architecture of the trabecular physes, to the dense, fiber-reinforced arrangement of the diaphyseal cortex. In addition, bone is both self healing and can adapt to changing environmental conditions by specific and highly organized structural adaptations. For instance, with heavy exercise, bones change in cross-sectional geometry to provide structures of increased load-bearing capacity (Jones et al., 1977; Woo et al., 1981). With aging and disuse, bone tissue is resorbed, resulting in dramatic losses of tissue stiffness and strength (Bergot et al., 1988; Burstein et al., 1976; Mosekilde, 1988; Mosekilde et al., 1987; Parfitt, 1984; Preteux et al., 1985). However, to compensate, the cortex expands both its periosteal and its endosteal diameters in an attempt to maintain a structure of approximately constant stiffness and strength (Hayes and Ruff, 1986; Lindahl and Lindgren, 1967; Ruff and Hayes, 1982).

Since the mid-19th century, it has also been noted that the form and structure of trabecular bone appear to be organized so as to optimally resist loads imposed by functional activities. While these form-function relationships have long been referred to as Wolff's Law [after the German anatomist Wolff (1892), who first called attention to the phenomenon], it should be noted that verified, mathematical formulations of this "law" are not available (Cheal et al., 1987; Cowin, 1986; Fyhrie and Carter, 1986; Hart et al., 1984; Hayes and Snyder, 1981; Huiskes et al., 1989). As a consequence, the magnitudes, frequencies and types of stresses necessary to maintain a viable trabecular architecture are not known. Moreover, the specific mechanisms or mechanical signals through which cells control bone architecture are not understood (Rubin et al., 1990). Understanding these stress-related, adaptive processes has been a central concern of mechanicians and bone physiologists for over a century. Interest in the problem has increased in the last several decades as it has become apparent that the altered stresses in bone associated with total joint replacement can influence bone remodeling (Huiskes and Nunamaker, 1984; Zimmerman et al., 1989) and thereby have profound effects on the long-term success of these procedures.

Beyond a basic scientific understanding of bone remodeling and its applications to total joint replacement, there is a variety of additional clinical issues for which the biomechanics of bone are directly relevant. For example, age-related fractures of the hip and spine are health care problems of crisis proportions in the U.S., with over 250,000 hip fractures and 500,000 vertebral fractures occurring annually. As a result, there is an urgent need to improve our understanding of their etiology, to identify patients most at risk, and to develop cost-effective interventions aimed at fracture prevention. To do so, however, requires an understanding of such mechanical factors as the relative importance of bone loss and trauma in fracture etiology, the role of trabecular vs. cortical bone in the strength of the hip and spine, the importance of fatigue damage accumulation in the etiology of spontaneous fractures, and the relationships between fracture risk and the different load regimes that occur both during the activities of daily living and in response to traumatic events such as falls.

To address these issues, one must perform analyses on specific whole bone structures subject to realistic external loads such as gait, or, for fracture etiology of the hip, a fall from standing height. Such analyses must be performed in three stages: first, the material behavior of the bone tissue which makes up the whole bone is determined; second, the geometric properties of the whole bone are determined; third, appropriate external loads are identified and a structural analysis is performed using both material and geometric property data. Thus, when discussing bone biomechanics, it is important to distinguish between bone as a material and bone as a structure. In this chapter, we focus on bone as a material. Our purpose is to provide an introductory survey of current knowledge of bone material properties. Whereas most surveys describe only the stiffness and strength properties of bone, we will also discuss the behavior of bone in response to repetitive loading (fatigue properties) and more complex loading (multiaxial properties) conditions which occur *in vivo*. Since fractures of whole bones and bone remodeling have been associated with damage accumulation in bone, we will also review the mechanisms of damage accumulation in bone and how the mechanical properties of bone are dependent on its microstructure.

Material vs. Structural Behavior

The material behavior of bone describes how bone *tissue* behaves mechanically, regardless of where that tissue is located in any particular whole bone. To determine this fundamental material behavior, mechanical tests are performed on standardized specimens under controlled mechanical and environmental conditions. These tests are designed to eliminate any behavior associated with specimen geometry. Consequently, data generated from these tests may be used to describe the mechanical behavior of a small unit of bone tissue anywhere in the skeleton. The single requirement for the validity of these data is that they be used only for bone with the same microstructure and in the same environment as the test specimens.

When forces are applied to any solid object, the object is deformed from its original dimensions. At the same time, internal forces are produced within the object. The relative deformations (change in length divided by original length) created at any point are referred to as the *strains* at that point. The internal force intensities (force divided by area) are referred to as the *stresses* at that point. When a bone is subjected to forces, these stresses and strains are introduced throughout the structure and can vary in a complex manner. To avoid some of these complexities and demonstrate some important mechanical concepts, it is useful to focus on a regular structure loaded under well-defined conditions (Fig. 1). Similar specimens are used to determine the material properties of bone tissue. In Fig. 1a, a cylindrical bar of length L and a constant cross-sectional area (A) is shown subjected to a pure compressive force (F). As load is applied, the cylinder begins to compress. This situation can be described by analogy to the simple equation which describes stretching of a spring

$$F = (k)x \qquad (1)$$

where F is the applied force, x is the change in length of the spring, and k is the spring constant or stiffness of the spring. Inverting this simple relationship (x = F/k) demonstrates that with a very stiff spring (high k), the elongation, x, is small for a given applied force. The analogous relation to Equation 1 for compression of the cylinder is

$$F = (AE/L)\Delta L \qquad (2)$$

where, F is the force, (ΔL) is the elongation of the cylinder, L is the original length, A is the cross-sectional area, and E is a factor (which we will subsequently define as the Young's modulus) that describes whether the material is rigid (such as with steel) or flexible (as with rubber). Analogous to the spring, the *structural stiffness* of the cylinder is defined as k = AE/L.

A plot of force against deformation (Fig. 1b) describes the *structural behavior* of this cylinder. The slope of the force-deformation plot, the structural stiffness, is directly proportional to both cross-sectional area and the quantity E, and inversely proportional to the length. Thus, if one were to test two cylinders made from the same material (E constant), and of equal lengths (L constant) but with different cross-sectional areas (A different), then the slopes of the force-deformation curves and thus the structural stiffnesses would be different for the two cylinders — even though they are both made from the same material. Similarly, two bones of equal quality bone (same E) but with different geometries will display different structural stiffnesses. Conversely, because whole bones have different cross-sectional areas and lengths, it is not possible to use force-deformation plots of different whole bones to compare the material behavior of the bone tissue within the bones.

To eliminate these geometric effects, force is divided by cross-sectional area (F/A) and elongation is divided by original length ($\Delta L/L$), producing the geometrically normalized measures of force and elongation, known as stress (σ) and strain (ϵ), respectively. Thus, the force-deformation plot (Fig. 1b) is transformed to a stress-strain plot (Fig. 1c). An important property of the stress-strain relationship is its independence of the specimen geometry. Consequently, this relationship describes only *material behavior*. The initial slope of the stress-strain plot actually defines the *Young's modulus* (E), so that

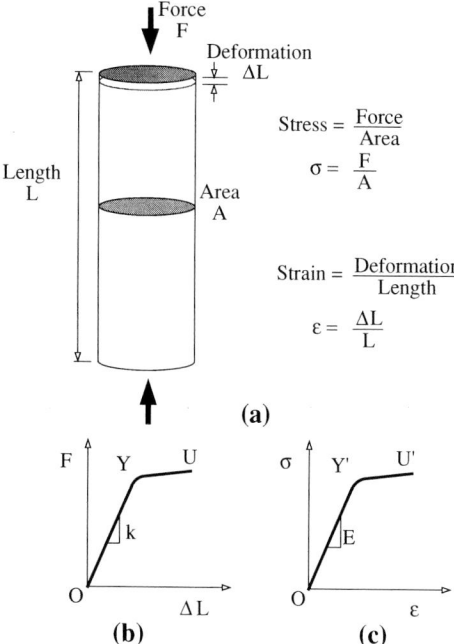

Fig. 1 (a) Cylindrical specimen used in uniaxial compression tests of human bone. Stress and strain are calculated from the force, deformation, and dimensions of the specimen. (b) The force-deformation plot describes the *structural behavior* of the specimen. The linear region (also known as the elastic region) is from O to Y. At Y, "yielding" occurs, with internal rearrangement of the structure, often involving damage to the material. In the region Y to U (also known as the post-yield region), nonelastic deformation occurs until finally, at U, fracture occurs. (c) The stress-strain plot describes the *material behavior* of the tissue which makes up the specimen. The elastic behavior occurs up to Y', and the postyield behavior occurs after Y'. The yield strength is at Y' and the ultimate strength is at U' where fracture occurs. The Young's modulus, E, is the slope of the linear region of this plot.

the slope of the stress-strain plot describes the inherent stiffness of a material. Since the units of strain are nondimensional, the units of modulus are the same as those of stress, MPa (10^6 N/m^2) or GPa (10^9 N/m^2). Thus, the parameter used to compare the stiffness of different materials is the Young's modulus. For example, stainless steel, oak, and polyvinylchloride (PVC) have Young's moduli of 200 GPa, 12 GPa, and 2 GPa, respectively. Cortical bone and relatively stiff trabecular bone have Young's moduli of approximately 17 and 1 GPa, respectively. We can see from these numbers that stainless steel is over ten times stiffer than cortical bone.

As a final example to illustrate how structural stiffness is dependent on geometric properties, consider the following. One can easily deform a paper clip, which is made from stainless steel, a very stiff material, but which is

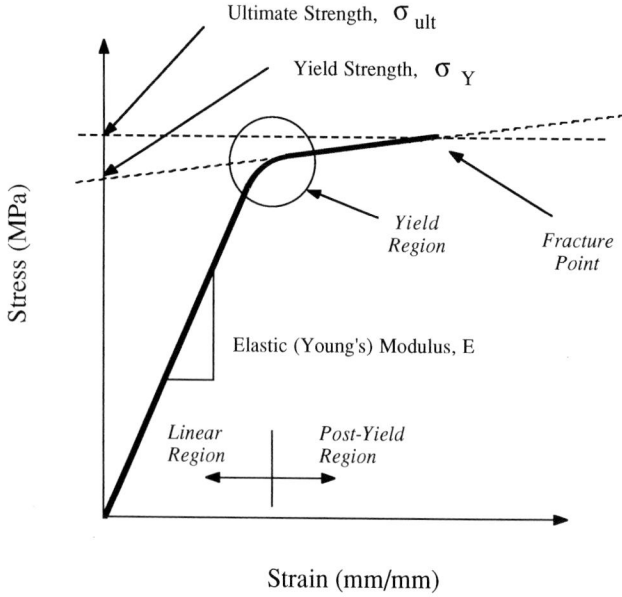

Strain (mm/mm)

Fig. 2. Typical stress-strain plot for compact bone in tension, showing the linear, yield, and postyield regions. Note that the yield and ultimate strengths are similar.

also very thin. However, one cannot easily deform a six inch cube of oak, which is made from a much more flexible material than stainless steel, but is much larger than the paper clip. It is much more difficult to deform the large wooden block than the tiny metal clip precisely because the structural stiffness of the block is so much greater than that of the paper clip. In summary, then, structural behavior includes the combined effects of geometry and material, whereas material behavior eliminates the effect of geometry.

Material Properties

Materials deform when loaded, and we have discussed how the modulus tells us something about how much a material will deform when loaded. However, materials also break if subjected to excessively large loads. Thus, material properties are described by both modulus and strength data. A generalized stress-strain curve is shown in Fig. 2 for wet cortical bone, obtained from the femoral diaphysis and tested in uniaxial tension. This stress-strain curve can be broken into three general regions: the initial linear region, the yield region, and the post-yield region. As we have discussed, the modulus is obtained from the linear region. In contrast, the strength properties are obtained from the yield and post-yield regions. We say that yielding occurs in the yield region, which is the junction of the linear and post-yield regions. Yielding occurs at the *yield strength*, which, for bone, represents the stress when some microstructural damage occurs within the bone (Burstein *et al.*, 1973, Fondrk *et al.*, 1988; Krajcinovic *et al.*, 1987). Fracture occurs when the *ultimate strength* is reached.

The most basic mechanical properties of bone are obtained from tests where standardized specimens are progressively loaded in one direction until fracture. Such tests (as shown schematically in Fig. 1) are called uniaxial, monotonic tests. If the bone is stretched, the test is called a tension test; if the bone is compressed, the test is a compression test. If the bone is twisted, the test is a torsion test. For a torsion test, the bone specimen shown in Fig. 1 would be twisted about its longitudinal axis. By recording the values of torsion and angular twist of the bone, one could plot a torsion-twist diagram, exactly analogous to the force-deformation plot for a compression or tension tension. Similarly, if one normalized the torsion and angular twist by the appropriate geometric parameters, one could derive a stress-strain plot, where stress is called the *shear stress*, and strain is called the *shear strain*. The slope of the shear stress-strain plot is called the *shear modulus* (G). Thus, the shear modulus, units MPa, is directly analogous to the Young's modulus.

Other, more complicated loading configurations may sometimes be used, where loads act simultaneously in different directions. These are called multiaxial tests. The strength properties of bone are different for multiaxial loading than for the simpler, uniaxial loading cases. Furthermore, the material properties of bone under multiple loading cycles (fatigue) are different from those for single, monotonic loads. Finally, all these properties depend on the rate of loading, the amount of time the loads act on the bone, and the age of the bone tissue.

Cortical and Trabecular Bone

Cortical and trabecular bone are distinguished from each other primarily by differences in porosity and, consequently, apparent density (Carter and Spengler, 1978). Apparent density is the ratio of the mass of mineralized bone tissue in a specimen to the bulk volume of the specimen (mineralized bone plus bone marrow spaces). Typically, mean values of apparent density of hydrated human femoral cortical bone and proximal tibial trabecular bone are 1.86 gm/cc (Snyder and Schneider, 1990) and 0.30 gm/cc (Carter and Hayes, 1977c), respectively. The respective standard deviations are typically 0.057 gm/cc ($\pm 3\%$ of the mean value) (Snyder and Schneider, 1990) and 0.09 gm/cc ($\pm 30\%$ of the mean value) (Carter and Hayes, 1977c). This indicates that two thirds of the apparent density values for cortical bone are in the range 1.80 to 1.91 gm/cc, while two thirds of the values for trabecular bone are in the range 0.21 to 0.39 gm/cc. While the magnitudes

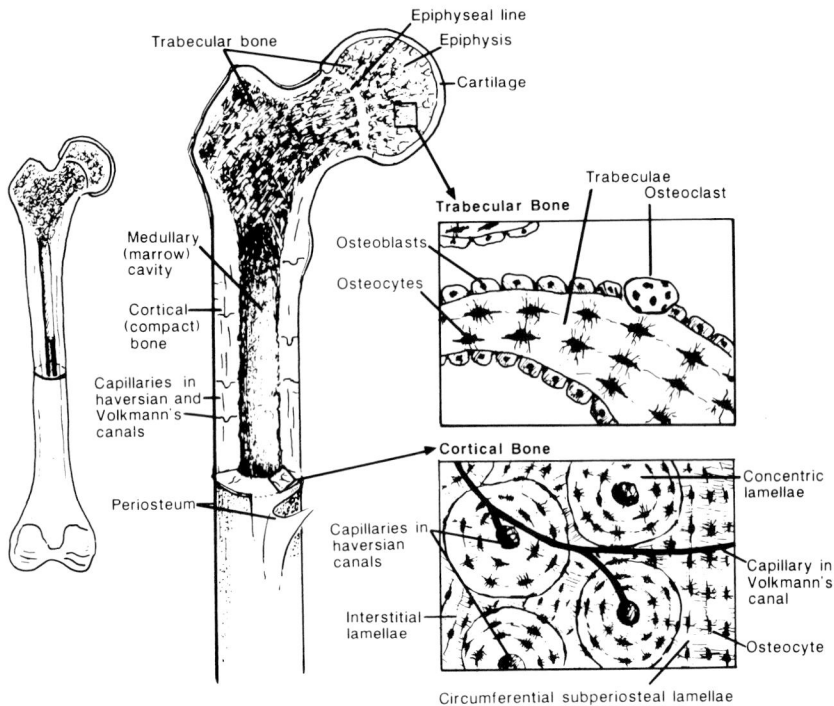

Fig. 3. Schematic diagram of cortical and trabecular bone showing the different microstructures. [From Hayes, W. C. (1991). In *Basic Orthopaedic Biomechanics*, Mow, V. C. and Hayes, W. C., eds., Raven Press, New York, 93–142. With permission.]

of these ranges are similar, the percentage deviations are much larger for trabecular bone. This is important because the material properties of trabecular bone are very sensitive to apparent density.

Since the densities of trabecular and cortical bone can overlap, cortical bone is usually defined as bone with less than approximately 30% porosity (Carter and Spengler, 1978). However, porosity is not the only difference between cortical and trabecular bone. Trabecular bone can also be distinguished from cortical bone by differences in bone architecture (Fig. 3). The architecture of cortical bone can be described as a solid containing a series of voids (Haversian canals, Volkmann's canals, lacunae, and canaliculi). The porosity of cortical bone tissue (typically 10%) is primarily a function of the density of these voids. However, for trabecular bone, the architecture can be described as a network of small, interconnected plates and rods of individual trabeculae (Amstutz and Sissons, 1969; Gibson, 1985; Whitehouse *et al.*, 1971; Whitehouse, 1975) with relatively large spaces between the trabeculae. Individual trabeculae contain only some of the voids (canaliculi, lacunae) which are contained in cortical bone. Therefore, the porosity of trabecular bone (typically 50 to 90%) is dominated by the spaces between individual trabeculae. It is the combination of differences in porosity and architecture which primarily differentiates cortical from trabecular bone and which accounts for their characteristic material properties.

Cortical Bone

Modulus

Elastic properties of *isotropic* materials do not depend on the orientation of the material with respect to the loading direction, and are characterized by a single modulus (Young's modulus). Most conventional engineering materials, such as the 316L stainless steels used for orthopedic implants, are isotropic. The other parameter necessary to fully characterize the elastic behavior of an isotropic material is called the *Poisson's ratio*. This parameter (typically 0.3 for metals) is also found from a uniaxial test, and is defined as the strain perpendicular to the loading direction divided by the strain along the loading direction. It is a measure of how much a material bulges when compressed, or of how much a material contracts when stretched.

The elastic properties of bone, however, depend on its orientation with respect to the loading direction (Ashman *et al.*, 1984; Cowin, 1989; Reilly and Burstein, 1975; Reilly *et al.*, 1974; Yoon and Katz, 1976). Materials with directional-dependent elastic properties are called *anisotropic* materials. However, the elastic properties of cortical bone display a certain degree of symmetry, reflecting its osteonal microstructure (Martin and Burr, 1989). Consequently, human cortical bone is usually considered to be a *transversely isotropic* material (Reilly and Burstein, 1975; Yoon and Katz, 1976) because its elastic properties for loading in one plane (transverse to the longitudinal axis) are approximately isotropic, and are substantially different from those for loading in the longitudinal direction. The longitudinal direction for human cortical bone is parallel to the axis of the osteons, i.e., along the longitudinal axis of the diaphysis.

Whereas only two parameters are necessary to describe the elastic properties of an isotropic material, five parameters are necessary for a transversely isotropic material: the longitudinal and transverse moduli, the shear modulus, and two Poisson's ratios (Table 1). In addition, the elastic properties of cortical bone are similar for tension and compression loading (Reilly *et al.*, 1974). The modulus of cortical bone in the longitudinal direction is approximately 1.5 times larger than its modulus in the transverse direction and over 5 times its shear modulus. Its relatively high Poissons' ratios, with values up to 0.6 (Cowin, 1989; Reilly and Burstein, 1975), indicate that cortical bone bulges more than metals when subjected to uniaxial compres-

Table 1.
Elastic Properties of Human Femoral
Cortical Bone

Longitudinal modulus (MPa)	17,000
Transverse modulus (MPa)	11,500
Shear modulus (MPa)	3,300
Longitudinal Poisson's ratio	0.46
Transverse Poisson's ratio	0.58

From Reilly, D. J. and Burstein, A. H.
(1975). *J. Biomech.*, **8**: 393–405. With
permission.

sion. Despite these anisotropic elastic properties, cortical bone is often modeled as an isotropic, elastic material to simplify analyses. In fact, this approach is valid for uniaxial loading conditions. In these cases, the modulus is usually assumed to be approximately 14 to 18 GPa, with a Poisson's ratio of approximately 0.3 (Hayes *et al.*, 1978).

Uniaxial Strength

The strength properties of cortical bone also depend on the loading direction (Cezayirlioglu *et al.*, 1985; Pope and Outwater, 1974; Reilly and Burstein, 1975). Consequently, cortical bone is anisotropic (transversely isotropic) from both modulus and strength perspectives. The strength of cortical bone also depends on whether the bone is loaded in tension, compression, or torsion. This represents an asymmetry in the strength properties, adding further complexity to the description of these properties. Therefore, it is not sufficient to specify the strength of cortical bone with a single number.

Fig. 4 shows typical stress-strain curves for cortical bone for uniaxial, monotonic tension and compression loading, both in the longitudinal and transverse loading directions. Because the strengths are higher in compression than in tension, cortical bone is strongest in compression (Table 2). For example, the tensile strength in longitudinal loading is approximately 133 MPa, while the corresponding compressive strength is 193 MPa (Reilly and Burstein, 1975). For transverse loading, the tensile strength is very low (51 MPa), while the compressive strength (133 MPa) is comparable to its tensile strength in longitudinal loading. This suggests that cortical bone has adapted to a situation where compressive loading is greater than tensile loading. This is consistent with the combined bending and axial compressive loads which are thought to act on the femoral diaphysis during everyday activities such as gait. Under these loading conditions, maximum compressive stresses are larger than maximum tensile stresses.

Fig. 4 also shows how the tensile and compressive yield strengths of cortical bone are approximately equal to their respective ultimate strengths.

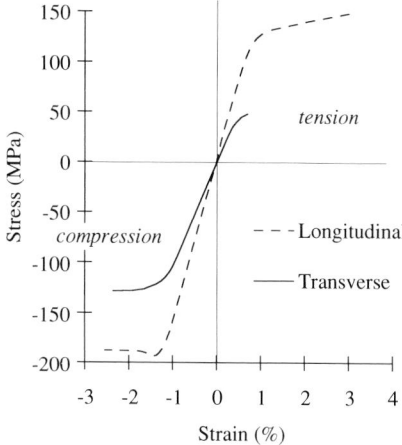

Fig. 4. Stress-strain plots for human cortical bone for tensile and compressive loading. Data are shown for both longitudinal and transverse loading directions. [From Gibson, L. J. and Ashby, M. F. (1988). *Cellular Solids: Structure and Properties*, Pergamon Press, New York. With permission.]

Table 2.
Ultimate Strength Properties of Human Femoral Cortical Bone

Longitudinal (MPa)	Tension	133
	Compression	193
Transverse (MPa)	Tension	51
	Compression	133
Shear (MPa)		68

From Reilly, D. J. and Burstein, A. H. (1975). *J. Biomech.*, **8**: 393–405. With permission.

Therefore, the maximum stresses which bone can sustain are close to its yield strength. Thus, if bone is loaded so that it is close to its yield point, it is also close to fracture. Furthermore, if bone is loaded by stresses which are just above its yield strength, the bone will deform by a relatively large amount compared to its elastic behavior. Therefore, cortical bone will undergo relatively large deformations just prior to fracture.

Energy Absorption, Ductility, and Brittleness

The total energy per unit volume absorbed by a material upon loading is equal to the total area under the stress-strain curve. Materials which absorb substantial energy before failure are classified as *tough* materials. Biomechanically, toughness is important in situations where bone is forced to absorb energy, such as in automobile accidents or falls from standing height.

If the energy delivered to the bone is greater than the energy the bone can absorb, then fracture will occur. Fig. 4 indicates that, for both tensile and compressive loading in the longitudinal direction, the strains which occur in cortical bone at failure (ultimate strains) are much larger than those which occur at yielding (yield strains). Therefore, for longitudinal loading, cortical bone is a tough material because it can absorb substantial energy before fracture. Furthermore, because the ultimate strain for longitudinal loading is substantially larger than the yield strain, cortical bone can be classified as a relatively *ductile* material for longitudinal loading. The stress-strain curve for transverse loading (Fig. 4) shows also that bone is tougher under compressive loads than under tensile loads. Consequently, bone has the lowest resistance to loading regimes which cause tensile stresses in the transverse direction. Such stresses, for example, can arise as "hoop" stresses when artificial implants are press-fit into the diaphysis of long bones. Because the ultimate strain is close to the yield strain for tension loading in the transverse direction, bone is relatively *brittle* for this loading condition. Thus, cortical bone can behave in a relatively ductile or brittle fashion, depending on the loading direction and whether tension or compression forces are applied.

Multiaxial Strength

While the uniaxial properties are the most basic, they only describe the response of bone to uniaxial loading conditions. However, because of the complexity of loading conditions *in vivo*, bone is often subjected to multiaxial loading conditions, particularly in strenuous activities which may result in bone fractures. Thus, the multiaxial strength properties of bone are important. The strength of most engineering materials depends on whether loads are applied in just one direction (uniaxial loading) or in more than one direction (multiaxial loading). For example, the strength of stainless steel is much less when loaded simultaneously by tension forces in three mutually perpendicular directions compared to the case when loaded by just one of the loads in a single direction. For most metals, the multiaxial strength can be predicted with knowledge of just the uniaxial strength. Unfortunately, this is not the case for cortical bone (Cezayirlioglu *et al.*, 1985; Cowin, 1989; Hayes and Wright, 1977; Reilly and Burstein, 1975). Therefore, experiments must be performed to find the strength of bone tissue under combinations of loads acting simultaneously in different directions. Once these multiaxial strength data are obtained, a mathematical relationship, called a *failure criterion*, can be established to predict failure for any combination of loads.

As a relatively simple example of how a multiaxial failure criterion is applied to a material, we consider the widely used von Mises yield criterion, as applied to an isotropic material such as stainless steel. The criterion predicts when yielding will occur for isotropic materials under multiaxial

$$\sigma_{\text{von Mises}} = \frac{1}{\sqrt{2}}\sqrt{(\sigma_1-\sigma_2)^2+(\sigma_1-\sigma_3)^2+(\sigma_3-\sigma_2)^2}$$

Von Mises Failure Criterion:

Failure occurs at $\sigma_{\text{von Mises}} = \sigma_Y$

Example:

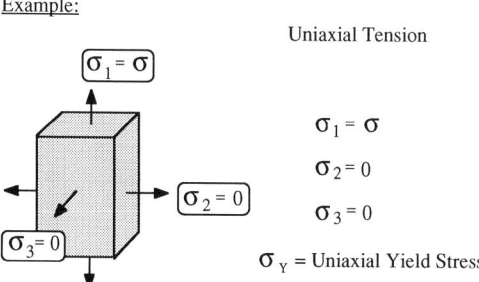

Uniaxial Tension

$\sigma_1 = \sigma$

$\sigma_2 = 0$

$\sigma_3 = 0$

σ_Y = Uniaxial Yield Stress

For Uniaxial Tension:

$\sigma_{\text{von Mises}} = \sigma$

Failure occurs at $\sigma = \sigma_Y$

Fig. 5. The von Mises yield criterion applied to an isotropic material. The mathematical expression of the von Mises stress, $\sigma_{\text{von Mises}}$, is shown in terms of the principal stresses, σ_1, σ_2, and σ_3. Failure occurs when the von Mises stress exceeds the uniaxial yield strength. For this simple case of uniaxial tension, failure is predicted when the applied stress, σ, equals the uniaxial yield strength, σ_Y.

loading. We will first describe its application to the simple case of uniaxial loading, and then describe its application to the more complicated case of multiaxial loading conditions. Fig. 5 shows a tensile force acting in the longitudinal direction on a cube. This loading produces a single stress, known as a principal stress (σ_1), in the longitudinal direction. The other two principal stresses are zero ($\sigma_2 = \sigma_3 = 0$). The von Mises stress is defined in terms of the principal stresses as shown in Fig. 5. The yield stress, σ_Y, is obtained experimentally from a uniaxial tension test, and is the only experimental strength parameter used in the von Mises yield criterion. For this trivial case of uniaxial loading, the von Mises criterion states that yielding will occur when the applied stress, σ, is equal to the uniaxial yield strength of the specimen, σ_Y. However, for some cases of multiaxial loading, the von Mises criterion predicts that yielding will occur when the largest component of the multiaxial stress state is actually less than the uniaxial yield stress.

Failure Stress

A. Biaxial Compression:

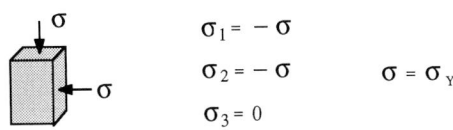

$\sigma_1 = -\sigma$

$\sigma_2 = -\sigma$ $\sigma = \sigma_Y$

$\sigma_3 = 0$

B. Triaxial Compression:

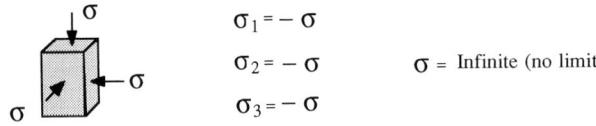

$\sigma_1 = -\sigma$

$\sigma_2 = -\sigma$ $\sigma = $ Infinite (no limit)

$\sigma_3 = -\sigma$

C. Biaxial Tension and Compression (Pure Shear):

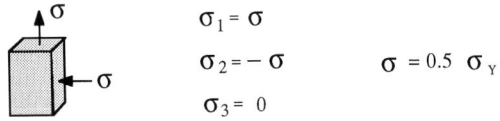

$\sigma_1 = \sigma$

$\sigma_2 = -\sigma$ $\sigma = 0.5 \ \sigma_Y$

$\sigma_3 = 0$

Fig. 6. Multiaxial loading and failure prediction using the von Mises yield criterion. Different states of multiaxial loading can result in relatively strong or weak behaviors when compared to uniaxial behavior. For biaxial compression (A), failure will occur when the magnitude of the applied stress equals the uniaxial yield strength; for triaxial compression (B), also known as hydrostatic compression, failure will never occur because the von Mises stress (see Fig. 5) is zero; for combined (biaxial) tension and compression (C), also known as pure shear, failure will occur when the magnitude of the applied stress equals one half of the uniaxial yield strength.

Fig. 6 shows the maximum stress which can be applied to the cube in the above example for some simple cases of multiaxial loading. For biaxial compression (Fig. 6a), the maximum stress is the uniaxial yield stress. For hydrostatic (same stress in each direction) compression (Fig. 6b), there is no limit on the applied stress (yielding will never occur!). For equal tension and compression in two directions (Fig. 6c), yielding will occur when the applied stress is just half the uniaxial yield stress. Therefore, depending on the type of multiaxial loading, the material may appear to be relatively strong or weak compared to its uniaxial behavior. This phenomenon occurs, not because the material is anisotropic or because of combined loading in the same direction, but because of the interaction of loading in different directions.

The von Mises criterion is just one of many yield criteria which are used to predict yielding of materials. For some materials, it is more appropriate to predict yielding based on the maximum stress in any one direction. For that criterion, yielding in the previous example would occur at the same stress level ($\sigma = \sigma_Y$) for each loading condition. This demonstrates how different yield criteria predict different multiaxial yield stresses for the same loading conditions. The von Mises yield criterion has been verified and is used for most ductile metals, while a failure criterion based on the maximum principal stress is useful for some brittle materials. Unfortunately, neither the von Mises nor the maximum principal stress criteria apply well to cortical bone.

A generalized failure criterion, applicable to almost all materials, is called the Tsai-Wu criterion (Tsai and Wu, 1971). While the uniaxial yield strength is the only material property necessary to fully characterize the (isotropic) von Mises yield criterion, up to 27 constants are necessary to fully characterize the most general version of the Tsai-Wu criterion. Fortunately, for a transversely isotropic (from a strength perspective) material such as cortical bone, only seven of these constants are independent. This simpler version of the Tsai-Wu criterion has been applied to cortical bone (Cezayirlioglu et al., 1985; Hayes and Wright, 1977) since it accounts for all the observed strength properties including directional dependence (anisotropy) and unequal values in tension and compression (asymmetry). Less general but simpler yield criteria have also been applied to cortical bone (Cezayirlioglu et al., 1985; Reilly and Burstein, 1975). These criteria either neglect anisotropy or asymmetry, but can be valid for certain loading conditions.

Fig. 7 illustrates the application of two failure criteria to human cortical bone. Specimens were loaded in either pure tension, pure compression, pure torsion, or combinations of either tension or compression with torsion (Cezayirlioglu et al., 1985). These data indicate that the maximum tensile or compressive stress that bone can sustain is reduced as shear stresses (due to torsion) are superimposed. For this relatively simple state of multiaxial stress, both the Tsai-Wu and a simpler criterion which neglects the asymmetry of strengths (the Hill criterion) provide comparable representations of the experimental data. However, a separate Hill criterion must be applied for tension and compression loading, illustrating that, while it can be used to fit data for certain loading conditions, it does not have the generality of the Tsai-Wu criterion.

As seen in Fig. 6, the major concept in the von Mises yield criterion is that the strength of a material is dependent on the type of multiaxial stress state in addition to the magnitudes of the stresses. While the von Mises failure criterion does not apply well to bone, it can be used to illustrate how multiaxial loading may be associated with the asymmetry of strengths for cortical bone. Consider the situation of the femoral diaphysis which has compressive bending stresses acting on the medial aspect, and tensile bending stresses acting on the lateral aspect (Fig. 8). Furthermore, a tensile circumferential (hoop) stress equal to half the magnitude of the bending

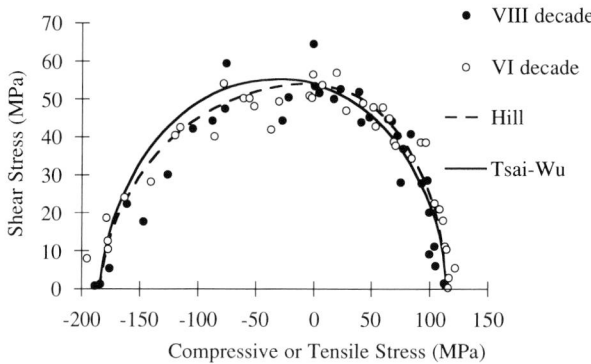

Fig. 7. Tension-torsion and compression-torsion yield stresses for human femoral cortical bone. Data are shown for two age groups. By convention, tensile stresses are positive while compressive stresses are negative. The Hill and Tsai-Wu criteria are both fitted to these data, illustrating that each of these criteria describe the multiaxial yield behavior for these relatively simple multiaxial loading cases. [From Cezayirlioglu, H., Bahniuk, E., Davy, D. T., and Heiple, K. G. (1985). *J. Biomech.*, **18**: 61–69. With permission.]

stress acts at both locations, and the radial stresses are zero. This situation could occur at the periosteal or endosteal surface of the femoral diaphysis during some strenuous activities. Fig. 8 shows that, to avoid yielding of the bone, the maximum bending stress can only be 75% of the uniaxial yield stress along the medial aspect, while it can be 115% of the uniaxial yield stress along the lateral aspect. For simplicity, assuming a uniaxial yield stress for cortical bone of 150 MPa, a bending stress of 112 MPa would cause yielding along the compressive side, while yielding would not occur along the lateral aspect until the bending stress is 172 MPa. This simple example indicates that, if bone were an isotropic material with equal strengths in tension and compression, it would be weaker along the medial aspect than along the lateral aspect. In reality, bone is stronger in compression (the medial aspect of the femur) than in tension (the lateral aspect). This asymmetry of strengths may be related to an adaption of bone strength for *in vivo* multiaxial loading.

Viscoelastic Behavior

A material is said to display *viscoelastic* behavior if any of its mechanical properties depend on time, i.e., on how fast (strain rate sensitivity) or how long (creep behavior) loads are applied to the material. Cortical bone displays viscous behavior because its mechanical properties are sensitive to both strain rate and the duration of the applied loads.

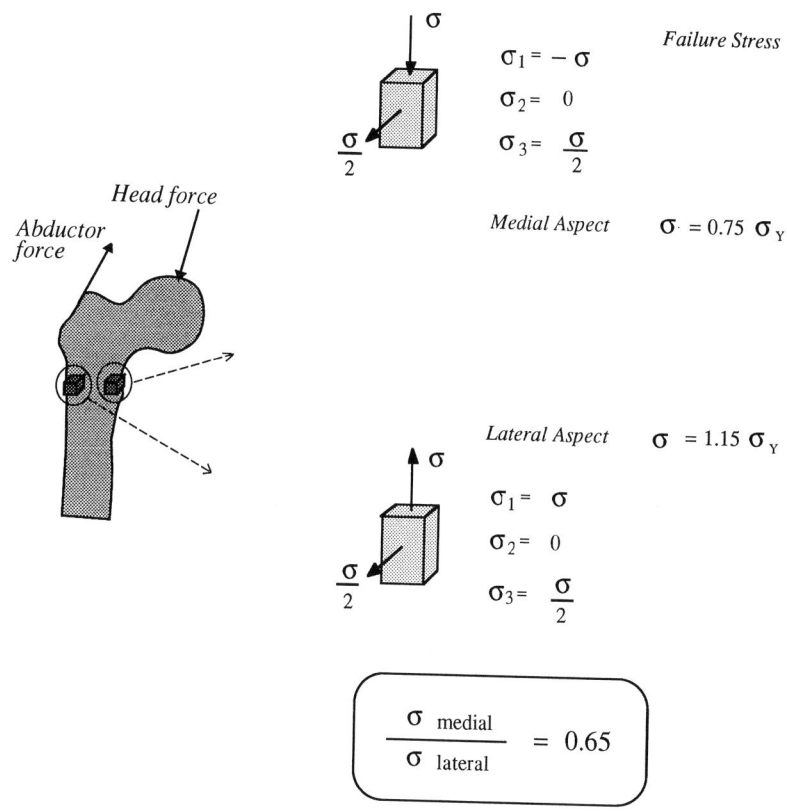

$$\sigma_1 = -\sigma$$

$$\sigma_2 = 0$$

$$\sigma_3 = \frac{\sigma}{2}$$

Failure Stress

Medial Aspect $\sigma = 0.75\ \sigma_Y$

Head force

Abductor force

Lateral Aspect $\sigma = 1.15\ \sigma_Y$

$$\sigma_1 = \sigma$$

$$\sigma_2 = 0$$

$$\sigma_3 = \frac{\sigma}{2}$$

$$\frac{\sigma\ \text{medial}}{\sigma\ \text{lateral}} = 0.65$$

Fig. 8. Multiaxial failure criteria and stresses in the proximal femur for strenuous exercise. The von Mises yield criterion predicts that bone should be weakest for compressive loading, which occurs mainly on the medial aspect. For this example, the maximum stress before yielding on the medial aspect is only 65% of the maximum stress on the lateral aspect. Therefore, bone may have adapted for multiaxial loads by developing extra strength for compressive loading.

Strain Rate Sensitivity

The *in vivo* strain rate for bone can vary by more than an order of magnitude in the course of daily activities such as slow walking (strain rate = 0.001 per second), brisk walking (strain rate = 0.01 per second), and slow running (strain rate = 0.03 per second) (Lanyon *et al.*, 1975, 1981, 1982; Nunamaker *et al.*, 1990; O'Connor *et al.*, 1982; Robertson and Smith, 1978). Other activities, such as a jump from the height of two stairs and a fall from standing height, might result in strain rates as high as those encountered during slow and fast running, respectively. Generally, strain rate increases as activity becomes more strenuous.

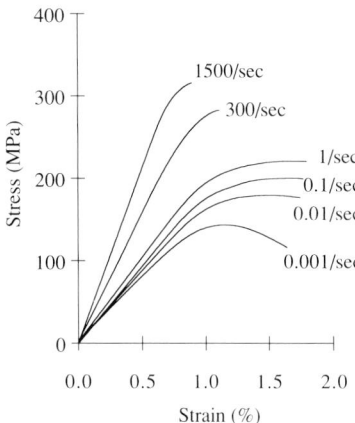

Fig. 9. Strain rate dependence of cortical bone material behavior. Both modulus and strength increase for increased strain rates. [From McElhaney, J. H. (1966). *J. Appl. Physiol.*, **21**: 1231–1236. With permission.]

The mechanical properties of cortical bone are sensitive to strain rate (Crowninshield and Pope, 1974; McElhaney, 1966; Saha and Hayes, 1976; Wright and Hayes, 1976b). Fig. 9 shows how the stress-strain behavior (for longitudinal compression of bovine bone) is sensitive to strain rate. Since the initial slope of the stress-strain plot increases as the strain rate increases, cortical bone has a higher modulus at higher strain rates. However, for typical daily activity (strain rates from 0.001 to 0.01 per second), the modulus only changes by approximately 15%, indicating that, for normal activities, strain rate does not affect modulus appreciably (Crowninshield and Pope, 1974; McElhaney, 1966; Wright and Hayes, 1976b).

Fig. 9 also shows how strength depends on strain rate. The yield and ultimate strengths of cortical bone increase as the strain rate increases over the complete range of strain rates. This indicates that cortical bone is stronger for more strenuous activity. Fig. 10 shows how the ultimate tensile strength is slightly more sensitive to strain rate than is modulus, since the same change in strain rate produces a relatively larger change in strength than in modulus. These data indicate that bone is approximately 20% stronger for brisk walking than for slow walking (Crowninshield and Pope, 1974; Wright and Hayes, 1976b).

As shown in Fig. 9, at very high strain rates (greater than 0.1 per second) representing high impact trauma, cortical bone becomes more brittle (ultimate strain decreases) for loading in the longitudinal direction (McElhaney, 1966; Saha and Hayes, 1976). Thus, cortical bone exhibits a ductile to brittle transition as the strain rate increases (Behiri and Bonfield, 1984; Carter and Caler, 1985; Wright and Hayes, 1980). However, for the range of strain rates typical of more normal activity (less than 0.1 per second),

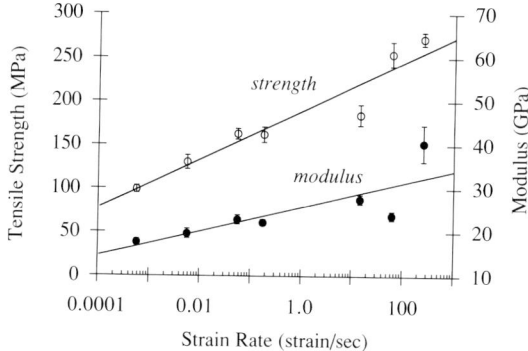

Fig. 10. Comparison of strain rate sensitivities for modulus and ultimate tensile strength of human cortical bone for longitudinal loading. Over the full range of strain rates, strength increases by about a factor of three, and modulus by a factor of two. [From Wright, T. M. and Hayes, W. C. (1976). *Med. Biol. Eng. Comput.* **14**: 671–680. With permission.]

ductility increases (ultimate strain increases) as strain rate increases. Based on the shapes of these stress-strain plots, and recalling that energy per unit volume is equal to the area below the stress-strain curve, there is an optimal range of strain rates for maximum energy absorption (strain rates from 0.01 to 0.1 per second). This suggests that bone has adapted to absorb energy from the impact which arises from relatively strenuous activities such as running.

Creep Behavior

If bone tissue is subjected to a constant stress for an extended period of time, it will continue to deform even though the stress is constant (Caler and Carter, 1989; Carter and Caler, 1983; 1985; Fondrk *et al.*, 1988). This phenomenon is called *creep* behavior. Fig. 11 shows a typical creep curve for adult human cortical bone under tensile loading. This curve, which is a plot of strain as a function of time for a constant stress level, indicates that the three characteristic stages of creep behavior exhibited by many conventional engineering materials are also exhibited by cortical bone (Caler and Carter, 1989; Carter and Caler, 1985). In the primary creep stage, there is continued specimen strain after loading with a gradually decreasing creep (increase in strain) rate. In the secondary creep stage, a lower, usually constant creep rate occurs. Finally, in the tertiary creep stage, there is a marked increase in the creep rate just before creep fracture occurs. This curve indicates that, if cortical bone is loaded for enough time, creep fracture will occur, even though the stress level is well below the yield and ultimate strengths. For example, the data in Fig. 11 indicate that creep fracture will occur if a

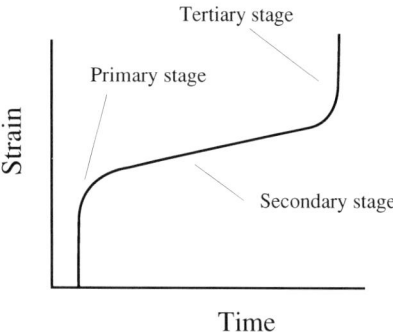

Fig. 11. Schematic diagram showing the three stages of creep behavior of human cortical bone. [From Carter, D. R. and Caler, W. E. (1985). *J. Orthop. Res.*, **3**: 84–90. With permission.]

tensile stress of approximately 60 MPa is applied for about 7 h. Recall that the longitudinal tension ultimate strength for cortical bone is approximately 133 MPa. Thus, creep fracture can occur at substantially lower levels of stress than monotonic fracture. In addition, Fig. 12 illustrates how the time required for creep fracture to occur decreases as the stress increases and how the resistance to creep fracture is greater for compression than for tension loading (Caler and Carter, 1989).

If creep occurs without fracture, and then the bone is fully unloaded, permanent deformations will develop (Fondrk *et al.*, 1988). For example, if creep occurs due to the action of relatively high tensile stresses held for several minutes, and the specimen is unloaded before creep fracture occurs, the specimen will have a permanent deformation so that it will be longer than its original length. This behavior is referred to as *viscoplastic* behavior, the viscosity due to the creep behavior during loading, and the plasticity due to permanent deformation after unloading. Furthermore, if the applied constant stress is above a threshold level (Fondrk *et al.*, 1988), which is approximately 70 MPa for human cortical for longitudinal tension loading, or 55% of its ultimate strength, then the rate at which creep deformation occurs and the magnitude of the permanent deformation after unloading both increase sharply (Fig. 13). Creep studies have not yet been performed for loading in the transverse direction.

To date, the mechanisms for creep behavior in cortical bone have not been determined and remain an open question. However, scanning electron micrographs of fractured surfaces have shown that osteon pullout is common for tensile loading, whereas fractures tend to cross through osteons for compressive loading (Caler and Carter, 1989). Thus, the creep mechanisms appear to be different for tensile and compressive loading. Studies on the viscoplastic behavior for tensile loading have suggested that damage occurs at the level of the collagen fibers because the creep behaviors of fully

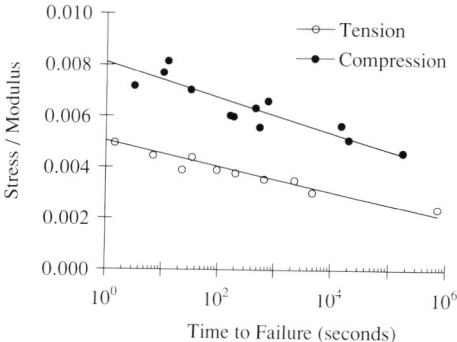

Fig. 12. Creep fracture stress for human cortical bone as a function of the time to failure. To account for variations in modulus between specimens, stress values have been normalized (divided) by the initial modulus (measured at the beginning of the experiment). These data indicate that resistance to creep fracture is greater for compressive loading. [From Caler, W. E. and Carter, D. R. (1989). *J. Biomech.*, **22**: 625–635. With permission.]

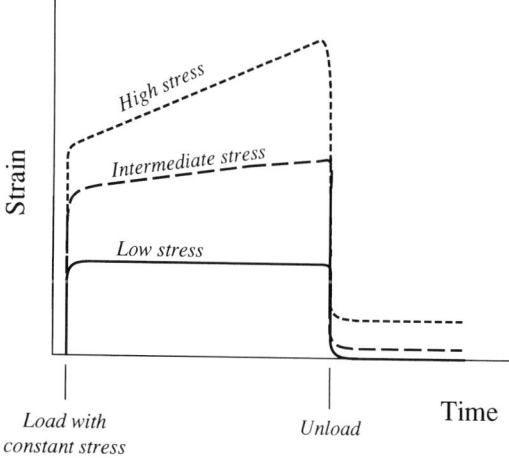

Fig. 13. Schematic of typical strain-time curves, illustrating the viscoplastic behavior of human cortical bone. In this experiment, the bone is loaded at a constant stress, and the strain is measured as a function of time. The specimen is then unloaded before creep fracture occurs. Typical behaviors are shown for different applied stresses. As the stress is increased, a creep threshold is reached, beyond which the creep rate (in the second stage of creep behavior) increases. The permanent deformation (strain after unloading) also increases as the applied stress is increased. [From Fondrk, M., Bahniuk, E., Davy, D. T., and Michaels, C. (1988). *J. Biomech.*, **21**: 623–630. With permission.] Interestingly, exactly similar behavior occurs for some glass-fiber composite materials at elevated temperatures.

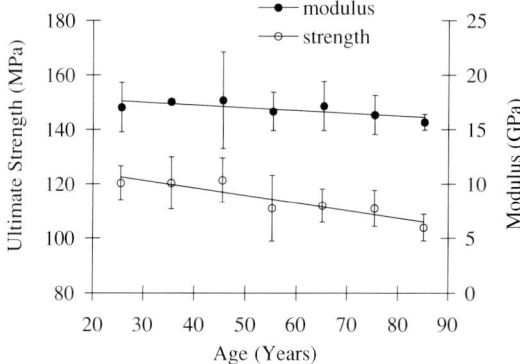

Fig. 14. Age-related effects on longitudinal modulus and ultimate tensile strength of human femoral cortical bone. [From Burstein *et al.* (1976). *J. Bone Jt. Surg.*, **58**: 82–86. With permission.]

secondary (many osteons) and predominantly primary (few osteons) bone are similar (Fondrk *et al.*, 1988).

Age Effects

With aging, both the modulus and strength properties of cortical bone progressively deteriorate (Burstein *et al.*, 1976; Currey, 1969; Lindahl and Lindgren, 1967), and these changes are similar for men and women (Burstein *et al.*, 1976). Fig. 14 shows that both the longitudinal modulus and tensile yield strength of cortical bone taken from the femoral middiaphysis decrease by approximately 2%/decade after age 20. For example, the ultimate tensile strength of bone (for longitudinal loading) decreases from approximately 140 to 120 MPa from the 3rd to 9th decades, respectively. Over the same period, the corresponding elastic moduli change from approximately 17 to 15.6 GPa, while the slope of the stress-strain curve after yielding actually increases by 8%/decade (Burstein *et al.*, 1976). Probably the most significant change from a fracture risk perspective is the reduction in energy absorption (area under the stress-strain curve) which occurs with aging. Energy absorption decreases by approximately 7%/decade (Burstein *et al.*, 1976), and is due mainly to reductions in the ultimate strain. Taken together, these data indicate that cortical bone material, at least in the human femur, becomes less stiff, less strong, and more brittle with aging.

Microstructure and Mechanical Properties

The age-related changes just described can vary for different long bones. For example, decreases in ultimate tensile strength and modulus are greater for the femur than for the tibia, while decreases in ultimate strain are similar for each bone (Burstein *et al.*, 1976). One explanation for this is that the rate of bone turnover in the tibia may be greater than in the femur, so that the mechanism which reduces both modulus and strength is inhibited as new osteons are formed (Burstein *et al.*, 1976). However, many parameters affect the mechanical properties of cortical bone.

In general, the parameters which have been investigated as determinants of the mechanical properties of cortical bone are apparent density (proportional to porosity) (Carter and Caler, 1981; Carter *et al.*, 1976; Currey, 1988a; Keller *et al.*, 1990; Schaffler and Burr, 1988; Snyder and Schneider, 1990), ash density (total mineral content divided by bulk volume) (Burstein *et al.*, 1975; Currey, 1988a; Keller *et al.*, 1990; Snyder and Schneider, 1990), histology (number of osteons, primary vs. secondary bone) (Carter *et al.*, 1976; Evans and Riolo, 1970; Evans and Vincentelli, 1974; Lipson and Katz, 1984), collagen composition and content (Burstein *et al.*, 1975; Lees and Davidson, 1977), orientation of the collagen fibers and mineral (Katz and Meunier, 1987; Sasaki *et al.*, 1989, 1991), composition of the cement lines (Burr *et al.*, 1988), bonding between the mineral and collagen phases (Bundy, 1985), and accumulation of microcracks in the bone matrix and osteons (Carter and Hayes, 1977b).

The difficulty in correlating these parameters with the mechanical properties of cortical bone is that the ranges of modulus and strength values for this tissue are relatively small. Consequently, many of these issues remain equivocal, and we only summarize the less controversial findings. The overall evidence is that many parameters contribute significantly to the mechanical properties of cortical bone. Modulus and ultimate strength are positively correlated with apparent density by a power law (Carter and Hayes, 1977c; Currey, 1988a; Keller *et al.*, 1990; Schaffler and Burr, 1988; Snyder and Schneider, 1990) with reported exponents for modulus ranging from 1.54 (Keller *et al.*, 1990) to 7.4 (Schaffler and Burr, 1988). Both monotonic and fatigue (see below) strengths are sensitive to the relative content of osteons (Carter *et al.*, 1976; Evans and Riolo, 1970; Evans and Vincentelli, 1974; Robertson and Smith, 1978). It has been shown that density and microstructure are correlated, suggesting that Haversian remodeling of primary bone is accompanied by a reduction in density (Carter *et al.*, 1976). Even so, microstructure has been shown to affect some mechanical properties after accounting for these changes in density (Carter *et al.*, 1976). Probably the most important determinant of modulus and strength is the ash density or mineral content. In a study on properties of cortical bone for a wide range of species, multiple regression analysis demonstrated that up to 88% of the variance in modulus and strength can be explained using a power law model with volume fraction (proportional to apparent density) and mineral content (proportional to ash density) as independent variables (Currey, 1988a). Wet bone, as found *in situ*, is also less stiff, less strong, and less brittle than fully dried bone (Currey, 1988b; Evans, 1973), although rewetting bone after it has been dried can almost fully restore the *in situ* behavior (Currey, 1988b). This indicates the importance of water content to the mechanical properties of cortical bone. Finally, collagen content has been shown to dominate the stiffness behavior after yielding has occurred (Burstein *et al.*, 1975).

Fatigue Properties

The strength properties described above characterize situations where there is a single application of force (monotonic loading). However, cortical bone is primarily exposed *in vivo* to repetitive, low-intensity loading, producing stress levels less than those required to fracture a bone specimen during monotonic loading. This cyclic loading of bone can result in damage at the microstructural level (Carter *et al.*, 1981; Carter and Hayes, 1977a; Schaffler *et al.*, 1989). For example, during gait, the proximal femur is loaded cyclically with each step. The rib cage is also cyclically loaded while breathing. Another type of cyclic loading, where the number of cycles per unit of time is less, is when the spine is cyclically loaded while lifting objects, raising from a chair, and bending over. Not all loads necessarily result in damage to bone. If damage does occur, however, and if the damage can accumulate over time, the strength of the bone is reduced (Carter and Hayes, 1977b). High levels of stress over shorter periods of time may also lead to fatigue damage, evidenced by the relatively frequent incidence of stress fractures in military recruits, active individuals, and race horses subjected to rigorous training programs (Nunamaker *et al.*, 1990; Orava and Hulkko, 1984; Tehranzadeh *et al.*, 1989). Thus, the major etiology of these fractures appears to be due to fatigue damage accumulation (Carter and Hayes, 1977a). The mechanical properties of bone under the action of cyclic, repetitive loading are called the *fatigue* properties of bone.

Besides being interesting for their role in stress fractures, fatigue properties of cortical bone are also of interest as a potential stimulus for strain-induced bone remodeling (Burr *et al.*, 1985; Carter and Hayes, 1977a; Martin and Burr, 1982). The fatigue properties of cortical bone have mainly been measured for devitalized bone specimens. Therefore, the effects of bone remodeling on the fatigue behavior of bone *in vivo* remain unknown. However, because physiologic levels of loading can induce fatigue damage and failure *in vitro* (Carter and Caler, 1981; Schaffler *et al.*, 1989), bone remodeling, which occurs continuously with bone *in vivo*, may repair the damage which occurs due to relatively low-intensity loading, such as gait (Carter and Caler, 1981; Martin and Burr, 1989). Indeed, studies have demonstrated that microcracks do occur *in vivo* (Burr *et al.*, 1985; Burr and Stafford, 1990; Frost, 1960). Thus, it has been hypothesized that bone remodeling occurs to repair microcracks which form in bone due to the repetitive loading of daily activity (Burr *et al.*, 1985; Carter and Hayes, 1977a; Lipson and Katz, 1984; Martin and Burr, 1982).

Up to 10 and over 50% of age-related hip and spine fractures, respectively, are classified as spontaneous because they occur without any obvious trauma. If fatigue cracks accumulate in bone due to years of repetitive loading, and there are age-related reduced rates of bone turnover to repair these cracks, bone strength may be compromised. Thus, it is feasible that the fatigue behavior of bone may be a factor in the etiology of spontaneous fractures. Consequently, the fatigue behavior of cortical bone is of interest from three perspectives: (1) as the major etiologic factor in stress fractures, (2) as a candidate stimulus for bone remodeling, and (3) as a possible etiologic factor in age-related spontaneous fractures.

There are two basic approaches to studying the fatigue properties of cortical bone. The more conventional approach is to use traditional concepts of stress and strain and apply them to cyclic loading conditions. The other approach is to use concepts of a more contemporary engineering discipline called *fracture mechanics* (Broek, 1986). In each approach, the objective is to describe how the strength of bone changes after loading for a given number of cycles. Again, these properties are material properties, and are independent of geometry.

Traditional Approach for Fatigue Life Prediction

To determine the fatigue properties of bone using traditional engineering techniques, standard specimens of bone are tested in controlled environments at a fixed level of stress (or, sometimes strain) and cyclically loaded to fracture. Using this method, the number of load cycles at fracture is recorded as the fatigue life corresponding to the specified stress level. Testing is performed for different stress levels and the corresponding fatigue life is found for each stress level. Results are usually presented as an S-N plot of stress level (S) vs. the logarithm of the fatigue life, or, number of cycles (N). Fig. 15 shows an idealized S-N curve for cortical bone. This curve indicates that fatigue fracture will occur at a given stress level if the number of load cycles is large enough. Conversely, one can think in terms of a fatigue life: under a given stress level, how many load cycles can be endured by the bone tissue before fracture. The important concept is that fatigue fracture, like creep fracture, can occur at stress levels which are substantially lower than the monotonic strength.

The fatigue life of bone is better correlated with strains than with stresses (Carter *et al.*, 1981), and in particular, with ranges of strains (defined as the difference between the maximum and minimum values of the applied cyclic strain). Fig. 16 shows how the *in vitro* fatigue life, for high cyclic strain ranges, depends on strain range for human bone. Strain ranges

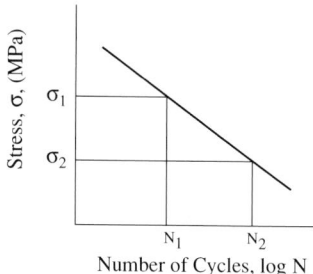

Fig. 15. Idealized fatigue S-N curve for cortical bone. Fatigue fracture occurs at stress σ_1 in N_1 cycles, or at stress level σ_2 at N_2 cycles. Note that the fatigue life (N) is shown on a log scale.

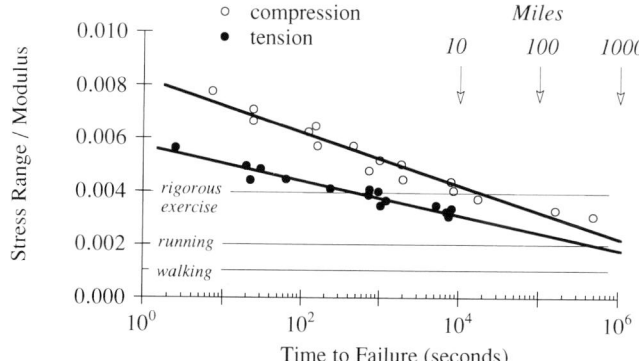

Fig. 16. Fatigue life curve as a function of strain-range (stress range/modulus) for human femoral cortical bone for compressive and tensile loading. Typical strain ranges for different activities are shown, and typical distances for walking and running are also shown. Values are extrapolated for less strenuous activities. Note that, as with creep behavior, resistance to fatigue fracture is greater for compressive loading. [From Carter, D. R. *et al.* (1981). *Acta Orthop. Scand.*, **52**: 481–490. With permission.]

representative of normal walking, mild exercise, and rigorous exercise are also shown. On average, approximately 5000 cycles of loading correspond to the number of steps in 10 miles of running, while one million cycles correspond to 1000 miles. The data in Fig. 16 indicate that a total running distance of less than 1000 miles could cause fracture of cortical bone (Carter *et al.*, 1981). This is consistent with stress fractures observed with military recruits who commonly undergo strenuous training programs of up to 1000 miles of running over a 6-week period.

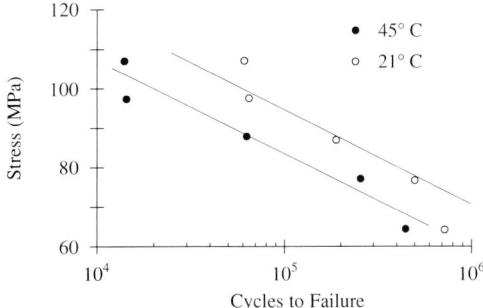

Fig. 17. Temperature dependence of fatigue life for bovine femoral cortical bone. Each data point represents the mean value for six specimens. The straight lines were statistically derived from all the specimen data. Fatigue life is reduced by a factor of three when temperature is increased from 21° to 45°C. [From Carter, D. R. and Hayes, W. C. (1976). *J. Biomech.*, **9**: 27–34. With permission.]

The fatigue life of bone is also dependent on temperature (Carter and Hayes, 1976). Fig. 17 shows the S-N curve for bovine cortical bone for two different temperatures (21° and 45°C). These data indicate that the fatigue life of cortical bone can be reduced by a factor of three as temperature is increased from room temperature to body core temperature. Foot skin temperatures of up to 43°C have been recorded in subjects walking briskly in a warm environment. Since deep tissue temperatures in the extremities can be within 2°C of skin temperatures, bone temperatures in the foot may vary from less than room temperature to a few degrees above body core temperature. Therefore, the temperature dependence of fatigue properties may have physiologic consequences. For example, military recruits may be at higher risk of stress fractures when training in hot, desert climates than in cooler climates. Similarly, jogging in cold weather may cause less fatigue damage in cortical bone than jogging in hot weather.

We have seen that increases in strain rate result in increases in the monotonic strength of cortical bone. However, for a fixed stress level, fatigue damage increases with increasing strain rate (Schaffler *et al.*, 1989). Therefore, more fatigue damage occurs for more strenuous exercise. Furthermore, for a fixed stress level, the fatigue life of cortical bone in uniaxial tension is less than in uniaxial compression (Caler and Carter, 1989). This indicates that regions of cortical bone which are in tension are at higher risk of fatigue failure than regions loaded in compression at the same magnitude. Indeed, studies have shown that the damage patterns for tension and compression loading are different, with mostly osteon debonding for tension and oblique cracking for compression (Carter and Hayes, 1977a). An important use of the curves shown in Fig. 16 is to estimate the damage which accumulates in the bone due to a number of cycles of loading at a particular strain-range level. One simple approach is to assume that there is a linear rate of damage accumulation at each strain-range level. From Fig. 16, we see that the *in vitro* fatigue life at a strain range of 0.002 is approximately 10^6 cycles. Therefore, a linear damage model (known as Miner's Rule) implies that 10^4 cycles at a strain range 0.002 (10 miles of running) uses up $10^4/10^6$ (one hundreth) of the fatigue life. In the absence of a biologic repair process, 100 of these 10-mile runs would use up all the fatigue life and cause fracture. Similarly, a few cycles of very high loads could substantially reduce the fatigue life, so that subsequent activities such as walking could cause fatigue fracture after, say, 10^6 cycles (approximately 1 year). Therefore, fatigue damage accumulation is likely an important etiologic factor in stress fractures (Carter and Hayes, 1977a).

Since most of the reported fatigue data has been derived from *in vitro* tests, little is known about *in vivo* fatigue damage accumulation and repair. Fatigue cracks do occur *in vivo* (Burr *et al.*, 1985; Burr and Stafford, 1990; Frost, 1960) and *in vivo* studies of bone remodeling have shown that dynamic loading (high strain rates) stimulates remodeling more than static loading (Rubin and Lanyon, 1987). The number of *in vivo* cracks also can increase with increasing loading rate (Burr *et al.*, 1985). Thus, it has been proposed that the osteonal remodeling process is associated with repair of fatigue damage. Furthermore, if the remodeling process is impaired due to aging or other reasons, fatigue damage accumulation in devitalized bone may approach that which occurs *in vivo*. In any case, the *in vitro* fatigue properties described above should present a lower bound on the *in vivo* properties.

Mechanisms

Since fatigue behavior is such an important aspect of the material properties of bone, much interest has developed in the actual mechanism of fatigue damage accumulation in cortical bone. It has been shown that the fatigue mechanism for cortical bone is similar to the mechanism for artificial, oriented, short-fiber composite materials (Carter and Hayes, 1977a; Martin and Burr, 1989; Wright and Hayes, 1976a). As with creep fracture, there are three characteristic stages of fatigue fracture, corresponding to crack initiation, crack growth (propagation), and final fracture. Since the modulus of the bone decreases as cracks form, these three stages can be demonstrated by a plot of modulus vs. number of cycles (Fig. 18). In the primary stage, crack initiation results in a small decrease in modulus. In the secondary stage, crack propagation results in a slow but steady decrease in modulus. Finally, in the tertiary stage, fracture is preceded by rapid decreases in modulus. The precise shape of these E-N curves depends on the magnitude and sign (tension vs. compression) of the applied load (Pattin, 1991).

For cortical bone, lacunae and canaliculi may act as crack initiators because these discontinuities in the bone microstructure can cause local

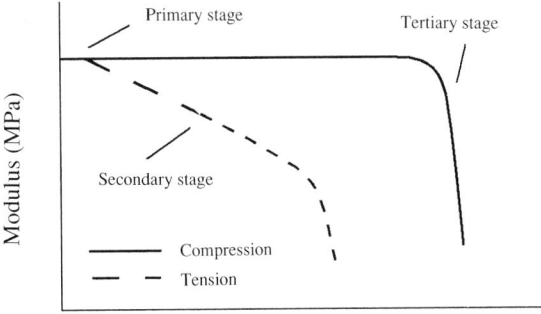

Fig. 18. Schematic diagram of the modulus degradation which occurs for human cortical bone with fatigue loading. Note the different behaviors for tensile and compressive loading. [From Pattin, C. A. G. (1991). Ph.D. dissertation, Stanford University, Palo Alto, CA. With permission.]

increases in stress (stress concentrations). Therefore, cracks are easily started in cortical bone. However, crack initiation, *per se,* is not necessarily detrimental to the structural integrity of cortical bone. Indeed, as mentioned above, these cracks may induce bone remodeling (Burr *et al.,* 1985). Furthermore, cortical bone has been shown to remodel so that stress concentrations about holes are reduced (Burstein *et al.,* 1972a). Therefore, bone not only repairs cracks, but may also remodel to reduce stresses about these cracks. What becomes important then is how well bone can stop the growth of cracks so that they remain small enough to be repaired by remodeling.

The second and most important stage of fatigue failure is the slow propagation of these microcracks. Cracks tend to join together once they progress beyond the initiation stage. These larger cracks then run into weak material interfaces (cement lines) between the osteons in the secondary Haversian systems (Burr *et al.,* 1988; Wright and Hayes, 1980). This causes two things to occur. First, some osteons debond from the matrix, contributing to the commonly observed "osteon pullout" phenomenon on fractured surfaces of cortical bone. Second, the direction of crack propagation is changed from being perpendicular to the loading direction to being parallel to the loading direction. Fig. 19 shows schematically how this has the effect of producing a stress at the crack tip which, instead of opening the crack, becomes parallel to the crack, and therefore harmless.

These effects, and possibly others, tend to stop cracks from progressing across bone in the transverse direction, thus increasing the resistance to propagation of transverse cracks under longitudinal loading. This mechanism occurs because there are many weak interfaces in bone which stop the progression of cracks. These include the interfaces between the osteons and

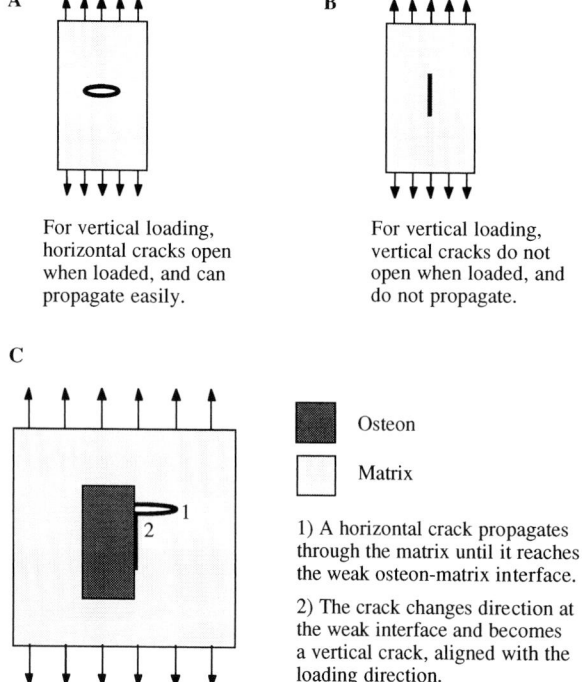

A

For vertical loading, horizontal cracks open when loaded, and can propagate easily.

B

For vertical loading, vertical cracks do not open when loaded, and do not propagate.

C

Osteon

Matrix

1) A horizontal crack propagates through the matrix until it reaches the weak osteon-matrix interface.

2) The crack changes direction at the weak interface and becomes a vertical crack, aligned with the loading direction.

Fig. 19. Schematic diagram showing how the cement line at the weak osteon interface can actually stop a crack from transversing across a whole bone. Transverse cracks, which would propagate easily for longitudinal loading in the absence of osteons (A), are converted into longitudinal cracks when they reach the weak osteon interface (C). Longitudinal cracks do not propagate easily for longitudinal loading (B). Thus, the osteonal microstructure of mature human cortical bone provides an effective mechanism to inhibit crack propagation.

the interstitial material, between adjacent lamellae in the interstitial material, or even between the interfaces within single osteons. Therefore, even if cracks are easily formed due to the presence of natural voids, other imperfections in the microstructure, namely the weak interfaces in the Haversian system, tend to stop their progression under loads typical of normal activity.

This second stage of fatigue damage only results in a slight reduction of modulus in bone (Martin and Burr, 1989; Pattin, 1991). However, because of damage accumulation, it reduces the fatigue life of bone. As damage accumulates in the specimen, the modulus gradually decreases. Eventually, the specimen fails as the final crack speeds across the specimen, resulting in a sharp decrease in modulus. Thus, the final stage of fatigue fracture occurs because cracks coalesce and become so large that the weak interfaces can no longer absorb them.

Fracture Mechanics Approach for Fatigue Life Prediction

The other, more-general approach to studying fatigue in bone makes use of engineering fracture mechanics (Bonfield, 1987; Broek, 1986). This approach assumes that there are flaws (cracks, holes, voids) in a material, and that cracks propagate from these flaws, resulting in fracture when the crack has extended across an entire cross-section. Fracture mechanics can quantify the resistance to fracture of a material, and can also quantify how fast cracks will propagate from existing flaws.

The most important parameter in fracture mechanics is the stress intensity factor (K), which is used to predict whether or not monotonic fracture will occur for a material containing a crack. K relates stresses at the crack tip to the nominal stress acting on the specimen, the crack length, and geometry:

$$K = \alpha\sigma\,\{\pi a\}^{0.5} \tag{3}$$

where α is a dimensionless function (sometimes of the crack length) which depends on geometry, σ is the nominal stress, and a is the crack length. The units of K are $N\ m^{-1.5}$ (usually given as $MN\ m^{-1.5}$ or $MPa\ m^{0.5}$). Standard values of α are documented in engineering handbooks for many specimen geometries. However, sophisticated structural analysis techniques such as the finite element method (Zienkiewicz, 1977) are necessary to find K for complicated geometries such as whole bones.

The fracture mechanics failure criterion is that fracture occurs when K is greater than the *critical stress intensity factor* (K_C), which is a material property analogous to ultimate strength. The critical stress intensity factor can be measured in the materials testing laboratory, though it is quite sensitive to the specimen geometry, loads, temperature, moisture content, and strain rate. Fig. 20 shows the relationship between the crack length which causes fracture a_c, (the critical crack length) and the applied nominal stress, σ, for a test specimen which contains a crack of a given length in one side (single edge notch, SEN, specimen). If one measures the product of the critical crack length times the applied stress, this product is constant for a given material. This constant is proportional to the critical stress intensity factor (K_C). Thus, the critical stress intensity factor is a measure of a material's resistance to fracture. Fig. 20 shows how, for a given nominal stress, the critical crack length increases as K_C increases. Materials with a high value of K_C are called tough materials because they can sustain a long crack before fracturing. For this reason, K_C is often called the *fracture toughness*.

Note that the fracture toughness (K_C) is different from what is sometimes referred to as toughness in the more traditional engineering literature. The latter term simply means the ability of a material to absorb energy (area under the stress-strain curve). This measure does not account for how the

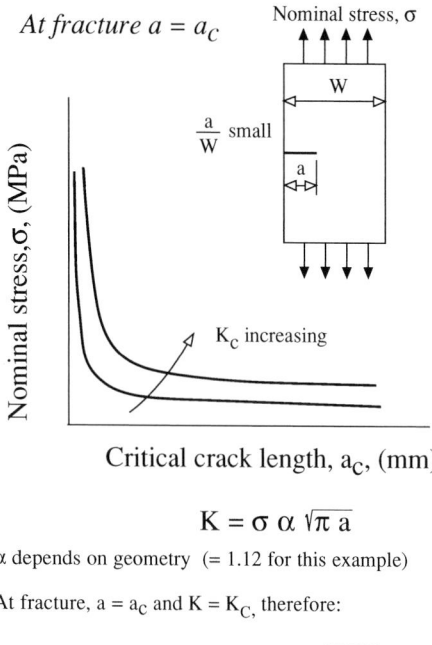

$$K = \sigma \, \alpha \, \sqrt{\pi \, a}$$

α depends on geometry (= 1.12 for this example)

At fracture, $a = a_c$ and $K = K_C$, therefore:

$$K_C = \sigma \, \alpha \, \sqrt{\pi \, a_c}$$

Fig. 20. Nominal stress, σ, vs. critical crack length, a_c, for a wide plate in uniaxial tensile loading. The stress intensity factor (K) is a function of nominal stress (σ), crack length (a), and specimen geometry (α), as shown. At fracture, the crack length is equal to the critical crack length, and the stress intensity factor is equal to the critical stress intensity factor (K_C). The plot of nominal stress vs. critical crack length indicates that, for a given nominal stress, materials with higher K_C values can sustain longer cracks before fracture than materials with lower K_C values.

presence of a crack reduces a material's resistance to fracture. Therefore, fracture toughness is a unique material property. However, high toughness materials (large energy absorption) generally have a high fracture toughness.

Values of K_C for cortical bone have been reported from 0.23 MN m$^{-1.5}$ (Bonfield *et al.*, 1978) to 15.9 MN m$^{-1.5}$ (Moyle and Gavens, 1986). Thus, the variation in reported values of K_C is considerable. In addition, cortical bone is tougher for cracks which propagate across bone in the transverse plane than for cracks which propagate along bone in the longitudinal direction (Bonfield, 1987; Pope and Outwater, 1972).

Like the other material properties of cortical bone, K_C is also sensitive to strain rate, density, and age. K_C increases as the strain rate increases (Behiri and Bonfield, 1984; Bonfield *et al.*, 1978; Robertson *et al.*, 1978), indicating that bone can better resist fracture for more traumatic loading rates. This is consistent with the observation that ultimate strength increases with increased strain rate. However, as mentioned earlier, bone exhibits a ductile-brittle transition, so that beyond a certain strain rate the fracture toughness (and energy absorption) decreases (Behiri and Bonfield, 1984; Wright and Hayes, 1980). Indeed, many metals also display this ductile-brittle transition as temperature is decreased. Thus, above a certain loading rate, fracture is catastrophic and sudden, while, below this threshold, fracture is slow and progressive (Behiri and Bonfield, 1984). For loading rates typical of a gunshot wound or vehicular accident, the fracture toughness can be quite low. Consequently, the optimal fracture toughness appears to be for relatively strenuous impact loading.

Fracture toughness increases with increased bone density (Behiri and Bonfield, 1984; Wright and Hayes, 1977). For example, a 5% decrease in bone density results in a 30% decrease in fracture toughness (Wright and Hayes, 1977). This indicates that osteoporosis, which manifests as a reduction in bone density, may considerably reduce fracture toughness. Similarly, K_C is reduced with aging (Bonfield, 1987; Pope and Outwater, 1972). The fracture toughness of human bone decreases by a factor of approximately two (4.5 to 2.5 MN m$^{-1.5}$) from ages 25 to 90 years (Bonfield, 1987). Thus, fracture mechanics indicates that cortical bone is less capable of sustaining cracks (has a lower resistance to fracture) in older people than in younger people.

These changes in K_C indicate how the fracture toughness of cortical bone tissue changes for monotonic loading conditions. Consequently, the effects of bone porosity and high loading rates on the integrity of bone under cyclic loading can be substantial. For example, the cortical bone in an elderly osteoporotic patient may have a much lower fracture toughness than in a young healthy patient. Recall that materials with low values of fracture toughness can tolerate only small cracks before fracture. Furthermore, cracks in bone occur as damage accumulation due to fatigue loading. Studies of fatigue damage accumulation in cortical bone specimens cyclically loaded *in vitro* have shown that increased damage accumulation can occur due to an increase in strain rate, and that this damage consists of an increase in the number of cracks, but not their average length (Schaffler *et al.*, 1989). However, it is feasible that the average crack length or the maximum crack length could increase as the loading level is increased (this experiment has not yet been done). Consider the case where the same fatigue damage has accumulated over time in both osteoporotic and healthy patients. Then, because the fracture toughness is lower for the osteoporotic patient, relatively strenuous activities such as stair ascent or raising from a chair may present a greater fracture risk in the osteoporotic than the healthy patient. As such, fatigue damage accumulation could play a role in the approximately 25,000 spontaneous hip fractures that occur annually in the U.S.

The fracture toughness, or critical stress intensity factor, does not indicate how the size of a crack increases per cycle of fatigue loading. This information would be useful in predicting how much damage accumulates in bone for different activities. Fortunately, fracture mechanics can also be used to quantify this crack growth rate given information on the size of an existing crack, and on the range of the stress intensity factor for cyclic loading. Experiments have shown that there is a power law relationship between the rate of crack propagation and the cyclic stress intensity factor (Wright and Hayes, 1976a):

$$da/dN = C\{\Delta K\}^n \tag{4}$$

where da/dN is the rate of crack propagation, C and n are constants, and ΔK is the range of K for cyclic loading (Fig. 21). The constants C and n, which have only been determined for bovine cortical bone (Wright and Hayes, 1976; 1980), are sensitive to strain rate and may also be sensitive to microstructure. In general, the fatigue characteristics of primary bone appear to be different than those of secondary Haversian bone (Carter et al., 1976; Evans and Riolo, 1970; Moyle and Bowden, 1984) so that it is not clear what the constants C and n are for adult human cortical bone.

The general relationship shown in Equation 4 is known as the Paris Law. This law is applicable to most conventional engineering materials, and quantifies how many cycles of fatigue life, N, remain for a crack of given length, a, under loads which result in a cyclic stress intensity factor, ΔK. That a Paris Law applies to cortical bone also implies that the rate of fatigue damage increases as the number of cycles increases. This is in contrast to a linear damage model (each load cycle produces the same amount of damage) such as Miner's Rule (see above). Nonlinear damage accumulation is shown clearly in Fig. 22, which is a graph of the fatigue crack length as a function of the number of load cycles for a controlled fatigue crack propagation experiment. Note that the crack length, which is related to the fatigue damage, increases more per cycle as the number of cycles is increased. Therefore, as cracks grow larger in bone, they become more damaging due to their increasing size.

In summary, both the traditional engineering and fracture mechanics approaches can be used to study the monotonic and fatigue properties of cortical bone. These approaches complement each other in terms of ease of application and generality of results. However, no matter what approach is used, it should be clear that cyclic and creep loading can reduce the strength of bone substantially. To reflect the importance of damage accumulation, models have been developed using traditional engineering concepts such as the S-N curve to account for both creep and fatigue damage (Carter and Caler, 1985; Currey, 1989). In addition, fracture mechanics indicates that

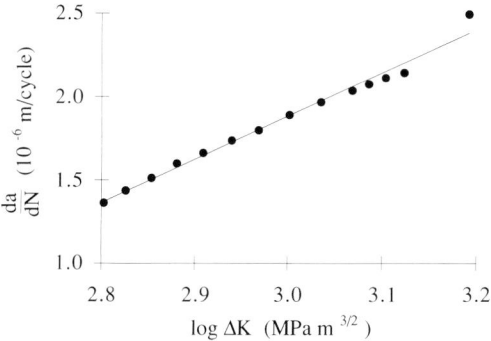

Fig. 21. Fatigue crack propagation in bovine femoral cortical bone. The straight line fit to the data confirms that the Paris Law (see text) is applicable for cortical bone, as it is for many conventional engineering materials. [From Wright, T. M. and Hayes, W. C. (1976). *J. Biomed. Mater. Res.*, **7**: 637–648. With permission.]

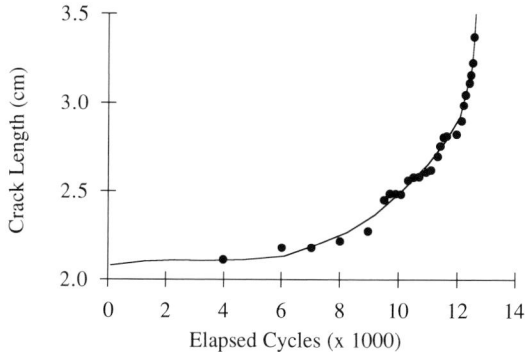

Fig. 22. Increase in crack length as a function of the number of cycles for a controlled crack propagation fatigue test on bovine femoral cortical bone. The data in Fig. 21 were derived from this curve. Note that there is more damage (the crack length increases more) toward the end of the life than at the start of the life. Therefore, damage accumulation is not a linear function of the number of cycles. [From Wright, T. M. and Hayes, W. C. (1976). *J. Biomed. Mater. Res.*, **7**: 637–648. With permission.]

as cracks become larger, the resistance to fracture is reduced. Thus, damage in cortical bone may be important as an etiologic factor in stress- and age-related fractures. We emphasize again that these approaches do not account for repair of fatigue or creep damage which can occur *in vivo*. Consequently, one must consider the fatigue and creep properties of devitalized bone as lower bounds on the *in vivo* properties.

Trabecular Bone

As noted earlier, there is a large variation in density for trabecular bone. Both spatial and temporal variations in trabecular bone density can occur due to changes in anatomic location and age, respectively. For example, trabecular bone material properties within the proximal tibia can vary by up to two orders of magnitude due to changes in density alone (Goldstein *et al.*, 1983). Reflecting the importance of particular anatomic sites, material properties for trabecular bone have been reported for a number of anatomic sites, including the cranium (McElhaney *et al.*, 1970a, 1970b), lumbar spine (Galante *et al.*, 1970; Hansson *et al.*, 1986; Keller *et al.*, 1989; Mosekilde *et al.*, 1987), iliac crest (Mosekilde and Mosekilde, 1986; Mosekilde *et al.*, 1985), proximal femur (Brown and Ferguson, 1980; Esses *et al.*, 1989; Lotz *et al.*, 1990; Martens *et al.*, 1983), distal femur (Ducheyne *et al.*, 1977), patella (Townsend *et al.*, 1975a), proximal tibia (Carter and Hayes, 1977c; Goldstein *et al.*, 1983; Hvid and Hansen, 1985), distal tibia (Aitken *et al.*, 1985; Jensen *et al.*, 1989), distal fibula and talus (Jensen *et al.*, 1988), and calcaneus (Jensen *et al.*, 1991; Weaver and Chalmers, 1966). In addition, noninvasive densitometric studies have shown that trabecular bone mineral density in the hip and spine decreases with age, reaching lower levels in women than men (Genant *et al.*, 1985; Mazess, 1982; Melton *et al.*, 1986; Riggs and Melton, 1986; Riggs *et al.*, 1982). Since it is well known from the above *in vitro* biomechanical studies of cadaveric material that the material properties of trabecular bone are very sensitive to apparent density, one cannot discuss the material properties of trabecular bone without reference to the anatomic location and the age of the tissue.

To further complicate matters, material properties also depend on the architecture of the trabecular bone, which, like density, is dependent on the anatomic site, and to a lesser extent, on age. While cortical bone is essentially a low-porosity solid, trabecular bone is best described as an open-celled porous foam (Gibson, 1985; Gibson and Ashby, 1988). Its architecture, made up of a series of interconnecting trabeculae, can be idealized as a combination of rod-rod, rod-plate, of plate-plate basic cellular structures where rods and plates represent thin and thick trabeculae, respectively (Fig. 23). Depending on the type and orientation of these basic cellular structures, i.e., depending on the architecture of the trabecular bone, the mechanical properties can vary by at least an order of magnitude (Brown and Ferguson, 1980; Ducheyne *et al.*, 1977; Evans, 1973; Galante *et al.*, 1970; Goldstein *et al.*, 1983; Hvid and Hansen, 1985; Jensen *et al.*, 1991; Martens *et al.*, 1983; Mosekilde and Mosekilde, 1988; Mosekilde *et al.*, 1985; Townsend *et al.*, 1975a). In the following discussion of trabecular bone material properties, we will describe the general properties of trabecular bone, and discuss the dependence of these properties on density and architecture in more detail.

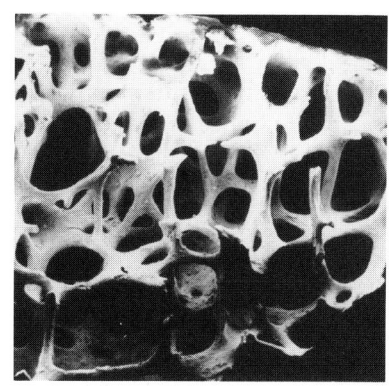

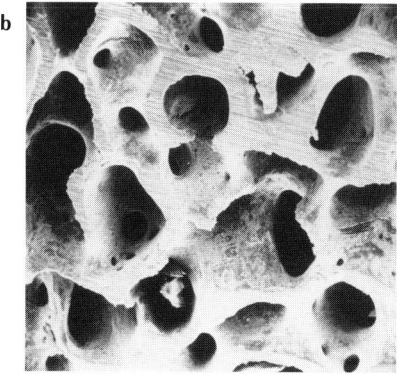

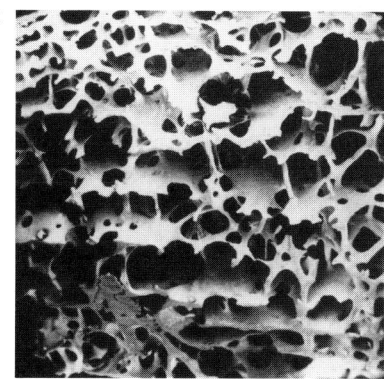

Fig. 23. Scanning electron micrographs showing the various basic cellular structures of human trabecular bone: (a) the rod-rod basic cellular structure, from the femoral head; (b) the more dense plate-plate cellular structure, also from the femoral head; (c) the plate-rod cellular structure, from the femoral condyle. [From Gibson, L. J. (1985). *J. Biomech.*, **18**: 317–328. With permission.]

Modulus

In general, the modulus of trabecular bone can vary from approximately 10 to 2000 MPa, depending on the anatomic site and age. Given that the modulus of cortical bone is approximately 17000 MPa, this indicates that trabecular bone is much more compliant than cortical bone. However, there are regions in the skeleton, such as the cranium, the subchondral plate in the proximal tibia, the metaphyseal shell in the proximal femur, and the endplates in vertebral bodies, where the distinction between cortical and trabecular bone is less clear. Mean values of the modulus in these regions have been measured in the range of 1150 to 9650 MPa (Choi *et al.*, 1990; Lotz *et al.*, 1989; McElhaney *et al.*, 1970b; Murray *et al.*, 1984). Since most research has focused on the material properties of the trabecular bone which is found in the metaphyses of long bones, we shall limit our attention to these regions.

Dependence on Apparent Density

As mentioned above, the material properties of trabecular bone are very sensitive to apparent density. In particular, it has been demonstrated (Carter and Hayes, 1976, 1977c; Gibson, 1985; Rice *et al.*, 1988) that the modulus of trabecular bone in any loading direction (E) is related to its apparent density (ρ) by a power-law relationship of the form

$$E = a + b\rho^c \qquad (5)$$

where a, b, and c are constants which depend on the architecture of the tissue (Gibson, 1985; Rice *et al.*, 1988). It has been shown that the intercept (a) in a pooled set of specimens of varying architectures has a value of approximately 70 MPa (Rice *et al.*, 1988). This implies that the zero apparent density datum is outside the range of this power-law relationship. If trabecular bone disappears once it reaches a minimum size, perhaps due to a minimum cross-sectional geometry necessary to contain lacunae, there would be a lower bound on apparent density. Consequently, any parameter which is a function of apparent density need not have a zero intercept, and the corresponding relationship will be valid only for the measured range of apparent density values.

As with any power law, the most important parameter in this relationship is the exponent c. By analogy with other cellular solids, the exponent primarily describes how density affects the modulus (Gibson, 1985). In general, the exponent has a value of approximately 2 (Fig. 24). Statistical analyses have shown that the best fit for the modulus of specimens pooled from a wide range of anatomical sites is obtained by a squared exponent (Rice *et al.*, 1988). Consequently, a 25% reduction in density, as has been observed

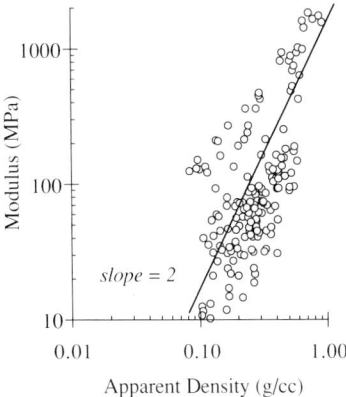

Fig. 24. Compressive modulus as a function of apparent density for trabecular bone. The orientation of the specimen is not controlled. In general, the modulus of trabecular bone, when taken from a wide range of species and anatomic location, varies as a power-law function of density with an exponent of approximately two.

in elderly cadaveric vertebrae (McBroom *et al.*, 1985; Mosekilde *et al.*, 1989), results in a 56% decrease in modulus. Theoretical models which treat trabecular bone as a porous foam predict a squared power-law relationship when the idealized architecture is primarily open celled (a network of connecting rods, as most human trabecular bone appears to be). The main mechanism of deformation in these open-celled foams is bending of individual trabeculae (Gibson, 1985; Gibson and Ashby, 1988), even though the bulk specimen is compressed without bending.

Dependence on Architecture

When the architecture is controlled, the variation in apparent density of trabecular bone can explain most of the variation of modulus. However, as can be seen from the scatter in modulus values for any particular value of apparent density (Fig. 24), other variables, namely the architecture, can also affect modulus. Scanning electron microscopes have been used successfully to illustrate the variation in trabecular architecture with different anatomic sites (Whitehouse, 1975; Whitehouse and Dyson, 1974; Whitehouse *et al.*, 1971). These studies clearly show how the architecture varies with anatomic location.

The architecture of trabecular bone describes both the shape of the trabecular basic cellular structure and its orientation. The basic cellular structure describes the general connectivity of the trabeculae, the mean thickness of the individual trabeculae, the mean spacing between trabeculae, and the number of trabeculae. Clearly, there is a relationship between the density

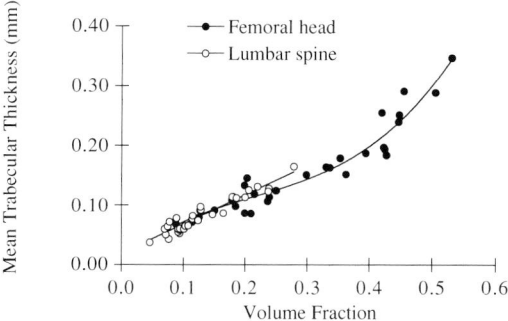

Fig. 25. Mean thickness of the trabeculae in the lumbar spine and the subcapital region of the proximal femur as a function of bone volume fraction, which is proportional to apparent density. [From Snyder, B. D. and Hayes, W. C. (1990). In *Biomechanics of Diarthrodial Joints*, Mow, V. C., Ratcliffe, A., and Woo, S. L. Y., eds., Springer-Verlag, New York, 31–59. With permission.]

of the bulk trabecular bone and both the number and mean thickness of the individual trabeculae (Snyder and Hayes, 1990). Indeed, for the lumbar spine, there is a strong linear relationship between density and these variables (Fig. 25). In the subcapital region of the proximal femur, however, there is a highly nonlinear relationship between mean trabecular thickness and density (Snyder and Hayes, 1990) (Fig. 25).

Apart from affecting the modulus, the shape of the basic cellular structure can also affect the Poisson's ratio of trabecular bone (Gibson and Ashby, 1988). For isotropic metals, Poisson's ratio must fall between 0.0 and 0.5. However, theoretical values of Poisson's ratio for open-celled foam materials such as trabecular bone may be negative (the material contracts when compressed) or well above unity, depending on the cell structure (Gibson and Ashby, 1988). For example, the Poisson's ratio for cork is approximately zero, allowing you to push a cork into a wine bottle without radial expansion of the cork. Mean values ($\pm$ standard deviation) of Poisson's ratio for trabecular bone have been reported in the range 0.06 ± 0.03 (Knauss, 1981) to 0.95 ± 1.29 (Snyder, 1991) (Table 3).

The other factor which relates to the architecture is the orientation of the basic cellular structures, reflected as the mean orientation of the trabeculae. The orientation of the individual trabeculae is controlled mainly by the direction of the applied forces to the skeleton, according to the well-known, but still qualitative, Wolff's Law (Wolff, 1892). Fig. 26 shows modulus as a function of apparent density for bovine trabecular bone in different orientations. These data indicate that there can be a ten-fold difference in modulus depending on the specimen orientation and that the sensitivity to density is higher for the longitudinal modulus than for the transverse modulus (Williams and Lewis, 1982).

Table 3.
Poisson's Ratio for Trabecular Bone

Study	Bone	Poisson's Ratio
McElhaney, 1970a	Femur (n = 28, age 37–86)	0.30 (± 0.06)
	Lumbar spine (n = 28, age 45–79)	0.14 (± 0.09)
Knauss, 1981	Femoral head (age 24–81)	0.06 (± 0.03)[a]
		0.16 (± 0.06)
Williams and Lewis, 1982	2D FEM proximal tibia (n = 2)	−0.07–0.52[b]
Beaupre and Hayes, 1985	3D FEM, idealized open cell model	0.08
Jasty et al., 1985	Distal femur and proximal tibia (n = 12)	0.081–0.845[b]
Klever et al., 1985	Proximal tibia (n = 27)	0.07–0.65[b]
Yahia et al., 1988	Lumbar spine (n = 30, age 25–35)	0.301 (± 0.270)[a]
		0.521 (± 0.443)
Snyder, 1991	Subcapital femur (n = 18, age 27–77)	0.156 (± 0.105)[a]
		0.652 (± 0.166)
		0.024–1.014[b]
	Lumbar spine (n = 12, age 62–81)	0.110 (± 0.087)[a]
		0.952 (± 1.286)
		−0.372–4.602[b]

We have not distinguished between different anisotropic Poisson's ratio values. FEM — finite element model prediction.

[a] More than one mean (standard deviation in parentheses) value is reported for those experiments which found all six Poisson's ratios. In these cases, only the maximum and minimum mean values are reported.
[b] Ranges are reported when these data are available.

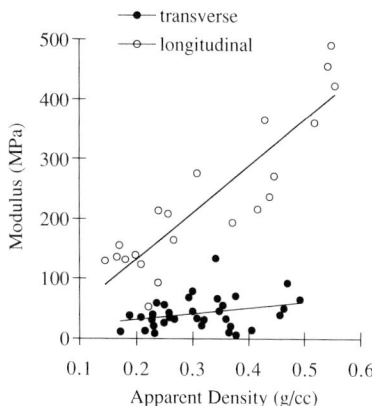

Fig. 26. Compressive modulus as a function of apparent density and loading direction for trabecular bone. Data are presented for specimens loaded in longitudinal and transverse directions, demonstrating the sensitivity of modulus to loading direction. [From Gibson, L. J. and Ashby, M. F. (1988). *Cellular Solids: Structure and Properties*, Pergamon Press, New York. With permission.]

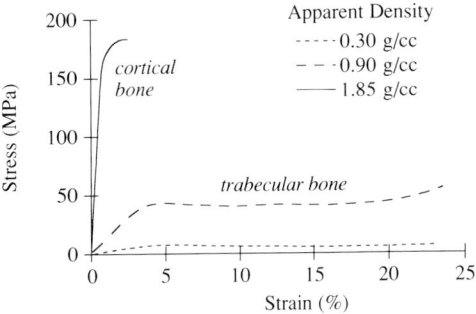

Fig. 27. Examples of typical compressive stress-strain behavior of trabecular and cortical bone for different apparent densities.

We have already discussed anisotropy (directional dependence) of the elastic properties of cortical bone. The different architectures which exist for trabecular bone result in an anisotropy of elastic properties for trabecular bone. However, in contrast to cortical bone, trabecular bone is nearly iso-tropic in some anatomic sites (proximal humerus) and highly anisotropic in others (elderly lumbar spine). Therefore, trabecular bone is both anisotropic and heterogeneous, so it is difficult to generalize about its elastic properties. In order to understand structure-anisotropy relations for trabecular bone, stereologic methods, which quantify the architecture (sometimes called the morphology) of trabecular bone, have recently been developed (Harrigan and Mann, 1984; Mosekilde, 1988; Mosekilde and Mosekilde, 1990; Snyder and Hayes, 1990). To develop structure-anisotropy relations, one must cor-relate the measured anisotropic mechanical properties of specimens of tra-becular bone with the stereologic descriptions of their architecture. The results from these studies indicate that there are excellent correlations be-tween architecture and the mechanical properties (Snyder and Hayes, 1990) and that multivariate (architecture and density) regressions provide mod-estly improved correlations with mechanical properties compared to the use of density alone. However, since these experiments are so difficult to perform, the results are sparse and cannot yet be generalized.

Uniaxial Strength

Much research has focused on the compressive strength of trabecular bone because it is believed that *in vivo* failure of trabecular bone is dominated by compressive loads. Fig. 27 shows typical stress-strain plots for specimens of trabecular bone with different apparent densities under uniaxial com-pressive loading (Carter and Hayes, 1977c; Gibson, 1985). Both the elastic and postyield behaviors are sensitive to apparent density. These characteristics are also displayed by artificial and natural porous foam materials such as aluminum honeycombs, cork, and balsa wood (Gibson and Ashby, 1988).

The stress-strain plots in Fig. 27 have three regions which represent distinct phases of material behavior (Carter and Hayes, 1977c; Gibson, 1985; Gibson and Ashby, 1988; Hayes and Carter, 1976). In the first stage, the material is in the linear region where individual trabeculae bend and compress as the bulk tissue is compressed. In the second stage, failure occurs by fracture of some trabeculae and buckling of others (Ducheyne *et al.*, 1977; Eurell and Kazarian, 1982; Gibson and Ashby, 1988; Hayes and Carter, 1976; Townsend *et al.*, 1975b; Turner, 1989). As more and more trabeculae fail, the strain increases until broken trabeculae begin to fill up the pores. As a result, the specimen stiffens in stage three. As seen in Fig. 27, lower-density specimens can deform more before the final stiffening phase than higher-density specimens. This ability to deform to compressive strains of over 50% highlights a unique feature of the trabecular bone: it can absorb considerable energy (area under the stress-strain curve) for large compressive loads (Hayes and Carter, 1976; Linde *et al.*, 1989) while maintaining a minimum mass.

As with modulus, the compressive strength of trabecular bone is also related to its apparent density primarily by a squared power-law relationship (Fig. 28) (Carter and Hayes, 1976, 1977c; Goldstein, 1987; Rice *et al.*, 1988). Indeed, many studies have demonstrated strong linear relationships between compressive strength and modulus (Brown and Ferguson, 1980; Ducheyne *et al.*, 1977; Goldstein *et al.*, 1983; Odgaard *et al.*, 1989; Turner, 1989; Williams and Lewis, 1982). Therefore, stiffer trabecular bone is also proportionally stronger. One consequence of this is that the main parameter which may control failure in trabecular bone is not the maximum level of stress, but the maximum level of strain (strain = stress divided by modulus). This is supported by the evidence that trabecular bone yields at strains in the range of 1 to 4%, with only a weak dependence on density (Brown and Ferguson, 1980; Linde *et al.*, 1989; Odgaard *et al.*, 1989; Turner, 1989).

These relationships between apparent density with both modulus and strength have important physiological and clinical consequences. First, it should be clear that bone can easily regulate its strength and stiffness by adjusting its apparent density. Second, subtle changes in bone apparent density result in large changes in strength and modulus. This indicates that an order of magnitude reduction in both trabecular bone strength and modulus can occur by the time density reductions of 30 to 50% are visible radiographically. Thus, conventional radiographic techniques used to assess fracture risk of whole bones are poor indicators of bone strength.

The tensile behavior of trabecular bone is much different from its compressive behavior (Carter *et al.*, 1980; Kaplan *et al.*, 1985; Stone *et al.*, 1983). Fig. 29 shows a typical stress-strain curve for trabecular bone under tensile

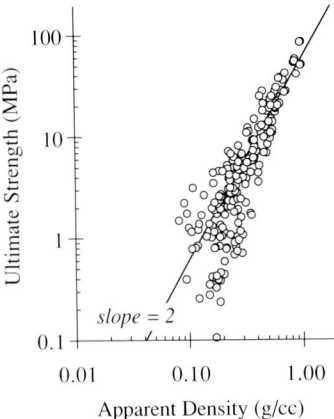

Fig. 28. Ultimate compressive strength as a function of apparent density for trabecular bone. In general, compressive strength varies as a power-law function of density, with an exponent of approximately two.

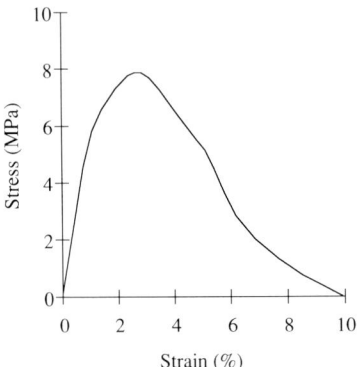

Fig. 29. Tensile stress-strain behavior for trabecular bone. Compare this with the compressive behavior shown in Fig. 27. [From Gibson, L. J. and Ashby, M. F. (1988). *Cellular Solids: Structure and Properties*, Pergamon Press, New York. With permission.]

loading. While the linear behavior is similar to that for compressive loading, the post-yield behavior is completely different. For tension loading, failure occurs by fracture of the individual trabeculae. As more trabeculae fracture, the specimen can take less and less load, until finally complete fracture occurs. This behavior is similar to that for fiber-reinforced concrete, and is typical of artificial materials which are designed to resist compressive forces.

Despite the substantial data available for the compressive uniaxial strength of trabecular bone, relatively few data have been reported for its tensile strength. Consequently, there is controversy concerning the magnitude of the tensile strength with respect to the compressive strength. While the weight of the evidence suggests that the tensile and compressive strengths are equal after adjusting for variations in apparent density (Bensusan *et al.*, 1983; Carter *et al.*, 1980; Neil *et al.*, 1983), there is some evidence that the tensile strength may be lower (Kaplan *et al.*, 1985; Stone *et al.*, 1983). It is possible that differences in trabecular bone architecture and experimental techniques account for these conflicting data.

By comparing the compressive and tensile behaviors of trabecular bone (Figs. 27 and 29), it is clear that the postyield load-carrying capacity of trabecular bone is high for compression, and almost negligible for tension. Therefore, if trabecular bone is loaded beyond the ultimate strength in compression, it can still carry substantial load. Consequently, it will not overload surrounding trabecular bone much, and thus failure will not spread to the surrounding tissue. However, for tension loading beyond the ultimate strength, no load can be carried by the tissue because it fractures. In this case, the surrounding tissue must carry the full load, and may thus be overloaded. If subsequent failure of that material occurs, a cascade effect could result where a crack could propagate across a whole bone causing fracture. Therefore, it is likely that local failure of trabecular bone in compression may not lead to failure of a whole bone, but that local failure in tension could have catastrophic consequences.

Multiaxial Strength

It is difficult to perform mechanical tests on trabecular bone because it is so heterogeneous. This places limitations on the size of the test specimen, making controlled mechanical testing difficult, even for uniaxial compression tests (Odgaard *et al.*, 1989; Odgaard and Linde, 1991). Further complexity arises because of the variation in density and architecture of trabecular bone between groups of specimens. Thus, results must always be expressed using correlations with density and architecture, demanding large sample sizes. Consequently, only limited data exist for multiaxial strength properties of trabecular bone, and these data exist only for bovine bone (Borchers, 1991; Stone *et al.*, 1983).

Fig. 30 shows data for biaxial loading of bovine trabecular bone. These data indicate that the maximum shear stress which can be sustained for combined tension and torsion loading is less than for pure torsion loading. In addition, more recent experiments have demonstrated that the mean stress (hydrostatic pressure component) can affect the strength of trabecular bone (Borchers, 1991). Thus, it appears that multiaxial failure criteria such as the von Mises criterion described earlier are not applicable to trabecular bone. Again, this is consistent with the behavior of many open-celled porous foam materials which show a sensitivity of multiaxial strength behavior to mean stress (Gibson and Ashby, 1988).

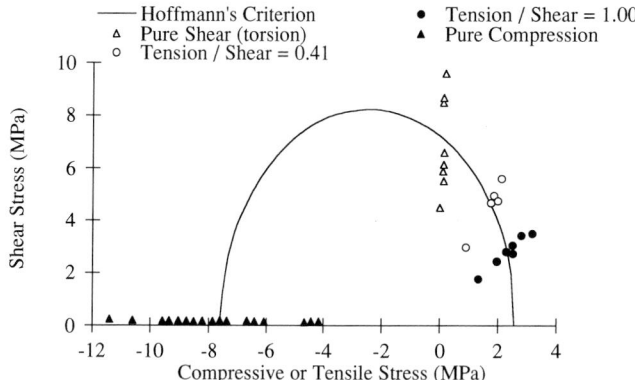

Fig. 30. Tension-torsion and compression-torsion yield stresses for bovine humeral trabecular bone. Tensile stresses are positive, compressive stresses are negative. Data are shown for different combinations of tension-shear loading. The Hoffmann isotropic yield criterion is applied to the data. Note that extrapolation of these data using the Hoffmann criterion suggests that the tensile strength of trabecular bone is approximately one third the compressive strength. [From Stone, J. L., Beaupre, G. S., and Hayes, W. C. (1983). *J. Biomech.*, **16**: 743–752. With permission.]

Viscoelastic Behavior

Very few experiments have been performed where constant loads have been held on trabecular bone for extended periods of time. Thus, the creep characteristics for trabecular bone remain obscure. By contrast, both modulus and strength of trabecular bone have been shown to be sensitive to strain rate (Carter and Hayes, 1976, 1977c; Ducheyne *et al.*, 1977; Linde *et al.*, 1991), though the dependence is weak. For most activities, the relationship between apparent density (ρ) and both modulus (E) and strength (σ_{ult}) can be expressed as a function of strain rate (γ) by power-law relationships which have the same exponent on the strain rate

$$E \ = a + h\gamma^{0.06} \rho^c \tag{6a}$$

$$\sigma_{ult} = m + n\gamma^{0.06} \rho^d \tag{6b}$$

where a, h, c, m, n, and d are constants (Carter and Hayes, 1977c). As discussed above, a squared exponent (c = d = 2) on ρ is a good representation of the general behavior of trabecular bone. The small exponent on γ implies that the sensitivities of both modulus and strength to strain rate are weak. For example, a 100-fold increase in strain rate from 0.001 (slow walking) to 0.1 (very strenuous exercise) would result in increases in both modulus and strength of approximately 30%. Again, it is interesting that the strength and modulus adjust equally to changes in strain rate, as they do for changes in density.

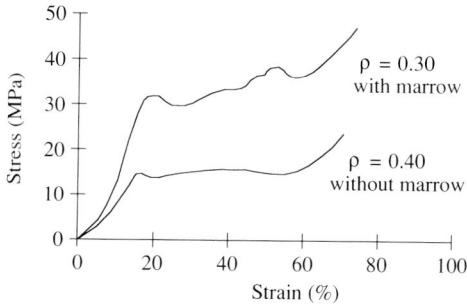

Fig. 31. Stress-strain curves for two specimens of trabecular bone, one with bone marrow, the other without marrow. The strain rate for this test was very high (10 s^{-1}), representative of severe traumatic loading. The modulus and strength are significantly higher for specimens with bone marrow. However, bone marrow only affects mechanical behavior at these high loading rates. [From Carter, D. R. and Hayes, W. C. (1977). *J. Bone Jt. Surg.*, **59**: 954–962. With permission.]

In addition to this strain rate affect which is due to the viscous behavior of the trabeculae, bone marrow can play a role in trabecular bone's load-carrying capacity, but only at very high strain rates (10 per second — gun shot wounds) (Carter and Hayes, 1976, 1977c). If the bone marrow is restricted from flowing through the intertrabecular spaces, as it is for very high strain rates, this restriction to flow can further enhance the mechanical properties (Fig. 31). Therefore, for severe, traumatic compressive loading, trabecular bone becomes stiffer, stronger, and can absorb more energy than for physiologic loading. Note, however, that at physiologic rates, the marrow plays no role in the viscous behavior (Carter and Hayes, 1976; Pugh *et al.*, 1973b).

Age Effects

Age-related fractures are an enormous clinical and social problem in the U.S., particularly for the spine, distal radius, and proximal femur, which are largely trabecular bone structures. We have discussed how both density and architecture can affect the material properties of trabecular bone. Both of these parameters change with aging, resulting in age-related trabecular bone fragility which has been associated with the large incidence of hip, spine, and radial fractures in the elderly (anonymous, 1984). Thus, a major research area in trabecular bone biomechanics is quantification of age-related changes in trabecular bone density and architecture.

Fig. 32 shows typical age-related changes in human trabecular bone. As the bone loses mass, its density reduces and its architecture changes. The reductions in density depend on a number of factors, including gender and anatomic site. In general, bone mineral density (which reflects density of

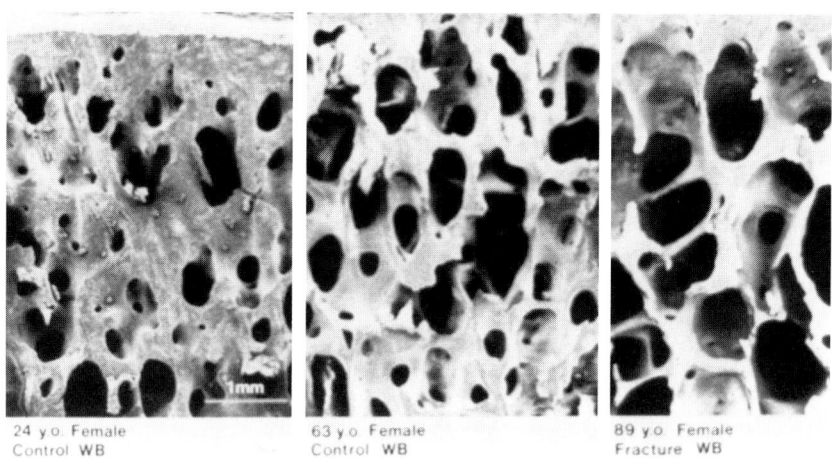

24 y.o. Female   63 y.o. Female   89 y.o. Female
Control WB   Control WB   Fracture WB

Fig. 32. Photograph showing age-related changes in apparent density and architecture of human trabecular bone from the femoral head. (Courtesy of Marc Grynpas, M.D. With permission.)

both trabecular and cortical bone for a particular cross-section) declines with age, reaching lower levels in females than males (Genant *et al.*, 1985; Mazess, 1982; Melton *et al.*, 1986; Riggs and Melton, 1986; Riggs *et al.*, 1982). Reflecting these gender-specific bone mineral density reductions, osteoporosis has been categorized as senile and postmenopausal osteoporosis. Senile osteoporosis is thought to affect females and, to a lesser extent, males, and to result in equal reductions in cortical and trabecular bone mass. Postmenopausal osteoporosis is thought to affect a relatively small subset of females, but is characterized by excessive and disproportionate trabecular bone loss. In the lumbar spine, direct measurements of trabecular bone density have shown a decrease in density of approximately 50% from ages 20 to 80 years (Mosekilde *et al.*, 1987).

Histomorphometric studies have also shown gender-specific changes in trabecular bone architecture due to aging (Aaron *et al.*, 1987; Bergot *et al.*, 1988; Mosekilde and Mosekilde, 1990). These studies have demonstrated that the number and thickness of the trabeculae decrease with decreasing density, while the size of the intertrabecular spaces increase (Bergot *et al.*, 1988; Mosekilde, 1988; Mosekilde and Mosekilde, 1990; Preteux *et al.*, 1985; Snyder, 1991; Snyder and Hayes, 1990). Three-dimensional stereologic studies have more recently demonstrated that, for the lumbar spine, the number of horizontal trabeculae is less than the number of vertical trabeculae, regardless of density, and that the number of vertical trabeculae decreases with decreasing density at twice the rate as the number of horizontal trabeculae (Fig. 33) (Snyder, 1991). Thus, contrary to the evidence from earlier two-dimensional histomorphometric studies (Arnold, 1980; Atkinson, 1967;

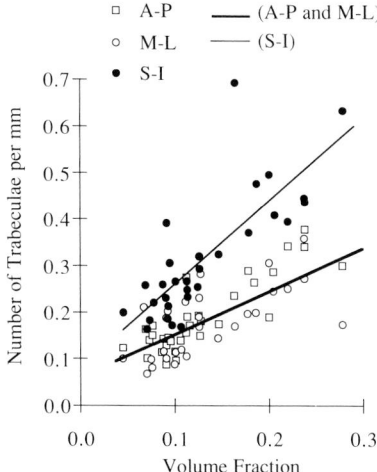

Fig. 33. Decrease in the number of vertical (S-I) and horizontal (M-L, A-P) trabeculae with decreasing volume fraction (proportional to density) for the human lumbar spine. The rate of loss of vertical trabeculae is twice that of the horizontal trabeculae. Even so, there are always more vertical than horizontal trabeculae (M-L, medial-lateral direction; S-I, superior-inferior direction, A-P, anterior-posterior direction). [From Snyder, B. D. and Hayes, W. C. (1990). In *Biomechanics of Diarthrodial Joints*, Mow, V. C., Ratcliffe, A., and Woo, S. L. Y., eds., Springer-Verlag, New York, 31–59. With permission.]

Parfitt, 1984), vertical trabeculae do not become thicker with aging, and preferential loss of horizontal trabeculae does not appear to occur for the lumbar spine. In fact, these three-dimensional data suggest that preferential loss of vertical trabeculae occurs with increasing age. It has also been noted that loss of trabeculae may be more damaging to the structural integrity of trabecular bone than mere thinning, because complete loss of a single trabecula is irreversible as lamellar new bone can be formed only on existing surfaces (Parfitt *et al.*, 1983).

Since the strength of trabecular bone depends on both apparent density and architecture, these age-related changes weaken trabecular bone. For example, failure by buckling of individual trabeculae is more likely to occur when trabeculae become fewer, thinner, and longer. (The length of trabeculae increases with age since intertrabecular spacing has been shown to increase with age.) This reduced resistance to failure by buckling of individual trabeculae has been referred to as a "triple jeopardy", since three independent factors (reduction in number, decrease in thickness, and increase in length) contribute to the weakening mechanism (Snyder and Hayes, 1990). In addition, we noted earlier that failure of individual trabecular may occur by fracture. A reduction in the number and thickness of the trabeculae would weaken the trabeculae by this mechanism (an analogous "double jeopardy").

To summarize this discussion on age effects, we note that the observed reductions in trabecular bone density are manifested as changes in the architecture which can be quite subtle. More importantly, because of the double and triple jeopardy mechanisms, the accompanying reductions in strength may be greater than those suggested by reductions in density alone. Obviously, the accelerated bone loss which occurs with postmenopausal osteoporosis further reduces the strength of trabecular bone. Thus, normal, age-related changes in trabecular bone coupled with pathological processes can produce substantial changes in the strength of trabecular bone. This weakening of trabecular bone must play a significant role in the etiology of age-related fractures of the hip and spine, particularly for the latter (Hayes et al., 1991).

Fatigue Properties

Fractures of individual trabeculae have been observed in the lumbar spine (Vernon-Roberts and Pirie, 1973), acetabulum (Ohtani and Azuma, 1984), femoral head (Benaissa et al., 1989; Dunstan et al., 1990; Freeman et al., 1974; McFarland and Frost, 1961; Todd et al., 1972; Urovitz et al., 1977; Wong et al., 1985), and proximal tibia (Pugh et al., 1973a) of post-mortem human specimens and in the proximal tibia of rabbits (Radin et al., 1973). Tiny cracks within individual trabeculae can be repaired by callus formation, similar to callus formation in fractures of long bones, resulting in the appearance of a "node" of new woven or lamellar bone about the original crack (Benaissa et al., 1989; Ohtani and Azuma, 1984; Radin et al., 1973; Todd et al., 1972; Urovitz et al., 1977; Wong et al., 1985). It has been suggested that these cracks are due to fatigue loading (Todd et al., 1972) and their possible role in bone remodeling (Pugh et al., 1973a), age-related fractures (Dunstan et al., 1990; Freeman et al., 1974; Urovitz et al., 1977; Wong et al., 1985), aseptic necrosis of the femoral head (McFarland and Frost, 1961), degenerative joint disease (Benaissa et al., 1989; Radin et al., 1973), and other bone disorders (Ohtani and Azuma, 1984) have been discussed.

Unfortunately, while much has been inferred about the fatigue behavior of trabecular bone, few controlled experiments have been performed. One reason for this lack of data is that the heterogeneity of trabecular bone (variations in density and architecture) results in large data scatter, confounding the precision of such analyses. As with the multiaxial strength data, the only fatigue data available for trabecular bone is for bovine bone. These data suggest that the uniaxial compressive strength of trabecular bone can be reduced by an order of magnitude by 10^6 cycles of loading (Fig. 34) (Michel et al., 1991). Furthermore, the resistance of trabecular bone to fatigue failure appears to be greater than for cortical bone. The mechanism

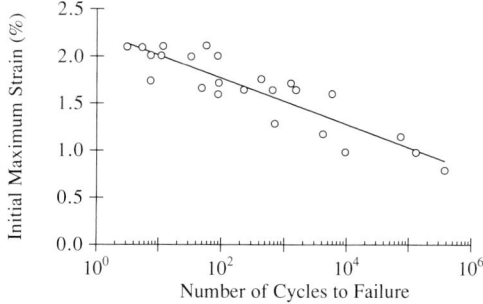

Fig. 34. Fatigue, strain-life curve for bovine distal femoral trabecular bone. This experiment was performed by cyclically compressing the bone specimens between upper and lower stress levels. For each specimen, this stress range was constant. The upper load level was varied for different specimens while the lower stress level was held constant. To account for variations in density, the loading is described here by dividing the upper stress level by the specimen modulus (obtained at the start of the experiment). Thus, we present initial maximum strain vs. number of cycles.

for fatigue damage in trabecular bone appears to involve fracture and buckling of individual trabeculae (Michel *et al.*, 1991) and as such differs from cortical bone where cracks accumulate within the bone matrix. This difference in mechanisms may account for the superior fatigue properties of trabecular bone.

Summary

In this chapter, we have surveyed the current literature on the material properties of both cortical and trabecular bone. Cortical bone is distinguished by its low porosity and osteonal microstructure, while trabecular bone is distinguished by its high porosity and open-celled architecture. An important characteristic of material properties (as opposed to structural properties) is that they are independent of the geometry of the bone from which the tissue is obtained.

Cortical bone is an anisotropic material, since its elastic properties are directional dependent. It is also anisotropic from a strength perspective, and its uniaxial strength depends on whether tensile, compressive, or torsional loads are applied. Multiaxial failure criteria for cortical bone have not yet been established. However, cortical bone becomes stiffer, stronger, and can absorb more energy as the loading rate is increased, until a threshold loading rate is reached after which these properties diminish. Stiffness and strength also diminish with aging.

Creep and fatigue loading of cortical bone can reduce both modulus and strength substantially. Both creep and fatigue loading of cortical bone produce microcracks which weaken the tissue. However, the osteonal microstructure of cortical bone resists the propagation of these cracks, so that cortical bone is a relatively tough material. There is evidence that the development of these microcracks is a stimulus for strain-induced bone remodeling.

Trabecular bone, compared to cortical bone, is relatively compliant and very heterogeneous. This heterogeneity makes it difficult to generalize about trabecular bone material properties, which are both age and anatomic location dependent. The high porosity of trabecular bone accounts for its compliance, and large variations in density and architecture account for its heterogeneity. Both modulus and strength are related to density by an approximately squared power law. Thus, subtle changes in density can result in relatively large changes in modulus and strength. Like cortical bone, trabecular bone is anisotropic both from modulus and strength perspectives. Its modulus and strength properties are weakly sensitive to loading rate.

Age effects are substantial for trabecular bone, whereby changes in density and architecture can change modulus and strength by an order of magnitude. As trabecular bone ages, its density is reduced, manifested by a reduction in the number and thickness of individual trabeculae, and an increase in intertrabecular spacing. These architectural changes accentuate strength reductions due to density alone. Finally, the multiaxial and fatigue behaviors of trabecular bone are not well understood, although the fatigue resistance of trabecular bone appears to be greater than cortical bone.

Acknowledgments

We gratefully acknowledge the support of grants from the National Institutes of Health (CA41295 and CCR103605), the Centers for Disease Control (CR102550), the National Cancer Institute (CA40211), the Maurice E. Mueller North American Foundation Scholar Support (TMK), and the Maurice E. Mueller Professorship in Biomechanics at Harvard Medical School (WCH). We also thank Jeanine Goodwin for her assistance in manuscript preparation.

References

Aaron, J. E., Makins, N. B., and Sagreiya, K. (1987). The microanatomy of trabecular bone loss in normal aging men and women. *Clin. Orthop.*, **215**: 260–271.
Aitken, G. K., Bourne, R. B., Finlay, J. B., Rorabeck, C. H., and Andreae, P. R. (1985). Indentation stiffness of the cancellous bone in the distal human tibia. *Clin. Orthop.*, **201**: 264–270.

Amstutz, H. C. and Sissons, H. A. (1969). The structure of the vertebral spongiosa. *J. Bone Jt. Surg.*, **51**: 540–550.

Anonymous (1984). Consensus conference: osteoporosis. *JAMA*, **252**: 799–802.

Arnold, J. S. (1980). Trabecular pattern and shapes in aging and osteoporosis. *Metab. Bone Dis. Rel. Res.*, **2**: 297–308.

Ashman, R. B., Cowin, S. C., VanBuskirk, W. C., and Rice, J. C. (1984). A continuous wave technique for the measurement of the elastic properties of cortical bone. *J. Biomech.*, **17**: 349–361.

Atkinson, P. J. (1967). Variation in trabecular structure of the vertebrae with age. *Calcif. Tissue Int.*, **1**: 24–32.

Beaupre, G. S. and Hayes, W. C. (1985). Finite element analysis of a three-dimensional open-celled model for trabecular bone. *J. Biomech. Eng.*, **107**: 249–256.

Behiri, J. C. and Bonfield, W. (1984). Fracture mechanics of bone: the effects of density, specimen thickness and crack velocity on longitudinal fracture. *J. Biomech.*, **17**: 25–34.

Benaissa, R., Uhthoff, H. K., and Mercier, P. (1989). Repair of trabecular fatigue fractures: cadaver studies of the upper femur. *Acta. Orthop. Scand.*, **60**: 585–589.

Bensusan, J. S., Davy, D. T., Heiple, K. G., and Verdin, P. J. (1983). Tensile, compressive and torsional testing of cancellous bone. *Trans. 29th Orthop. Res. Soc.*, **8**: 132.

Bergot, C., Laval-Jeantet, A.-M., Preteux, F., and Meunier, A. (1988). Measurement of anisotropic vertebral trabecular bone loss during aging by quantitative image analysis. *Calcif. Tissue Int.*, **43**: 143–149.

Bonfield, W. (1987). Advances in the fracture mechanics of cortical bone. *J. Biomech.*, **20**: 1071–1081.

Bonfield, W., Grynpas, M. D., and Young, R. J. (1978). Crack velocity and the fracture of bone. *J. Biomech.*, **11**: 473–479.

Borchers, R. E. (1991). *Multiaxial Failure Criteria for Trabecular Bone*. Master's thesis, Massachusetts Institute of Technology, Cambridge.

Broek, D. (1986). *Elementary Engineering Fracture Mechanics*. Martinus Nijhoff, Dordrecht.

Brown, T. D. and Ferguson, A. B. (1980). Mechanical property distributions in the cancellous bone of the human proximal femur. *Acta. Orthop. Scand.*, **51**: 429–437.

Bundy, K. J. (1985). Determination of mineral-organic bonding effectiveness in bone: theoretical considerations. *Ann. Biomed. Eng.*, **13**: 119–135.

Burr, D. B., Martin, R. B., Schaffler, M. B., and Radin, E. L. (1985). Bone remodeling in response to *in vivo* fatigue microdamage. *J. Biomech.*, **18**: 189–200.

Burr, D. B., Schaffler, M. B., and Frederickson, R. G. (1988). Composition of the cement line and its possible mechanical role as a local interface in human compact bone. *J. Biomech.*, **21**: 939–945.

Burr, D. B. and Stafford, T. (1990). Validity of the bulk-staining technique to separate artifactual from *in vivo* bone microdamage. *Clin. Orthop.*, **260**: 305–308.

Burstein, A. H., Currey, J. D., Frankel, V. H., Heiple, K. G., Lunseth, P., and Vessely, J. C. (1972a). Bone strength: the effect of screw holes. *J. Bone Jt. Surg.*, **54**: 1143–1156.

Burstein, A. H., Currey, J. D., Frankel, V. H., and Reilly, D. T. (1972b) The ultimate properties of bone tissue: the effects of yielding. *J. Biomech.*, **5**: 35–44.

Burstein, A. H., Reilly, D. T., and Martens, M. (1976). Aging of bone tissue: mechanical properties. *J. Bone Jt. Surg.*, **58**: 82–86.

Burstein, A. H., Reilly, D. T., and Frankel, V. H. (1973) Failure characteristics of bone and bone tissue. In: *Perspectives in Biomedical Engineering*. Kenedi, R. M., Ed., University Press, Baltimore, 131–134.

Burstein, A. H., Zika, J. M., Heiple, K. G., and Klein, L. (1975). Contribution of collagen and mineral to the elastic-plastic properties of bone. *J. Bone Jt. Surg.*, **57**: 956–961.

Caler, W. E. and Carter, D. R. (1989). Bone creep-fatigue damage accumulation. *J. Biomech.*, **22**: 625–635.

Carter, D. R. and Caler, W. E. (1981). Uniaxial fatigue of human cortical bone. The influence of tissue physical characteristics. *J. Biomech.*, **14**: 461–470.

Carter, D. R. and Caler, W. E. (1983). Cycle-dependent and time-dependent bone fracture with repeated loading. *J. Biomech. Eng.*, **105**: 166–170.

Carter, D. R. and Caler, W. E. (1985). A cumulative damage model for bone fracture. *J. Orthop. Res.*, **3**: 84–90.

Carter, D. R., Caler, W. E., Spengler, D. M., and Frankel, V. H. (1981). Fatigue behavior of adult cortical bone: the influence of mean strain and strain range. *Acta. Orthop. Scand.*, **52**: 481–490.

Carter, D. R. and Hayes, W. C. (1976). Fatigue life of compact bone. I. Effects of stress amplitude, temperature and density. *J. Biomech.*, **9**: 27–34.

Carter, D. R. and Hayes, W. C. (1977a). Compact bone fatigue damage. II. A microscopic examination. *Clin. Orthop.*, **127**: 265–274.

Carter, D. R. and Hayes, W. C. (1977b). Compact bone fatigue damage. I. Residual strength and stiffness. *J. Biomech.*, **10**: 325–327.

Carter, D. R. and Hayes, W. C. (1977c). The compressive behavior of bone as a two-phase porous structure. *J. Bone Jt. Surg.*, **59**: 954–962.

Carter, D. R., Hayes, W. C., and Schurman, D. J. (1976). Fatigue life of compact bone. II. Effects of microstructure and density. *J. Biomech.*, **9**: 211–218.

Carter, D. R., Schwab, G. H., and Spengler, D. M. (1980). Tensile fracture of cancellous bone. *Acta. Orthop. Scand.*, **51**: 733–741.

Carter, D. R. and Spengler, D. M. (1978). Mechanical properties and composition of cortical bone. *Clin. Orthop.*, **135**: 192–217.

Cezayirlioglu, H., Bahniuk, E., Davy, D. T., and Heiple, K. G. (1985). Anisotropic yield behavior of bone under combined axial force and torque. *J. Biomech.*, **18**: 61–69.

Cheal, E. J., Snyder, B. D., Nunamaker, D. M., and Hayes, W. C. (1987). Trabecular bone remodeling around smooth and porous implants in an equine patellar model. *J. Biomech.*, **20**: 1121–1134.

Choi, K., Kuhn, J. L., Ciarelli, M. J., and Goldstein, S. A. (1990) The elastic moduli of human subchondral, trabecular, and cortical bone tissue and the size-dependency of cortical bone modulus. *J. Biomech.*, **23**: 1103–1113.

Cowin, S. C. (1986). Wolff's Law of trabecular architecture at remodeling equilibrium. *J. Biomech. Eng.*, **108**: 83–88.

Cowin, S. C. (1989). *Bone Mechanics*. CRC Press, Boca Raton, FL.

Crowninshield, R. and Pope, M. (1974). The response of compact bone in tension at various strain rates. *Ann. Biomed. Eng.*, **2**: 217–225.

Currey, J. D. (1969) The mechanical consequences of variation in the mineral content of bone. *J. Biomech.*, **2**: 1–11.

Currey, J. D. (1988a). The effect of porosity and mineral content on the Young's modulus of elasticity of compact bone. *J. Biomech.*, **12**: 131–139.

Currey, J. D. (1988b). The effects of drying and re-wetting on some mechanical properties of cortical bone. *J. Biomech.* **21**: 439–441.

Currey, J. D. (1989). Strain rate dependence of the mechanical properties of reindeer antler and the cumulative damage model of bone fracture. *J. Biomech.*, **22**: 469–475.

Ducheyne, P., Heymans, L., Martens, M., Aernoudt, E., Meester, P. d. e., and Mulier, J. C. (1977). The mechanical behavior of intracondylar cancellous bone of the femur at different loading rates. *J. Biomech.*, **10**: 747–762.

Dunstan, C. R., Evans, R. A., Hills, E., Wong, S. Y. P., and Higgs, R. J. E. D. (1990). Bone death in hip fracture in the elderly. *Calcif. Tissue Int.*, **47**: 270–275.

Esses, S. I., Lotz, J. C., and Hayes, W. C. (1989). Biomechanical properties of the proximal femur determined *in vitro* by single energy quantitative computed tomography. *J. Bone Miner. Res.*, **4**: 715–722.

Eurell, J. C. and Kazarian, L. E. (1982). The scanning electron microscopy of compressed vertebral bodies. *Spine*, **7**: 123–128.

Evans, F. G. (1973). *Mechanical Properties of Bone*. Charles C Thomas, Springfield, IL.

Evans, F. G. and Riolo, M. L. (1970). Relations between the fatigue life and histology of adult human cortical bone. *J. Bone Jt. Surg.* **52**: 1579–1586.

Evans, F. G. and Vincentelli, R. (1974). Relations of the compressive properties of human cortical bone to histological structure and calcification. *J. Biomech.*, **7**: 1–10.

Fondrk, M., Bahniuk, E., Davy, D. T., and Michaels, C. (1988). Some viscoplastic characteristics of bovine and human cortical bone. *J. Biomech.* **21**: 623–630.

Freeman, M. A. R., Todd, R. C., and Pirie, C. J. (1974). The role of fatigue in the pathogenesis of senile femoral neck fracture. *J. Bone Jt. Surg.*, **56**: 698–702.

Frost, H. M. (1960). Presence of microscopic cracks *in vivo* in bone. *Henry Ford Hosp. Bull.*, **8**: 25–35.

Fyhrie, D. P. and Carter, D. R. (1986). A unifying principle relating stress to trabecular bone morphology. *J. Orthop. Res.*, **4**: 304–317.

Galante, J., Rostoker, W., and Ray, R. D. (1970). Physical properties of trabecular bone. *Calcif. Tissue Res.*, **5**: 236–246.

Genant, H. K., Ettinger, B., Cann, C. E., Reiser, U., Gordan, G. S., and Kolb, F. O. (1985). Osteoporosis: assessment by quantitative computed tomography. *Orthop. Clin. North Am.*, **16**: 557–568.

Gibson, L. J. (1985). The mechanical behavior of cancellous bone. *J. Biomech.*, **18**: 317–328.

Gibson, L. J. and Ashby, M. F. (1988). *Cellular Solids: Structure & Properties*. Pergamon Press, Elmsford, New York.

Goldstein, S. A. (1987). The mechanical properties of trabecular bone: dependence on anatomic location and function. *J. Biomech.*, **20**: 1055–1061.

Goldstein, S. A., Wilson, D. L., Sonstegard, D. A., and Matthews, L. S. (1983). The mechanical properties of human tibial trabecular bone as a function of metaphyseal location. *J. Biomech.*, **16**: 965–969.

Hansson, T. H., Keller, T. S., and Panjabi, M. M. (1986). A study of the compressive properties of lumbar vertebral trabeculae: effects of tissue characteristics. *Spine*, **11**: 56–62.

Harrigan, T. P. and Mann, R. W. (1984). Characterization of microstructural anisotropy in orthotropic materials using a second rank tensor. *J. Mater. Sci.*, **19**: 761–767.

Hart, R. T., Davy, D. T., and Heiple, K. G. (1984). Mathematical modeling and numerical solutions for functionally dependent bone remodeling. *Calcif. Tissue Int.*, **36**(suppl.): 104–109.

Hayes, W. C. (1991). Biomechanics of cortical and trabecular bone: implications for assessment of fracture risk. In: *Basic Orthopaedic Biomechanics*. Mow, V. C. and Hayes, W. C., Eds., Raven Press, New York, 93–142.

Hayes, W. C. and Carter, D. R. (1976). Post-yield behavior of subchondral trabecular bone. *J. Biomed. Mat. Res. [Symp.]*, **7**: 537–544.

Hayes, W. C., Piazza, S. J., and Zysset, P. K. (1991). Biomechanics of fracture risk prediction of the hip and spine by quantitative computed tomography. In: *Radiologic Clinics of North America*. Vol. 29, Rosenthal, D. I., Ed., W. B. Saunders, Philadelphia, 1–18.

Hayes, W. C. and Ruff, C. B. (1986). Biomechanical compensatory mechanisms for age-related changes in cortical bone. In: *Twelfth Annual Applied Basic Sciences Course*. Uhthoff, H. K. and Jaworski, Z. F. G., Eds., University of Ottawa, Canada, 371–377.

Hayes, W. C. and Snyder, B. D. (1981). Toward a quantitative formulation of Wolff's Law in trabecular bone. In: *Symp. on the Mechanical Properties of Bone*. Cowin, S. C., Ed., American Society of Mechanical Engineers, Boulder, 43–68.

Hayes, W. C., Swenson, L. W., and Schurman, D. J. (1978). Axisymmetric finite element analysis of the lateral tibial plateau. *J. Biomech.*, **11**: 21–33.

Hayes, W. C. and Wright, T. M. (1977). An empirical strength theory for compact bone. *Fracture*, **3**: 1173–1179.

Huiskes, R. and Nunamaker, D. (1984). Local stresses and bone adaption around orthopedic implants. *Calcif. Tissue Int.*, **36**(suppl.): 110–117.

Huiskes, R., Weinans, H., and Dalstra, M. (1989). Adaptive bone remodeling and biomechanical design considerations. *Orthopedics*, **12**: 1255–1267.

Hvid, I. and Hansen, S. L. (1985). Trabecular bone strength patterns at the proximal tibial epiphysis. *J. Orthop. Res.*, **3**: 464–472.

Jasty, M., Harrigan, T. M., Greer, J. A., Chen, J., and Harris, W. H. (1985). Prediction of directional variations in material properties of human cancellous bone using 3-D stereologic technique. *Trans. 31st O.R.S.*, **10**: 352.

Jensen, N. C., Hvid, I., and Kroner, K. (1988). Strength patterns of cancellous bone at the ankle joint. *Eng. Med.*, **17**: 71–76.

Jensen, N. C., Madsen, L. P., and Linde, F. (1991). Topographical distribution of trabecular bone strength in the human os calcanei. *J. Biomech.*, **24**: 49–55.

Jones, H. H., Priest, J. D., Hayes, W. C., Tichenor, C. C., and Nagel, D. A. (1977). Humeral hypertrophy in response to exercise. *J. Bone Jt. Surg.*, **59**: 204–208.

Kaplan, S. J., Hayes, W. C., Stone, J. L., and Beaupre, G. S. (1985). Technical note: tensile strength of bovine trabecular bone. *J. Biomech.*, **18**: 723–727.

Katz, J. L. and Meunier, A. (1987). The elastic anisotropy of bone. *J. Biomech.*, **20**: 1063–1070.

Keller, T. S., Hansson, T. H., Abram, A. C., Spengler, D. M., and Panjabi, M. M. (1989). Regional variations in the compressive properties of lumbar vertebral trabeculae. Effects of disc degeneration. *Spine*, **14**: 1012–1019.

Keller, T. S., Mao, Z., and Spengler, D. M. (1990). Young's modulus, bending strength, and tissue physical properties of human compact bone. *J. Orthop. Res.*, **8**: 592–603.

Knauss, P. (1981). Materials properties and strength behavior of spongy bone tissue at the coxal human femur. I. *Biomed. Tech.*, **26**: 200–210.

Krajcinovic, D., Trafimow, J., and Sumarac, D. (1987). Simple constitutive model for a cortical bone. *J. Biomech.*, **20**: 779–784.

Lanyon, L. E., Goodship, A. E., Pye, C. J., and MacFie, J. H. (1982). Mechanically adaptive bone remodelling. *J. Biomech.*, **15**: 141–154.

Lanyon, L. E., Hampson, W. G. J., Goodship, A. E., and Shah, J. S. (1975). Bone deformation recorded *in vivo* from strain gages attached to the human tibial shaft. *Acta. Orthop. Scand.*, **46**: 256–268.

Lanyon, L. E., Paul, I. L., Rubin, C. T., Thrasher, E. L., DeLaura, R., Rose, R. M., and Radin, E. L. (1981). *In vivo* strain measurements from bone and prosthesis following total hip replacement. *J. Bone Joint Surg.*, **63**: 989–1001.

Lees, S. and Davidson, C. L. (1977). The role of collagen in the elastic properties of calcified tissues. *J. Biomech.*, **10**: 473–86.

Lindahl, O. and Lindgren, A. G. H. (1967). Cortical bone in man. I. Variation in the amount and density with age and sex. II. Variation in tensile strength with age and sex. *Acta. Orthop. Scand.*, **38**: 133–147.

Linde, F., Hvid, I., and Pongsoipetch, B. (1989). Energy absorptive properties of human trabecular bone specimens during axial compression. *J. Orthop. Res.*, **7**: 432–439.

Linde, F., Norgaard, P., Hvid, I., Odgaard, A., and Soballe, K. (1991). Mechanical properties of trabecular bone dependency on strain rate. *J. Biomech.*, **24**: 803–809.

Lipson, S. F. and Katz, J. L. (1984). The relationship between elastic properties and microstructure of bovine cortical bone. *J. Biomech.*, **17**: 231–240.

Lotz, J. C., Gerhart, T. N., and Hayes, W. C. (1989). Mechanical properties of metaphyseal bone in the proximal femur. *J. Biomech.*, **24**: 317–329.

Lotz, J. C., Gerhart, T. N., and Hayes, W. C. (1990). Mechanical properties of trabecular bone from the proximal femur: a quantitative CT study. *J. Comput. Assist. Tomogr.*, **14**: 107–114.

Martens, M., van Audekercke, R., Delport, P., De Meester, P., and Mulier, J. C. (1983). The mechanical characteristics of cancellous bone at the upper femoral region. *J. Biomech.*, **16**: 971–983.

Martin, R. B. and Burr, D. B. (1982). A hypothetical mechanism for the stimulation of osteonal remodelling by fatigue damage. *J. Biomech.*, **15**: 137–139.

Martin, R. B. and Burr, D. B. (1989). *Structure, Function, and Adaptation of Compact Bone*. Raven Press, New York.

Mazess, R. B. (1982). On aging bone loss. *Clin. Orthop.*, **165**: 239–252.

McBroom, R. J., Hayes, W. C., Edwards, W. T., Goldberg, R. P., and White, A. A., III (1985). Prediction of vertebral body compressive fracture using quantitative computed tomography. *J. Bone Jt. Surg.*, **67**: 1206–1214.

McElhaney, J. H. (1966). Dynamic response of bone and muscle tissue. *J. Appl. Physiol.*, **21**: 1231–1236.

McElhaney, J. H., Alem, N., and Roberts, V. (1970a). A Porous Block Model for Cancellous Bone. *ASME Technical Publication*, 70-WA/BHF-2.

McElhaney, J. H., Fogle, J. L., Melvin, J. W., Haynes, R. R., Roberts, V. L., and Alem, N. M. (1970b). Mechanical properties of cranial bone. *J. Biomech.*, **3**: 495–511.

McFarland, P. H. and Frost, H. M. (1961). A possible new cause for aseptic necrosis of the femoral head. *Henry Ford Hosp. Med. Bull.*, **9**: 115–122.

Melton, L. J., Wahner, H. W., Richelson, L. S., O'Fallon, W. M., and Riggs, B. L. (1986). Osteoporosis and the risk of hip fracture. *Am. J. Epidemiol.*, **124**: 254–261.

Michel, M. C., Zysset, P. K., and Hayes, W. C. (1991). Fatigue behavior of trabecular bone. *Trans. 37th Orthop. Res. Soc.*, **16**: 156.

Mosekilde, L. (1988). Age-related changes in vertebral trabecular bone architecture — assessed by a new method. *Bone*, **9**: 247–250.

Mosekilde, L., Bentzen, S. M., Ortoft, G., and Jorgensen, J. (1989). The predictive value of quantitative computed tomography for vertebral body compressive strength and ash density. *Bone*, **10**: 465–470.

Mosekilde, L. and Mosekilde, L. (1986). Normal vertebral body size and compressive strength: relations to age and to vertebral and iliac trabecular bone compressive strength. *Bone*, **7**: 207–212.

Mosekilde, L. and Mosekilde, L. (1988). Iliac crest trabecular bone volume as predictor for vertebral compressive strength, ash density and trabecular bone volume in normal individuals. *Bone*, **9**: 195–199.

Mosekilde, L. and Mosekilde, L. (1990). Sex differences in age-related changes in vertebral body size, density and biomechanical competence in normal individuals. *Bone*, **11**: 67–73.

Mosekilde, L., Mosekilde, L., and Danielsen, C. C. (1987). Biomechanical competence of vertebral trabecular bone in relation to ash density and age in normal individuals. *Bone*, **8**: 79–85.

Mosekilde, L., Viidik, A., and Mosekilde, L. (1985). Correlations between the compressive strength of iliac and vertebral trabecular bone in normal individuals. *Bone*, **6**: 291–295.

Moyle, D. D. and Bowden, R. W. (1984). Fracture of human femoral bone. *J. Biomech.*, **17**: 203–213.

Moyle, D. D. and Gavens, A. J. (1986). Fracture properties of bovine tibial bone. *J. Biomech.*, **19**: 919–927.

Murray, R. P., Hayes, W. C., Edwards, W. T., and Harry, J. D. (1984). Mechanical properties of the subchondral plate and the metaphyseal shell. *Trans. 30th Orthop. Res. Soc.*, **9**: 197.

Neil, J. L., Demos, T. C., Stone, J. L., and Hayes, W. C. (1983). Tensile and compressive properties of vertebral trabecular bone. *Trans. 30th Orthop. Res. Soc.*, **8**: 344.

Nunamaker, D. M., Butterweck, D. M., and Provost, M. T., (1990). Fatigue fractures in thoroughbred racehorses: relationships with age, peak bone strain, and training. *J. Orthop. Res.*, **8**: 604–611.

O'Connor, J. A., Lanyon, L. E., and MacFie, H. (1982). The influence of strain rate on adaptive bone remodelling. *J. Biomech.*, **15**: 767–781.

Odgaard, A., Hvid, I., and Linde, F. (1989). Compressive axial strain distributions in cancellous bone specimens. *J. Biomech.*, **22**: 829–835.

Odgaard, A. and Linde, F. (1991). The underestimation of Young's modulus in compressive testing of cancellous bone specimens. *J. Biomech.*, **24**: 691–698.

Ohtani, T. and Azuma, H. (1984). Trabecular microfractures in the acetabulum: histologic studies in cadavers. *Acta. Orthop. Scand.*, **55**: 419–422.

Orava, S. and Hulkko, A. (1984). Stress fracture of the mid-tibial shaft. *Acta. Orthop. Scand.*, **55**: 35–37.

Parfitt, A. M. (1984). Age-related structural changes in trabecular and cortical bone: cellular mechanisms and biomechanical consequences. *Calcif. Tissue Int.*, **36**(suppl): 123–128.

Parfitt, A. M., Mathews, C. H. E., Villanueva, A. R., Kleerekoper, M., Frame, B., and Rao, D. S. (1983). Relationships between surface, volume, and thickness of iliac trabecular bone in aging and in osteoporosis. Implications for the microanatomic and cellular mechanisms of bone loss. *J. Clin. Invest.*, **72**: 1396–1409.

Pattin, C. A. G. (1991). Cyclic Mechanical Property Degradation in Bone during Fatigue Loading. Ph.D. dissertation, Stanford University, Palo Alto, CA.

Pope, M. H. and Outwater, J. O. (1972). The fracture characteristics of bone substance. *J. Biomech.*, **5**: 457–465.

Pope, M. H. and Outwater, J. C. (1974). Mechanical properties of bone as a function of position and orientation. *J. Biomech.*, **7**: 61–66.

Preteux, F., Bergot, C., and Laval-Jeantet, A. M. (1985). Automatic quantification of vertebral cancellous bone remodeling during aging. *Anat. Clin.*, **7**: 203–208.

Pugh, J. W., Rose, R. M., and Radin, E. L. (1972). Techniques for the study of structure of bone. *Microstructures*, **3**: 23–27.

Pugh, J. W., Rose, R. M., and Radin, E. L. (1973a). A possible mechanism of Wolff's Law: trabecular microfractures. *Arch. Int. Physiol. Biochim.*, **81**: 27–40.

Pugh, J. W., Rose, R. M., and Radin, E. L. (1973b). Elastic and viscoelastic properties of trabecular bone: dependence on structure. *J. Biomech.*, **6**: 475–485.

Pugh, J. W., Rose, R. M., and Radin, E. L. (1973c). A structural model for the mechanical behavior of trabecular bone. *J. Biomech.*, **6**: 657–670.

Radin, E. L., Parker, H. G., Pugh, J. W., Steinberg, R. S., Paul, I. L., and Rose, R. M. (1973). Response of joints to impact loading. III. Relationship between trabecular microfractures and cartilage degeneration. *J. Biomech.*, **6**: 51–57.

Reilly, D. T. and Burstein, A. H. (1974). The mechanical properties of cortical bone. *J. Bone Jt. Surg.*, **56**: 1001–1022.

Reilly, D. T. and Burstein, A. H. (1975). The elastic and ultimate properties of compact bone tissue. *J. Biomech.*, **8**: 393–405.

Reilly, D. T., Burstein, A. H., and Frankel, V. H. (1974). The elastic modulus for bone. *J. Biomech.*, **7**: 271–275.

Rice, J. C., Cowin, S. C., and Bowman, J. A. (1988). On the dependence of the elasticity and strength of cancellous bone on apparent density. *J. Biomech.*, **21**: 155–168.

Riggs, B. L. and Melton, L. J., III (1986). Involutional osteoporosis. *N. Engl. J. Med.*, **314**: 1676–1686.

Riggs, B. L., Wahner, H. W., Seeman, E., Offord, K. P., Dunn, W. L., Mazess, R. B.,Johnson, K. A., and Melton, L.J., III (1982). Changes in bone mineral density of the proximal femur and spine with aging. Differences between the postmenopausal and senile osteoporosis syndromes. *J. Clin. Invest.*, **70**: 716–723.

Robertson, D. M., Robertson, D., and Barrett, C. R. (1978). Fracture toughness, critical crack length and plastic zone size in bone. *J. Biomech.*, **11**: 359–364.

Robertson, D. M. and Smith, D. C. (1978). Compressive strength of mandibular bone as a function of microstructure and strain rate. *J. Biomech.*, **11**: 455–471.

Rubin, C. T. and Lanyon, L. E. (1987). Osteoregulatory nature of mechanical stimuli: function as a determinant for adaptive remodeling in bone. *J. Orthop. Res.*, **5**: 300–310.

Rubin, C. T., McLeod, K. J., and Bain, S. D. (1990). Functional strains and cortical bone adaptation: epigenetic assurance of skeletal integrity. *J. Biomech.*, **23**: 43–60.

Ruff, C. B. and Hayes, W. C. (1982). Subperiosteal expansion and cortical remodeling of the human femur and tibia with aging. *Science*, **217**: 945–948.

Saha, S. and Hayes, W. C. (1976). Tensile impact properties of human compact bone. *J. Biomech.*, **9**: 243–251.

Sasaki, N., Ikawa, T., and Fukuda, A. (1991). Orientation of mineral in bovine bone and the anisotropic mechanical properties of plexiform bone. *J. Biomech.*, **24**: 57–61.

Sasaki, N., Matsushima, N., Ikawa, T., Yamamura, H., and Fukuda, A. (1989). Orientation of bone mineral and its role in the anisotropic mechanical properties of bone: transverse anisotropy. *J. Biomech.*, **22**: 157–164.

Schaffler, M. B. and Burr, D. B. (1988). Stiffness of compact bone: effects of porosity and density. *J. Biomech.*, **21**: 13–16.

Schaffler, M. B., Radin, E. L., and Burr, D. B. (1989). Mechanical and morphological effects of strain rate on fatigue of compact bone. *Bone*, **10**: 207–214.

Snyder, B. D. (1991). Anisotropic Structure-Property Relations for Trabecular Bone. Ph.D. dissertation, University of Pennsylvania, Philadelphia.

Snyder, B. D. and Hayes, W. C. (1990). Multiaxial structure-property relations in trabecular bone. In: *Biomechanics of Diarthrodial Joints*. Mow, V. C., Ratcliffe, A., and Woo, S. L.-Y., Eds., Springer-Verlag, New York, 31–59.

Snyder, S. M. and Schneider, E. (1991). Estimation of mechanical properties of cortical bone by computed tomography. *J. Orthop. Res.*, **9**: 422–431.

Stone, J. L., Beaupre, G. S., and Hayes, W. C. (1983). Multiaxial strength characteristics of trabecular bone. *J. Biomech.*, **16**: 743–752.

Tehranzadeh, J., Serafini, A. N., and Pais, M. J. (1989). *Avulsion and Stress Injuries of the Musculoskeletal System*. S. Karger, Basel.

Todd, R. C., Freeman, M. A., and Pirie, C. J. (1972). Isolated trabecular fatigue fractures in the femoral head. *J. Bone Jt. Surg.*, **54**: 723–728.

Townsend, P. R., Raux, P., Rose, R. M., Miegel, R. E., and Radin, E. L. (1975a). The distribution and anisotropy of stiffness of cancellous bone in the human patella. *J. Biomech.*, **8**: 363–367.

Townsend, P. R., Rose, R. M., and Radin, E. L. (1975b). Buckling studies of single human trabeculae. *J. Biomech.*, **8**: 199–201.

Tsai, S. and Wu, E. (1971). A general theory for strength of anisotropic materials. *J. Composite Mater.*, **5**: 58–80.

Turner, C. H. (1989). Yield behavior of bovine cancellous bone. *J. Biomech. Eng.*, **111**: 256–260.

Urovitz, E. P., Fornasier, V. L., Risen, M. I., and MacNab, I. (1977). Etiological factors in the pathogenesis of femoral trabecular fatigue fractures. *Clin. Orthop.*, **127**: 275–280.

Vernon-Roberts, B. and Pirie, C. J. (1973). Healing trabecular microfractures in the bodies of lumbar vertebrae. *Ann. Rheum. Dis.*, **32**: 406–412.

Weaver, J. K. and Chalmers, J. (1966). Cancellous bone: its strength and changes with aging and an evaluation of some methods for measuring mineral content. *J. Bone Jt. Surg.*, **48**: 289–298.

Whitehouse, W., Dyson, E., and Jackson, C. (1971). The scanning electron microscope in studies of trabecular bone from a human vertebral body. *J. Anat.*, **108**: 481–496.

Whitehouse, W. J. (1975). Scanning electron micrographs of cancellous bone from the human sternum. *J. Pathol.*, **116**: 213–223.

Whitehouse, W. J. and Dyson, E. D. (1974). Scanning electron microscope studies of trabecular bone in the proximal end of the human femur. *J. Anat.*, **118**: 417–444.

Williams, J. L. and Lewis, J. L. (1982). Properties and an anisotropic model of cancellous bone from the proximal tibial epiphysis. *J. Biomech. Eng.*, **104**: 50–56.

Wolff, J. (1892). *Das Gesetz der Transformation der Knochen*. Hirschwald, Berlin.

Wong, S. Y. P., Kariks, J., Evans, R. A., Dunstan, C. R., and Hills, E. (1985). The effect of age in bone composition and viability in the femoral head. *J. Bone Jt. Surg.*, **67**: 274–283.

Woo, S.L.-Y., Kuei, S. C., Amiel, D., Gomez, M. A., Hayes, W. C., White, F. C., and Akeson, W. H. (1981). The effect of prolonged physical training on the properties of long bone: a study of Wolff's Law. *J. Bone Jt. Surg.*, **63**: 780–787.

Wright, T. M. and Hayes, W. C. (1976a). The fracture mechanics of fatigue crack propagation in compact bone. *J. Biomed. Mater. Res. Symp.*, **7**: 637–648.

Wright, T. M. and Hayes, W. C. (1976b). Tensile testing of bone over a wide range of strain rates: effects of strain rate, micro-structure and density. *Med. Biol. Eng. Comput.*, **14**: 671–680.

Wright, T. M. and Hayes, W. C. (1977). Fracture mechanics parameters for compact bone. Effects of density and specimen thickness. *J. Biomech.*, **10**: 419–430.

Wright, T. M. and Hayes, W. C. (1980). Mechanics of fracture and fracture propagation. In: *Scientific Foundations of Orthopaedics*. Goodfellow, O., Ed.,William Heinemann Medical Books, London, 252–258.

Yoon, H. A. and Katz, J. L. (1976). Ultrasonic wave propagation in human cortical bone. I. Theoretical considerations for hexagonal symmetry. *J. Biomech.*, **9**: 407–412.

Zienkiewicz, O. C. (1977). *The Finite Element Method.* McGraw Hill, London.

Zimmerman, M. C., Meunier, A., Katz, J. L., Christel, P., and Sedel, L. (1989). The evaluation of bone remodeling about orthopaedic implants with ultrasound. *J. Orthop. Res.*, **7**: 607–611.

Index

A

accutane, 218
ACE, *see* acetazolamide
acetaminophen, 181
acetazolamide (ACE), 195, 207, 208, 209, 210
acetylsalicylic acid (aspirin), 180, 182
achondroplasia, 172
acid phosphatase, 196
actidione, 204
actinobolin, 204
adaptation, 133, 135–140
adaptive remodeling, 27
adenine, 220
adenine arabinoside, 191
adenocarcinoma, 180
adriamycin, 204
aging, 245–276
　　cortical bone in, 306, 317
　　in extinct species, 267–268
　　growth marks in, *see* growth marks
　　histological, 272–276
　　individual variability in, 276
　　interpopulational variability in, 265, 276
　　microanatomical criteria in, 269–276
　　morphology and, 269–276
　　populational variability in, 265, 276
　　practical use of growth marks and, 258–265
　　skeletochronology and, *see* skeletochronology
　　synostosis and, 269–271
　　trabecular bone in, 331–334
L-alanosine, 204
alkaline phosphatase, 41
alkylating agents, 196–199, *see also* specific types
allometry, 96, 97, 108–109
　　cranial, 111–114, 115–120
　　dog breeds and, 111–115
　　limb, 114–115, 116–117, 120
　　ontogenetic, *see* ontogenetic allometry
　　primate evolution and, 146–151, 153
　　wild canid species and, 111–115
ametantrone acetate, 204

amiloride, 207
6-amino-nicotinamide, 204
aminopterin, 199
2-amino-1,3,4-thiadiazole, 205
amitriptyline, 213
analgesics, 180–183, *see also* specific types
anemia, 166–169
anesthetics, 183–185, *see also* specific types
anisotropy, 293, 326
annuli growth marks, 253, 263, 264
antianxiety agents, 211–214, *see also* specific types
antibiotics, 180, 189, 190, 204, *see also* specific types
anticonvulsants, 185–188, *see also* specific types
antidepressants, 213, 216–217, *see also* specific types
antifungal agents, 195, *see also* specific types
antihelmintic agents, 193–195, *see also* specific types
antihistamines, 180, *see also* specific types
anti-Hodgkin agents, 197, *see also* specific types
anti-infective agents, 188–189, *see also* specific types
antileukemic agents, 197, *see also* specific types
antimalarial agents, 192–193, *see also* specific types
antimetabolites, 199–204, *see also* specific types
antinomycin C, 204
antiparasitic agents, 192–195, *see also* specific types
antipsychotic agents, 214–216, *see also* specific types
antipyretic agents, 181, *see also* specific types
antitumor agents, 197, *see also* chemotherapeutic agents; specific types
antiviral agents, 191–192, *see also* specific types